AF846933

Energy Balance and Cancer

Volume 14

Series Editor:
Nathan A. Berger,
Case Western Reserve University, School of Medicine,
Cleveland, OH, USA

More information about this series at http://www.springer.com/series/8282

Elizabeth A. Platz • Nathan A. Berger
Editors

Energy Balance and Prostate Cancer

Springer

Editors
Elizabeth A. Platz
Department of Epidemiology
Johns Hopkins Bloomberg School of Public Health
Baltimore, MD, USA

Nathan A. Berger
Center for Science, Health and Society
Case Western Reserve University
Cleveland, OH, USA

ISSN 2199-2622 ISSN 2199-2630 (electronic)
Energy Balance and Cancer
ISBN 978-3-319-64939-9 ISBN 978-3-319-64940-5 (eBook)
DOI 10.1007/978-3-319-64940-5

Library of Congress Control Number: 2017952305

© Springer International Publishing AG 2018
This work is subject to copyright. All rights are reserved by the Publisher, whether the whole or part of the material is concerned, specifically the rights of translation, reprinting, reuse of illustrations, recitation, broadcasting, reproduction on microfilms or in any other physical way, and transmission or information storage and retrieval, electronic adaptation, computer software, or by similar or dissimilar methodology now known or hereafter developed.
The use of general descriptive names, registered names, trademarks, service marks, etc. in this publication does not imply, even in the absence of a specific statement, that such names are exempt from the relevant protective laws and regulations and therefore free for general use.
The publisher, the authors and the editors are safe to assume that the advice and information in this book are believed to be true and accurate at the date of publication. Neither the publisher nor the authors or the editors give a warranty, express or implied, with respect to the material contained herein or for any errors or omissions that may have been made. The publisher remains neutral with regard to jurisdictional claims in published maps and institutional affiliations.

Printed on acid-free paper

This Springer imprint is published by Springer Nature
The registered company is Springer International Publishing AG
The registered company address is: Gewerbestrasse 11, 6330 Cham, Switzerland

Preface

Prostate cancer is the most common cancer in American men with an age adjusted incidence of 123.2 per 100,000 men per year and 20 deaths per 100,000 per year. In 2017, it is estimated that there will be more than 161,360 new cases diagnosed and 26,730 deaths, making prostate cancer the third leading cause of cancer deaths in American men. Overall, it is estimated that 14% of men will be diagnosed with prostate cancer at some time during their lifetime and that the total number of US men living with some stage of prostate cancer reaches about 2.8 million.

All aspects of prostate cancer including incidence, screening, diagnostic procedures, comorbid conditions, approach and response to therapeutic options including surgery, radiation therapy, chemotherapy, hormone therapy as well as quality of life may be profoundly affected by overweight and obesity which is currently at pandemic proportions, affecting 60–70% of the adult population. Overweight and obesity is particularly prevalent in the older adult population, where the peak incidence of prostate cancer is noted to be in 66-year-old men.

The confluence of obesity with prostate cancer in older men has profound implications for healthcare planning and has been the target of intense fundamental, epidemiologic, and clinical research. In addition to obesity, the course of prostate cancer and its comorbidities may be significantly affected by other aspects of energy balance including physical activity and sleep.

The overall goal of this volume will be to explore areas of research linking energy balance to prostate cancer, identify impact on understanding implications for prostate cancer prevention, clinical care, and mitigation, and manage men with prostate cancer as well as indications of future needs. The volume initially focuses on epidemiology of prostate cancer and its relation to energy balance in terms of incidence, recurrence, mortality, race, and genetics as well as mechanisms by which energy balance impacts prostate cancer and associated comorbidities. Subsequent chapters will concentrate on research trials and their clinical implications to prevent and/or enhance effects of energy balance in men with prostate cancer. This volume provides a comprehensive treatise on the latest studies concerning the interface of prostate cancer and energy balance which together constitute major challenges and opportunities for research scientist, clinicians, and healthcare planners, especially those dealing with the expanding geriatric population.

We are pleased to have an international group of expert physicians and scientists to author these chapters on Energy Balance and Prostate Cancer. In Chap. 1, Nikos Papadimitriou, University of Ioannina, Ioannina, Greece; Elena Critselis, Academy of Athens, Athens, Greece; and Konstantinos K. Tsilidis, University of Ioannina, Ioannina, Greece, and the School of Public Health, Imperial College London, London, United Kingdom, provide an epidemiologic overview and critical appraisal of the literature indicating an association of obesity with prostate cancer, its apparent association with advanced and fatal prostate cancer, and research needed to further define this relation. Chapter 2, by David S. Lopez, University of Texas, Houston TX, reviews racial and ethnic influences on lifestyle factors affecting prostate cancer. In Chap. 3, Jeanette M. Schenk and Jonathan L. Wright, Fred Hutchinson Cancer Research Center and University of Washington, Seattle, WA, review the relationship between common obesity-related comorbidities and the impact of their therapy on prostate cancer. Cheryl L. Thompson and Mackenzie Reece, Case Western Reserve University, Cleveland OH, in Chap. 4 discuss mechanisms by which adipokines mediate the association between obesity and prostate cancer risk and aggressiveness. In Chap. 5, Mieke Van Hemelrijck, King's College London, UK, and Sabine Rohrmann, University of Zurich, Zurich, Switzerland, collaborate to discuss cross-sectional and intervention studies to evaluate how alterations in energy metabolism potentially affect mediators of prostate cancer progression. Chapter 6, written by Daniel S. Han and J. Kellogg Parsons, University of California San Diego Health, CA, discusses the complex influence of obesity on cancer screening, diagnosis, and management. In Chap. 7, Grace Huang and Shehzad Basaria, Harvard Medical School, Boston MA, discuss the important interaction and risks associated with obesity and androgen deprivation therapy in men with prostate cancer. In Chap. 8, Ciaran M. Fairman, the Ohio State University, Columbus, OH; Alexander R. Lucas, Wake Forest School of Medicine, Winston Salem, NC; Elizabeth Grainger, Steven K. Clinton, and Bryan C. Focht, the Ohio State University, Columbus, OH, provide an in-depth analysis of dietary intervention and exercise in men with prostate cancer, and in Chap. 9, Yonaira M. Rivera and Katherine Clegg Smith, Johns Hopkins Bloomberg School of Public Health, Baltimore, MD, discuss strategies and benefits of energy balance interventions in patients with prostate cancer. An important area of concern, not covered in this volume due to lack of information, is the influence of obesity on decision making and on outcomes of Active Surveillance, all of which forms an important focus for future research.

Overall, this volume provides a comprehensive treatise on the latest studies linking prostate cancer with energy balance, which together constitute a major challenge and opportunity for research scientists and clinicians especially those dealing with the expanding population of older men confronted with obesity and associated comorbidities. This volume should be a valuable resource to physicians, oncologists, urologists, endocrinologists, nurses, nutritionists, dieticians, and exercise therapists dealing with men with energy balance issues and/or questions regarding the linkage between energy balance and cancer. Moreover, this volume should serve as an important resource for cancer researchers, especially for scientists studying lifestyle modification and prevention strategies to better understand and disrupt the linkage between obesity and cancer.

Baltimore, MD, USA Elizabeth A. Platz
Cleveland, OH, USA Nathan A. Berger

Contents

List of Contributors

Shehzad Basaria Brigham and Women's Hospital, Harvard Medical School, Boston, MA, USA

Steven K. Clinton Division of Medical Oncology, College of Medicine, The Ohio State University, Columbus, OH, USA

Elena Critselis Biomedical Research Foundation of the Academy of Athens, Athens, Greece

Ciaran M. Fairman Kinesiology, Department of Human Sciences, The Ohio State University, Columbus, OH, USA

Brian C. Focht Kinesiology, Department of Human Sciences, OSU Comprehensive Cancer Center, The Ohio State University, Columbus, OH, USA

Elizabeth Grainger Division of Medical Oncology, College of Medicine, The Ohio State University, Columbus, OH, USA

Daniel S. Han Moores Cancer Center, University of California San Diego Health, La Jolla, CA, USA

Mieke Van Hemelrijck Division of Cancer Studies, King's College London, Guy's Hospital, London, UK

Grace Huang Section on Men's Health, Aging and Metabolism, Brigham and Women's Hospital, Harvard Medical School, Boston, MA, USA

David S. Lopez Division of Epidemiology, Human Genetics and Environmental Sciences, University of Texas School of Public Health, Houston, TX, USA

Division of Urology, University of Texas-Medical School at Houston, Houston, TX, USA

Alexander R. Lucas Department of Social Sciences and Health Policy, Wake Forest School of Medicine, Medical Center Boulevard, Winston, Salem, NC, USA

Nikos Papadimitriou Department of Hygiene and Epidemiology, University of Ioannina School of Medicine, University Campus, Ioannina, Greece

J. Kellogg Parsons Moores Cancer Center, University of California San Diego Health, La Jolla, CA, USA

MacKenzie Reece Department of Anatomy, Case Western Reserve University, Cleveland, OH, USA

Yonaira M. Rivera Department of Health, Behavior and Society, Johns Hopkins Bloomberg School of Public Health, Baltimore, MD, USA

Sabine Rohrmann Division of Chronic Disease Epidemiology, Epidemiology, Biostatistics and Prevention Institute, University of Zurich, Zurich, Switzerland

Jeannette M. Schenk Cancer Prevention Program, Fred Hutchinson Cancer Research Center, Seattle, WA, USA

Katherine Clegg Smith Department of Health, Behavior and Society, Johns Hopkins Bloomberg School of Public Health, Baltimore, MD, USA

Cheryl L. Thompson Department of Nutrition, Case Western Reserve University, Cleveland, OH, USA

Konstantinos K. Tsilidis Department of Hygiene and Epidemiology, University of Ioannina School of Medicine, Ioannina, Greece

Department of Epidemiology and Biostatistics, Imperial College London, School of Public Health, London, UK

Jonathan L. Wright Department of Urology, University of Washington, Seattle, WA, USA

Epidemiology Program, Fred Hutchinson Cancer Research Center, Seattle, WA, USA

Chapter 1
Epidemiology, Energy Balance and Prostate Cancer Incidence and Mortality

Nikos Papadimitriou, Elena Critselis, and Konstantinos K. Tsilidis

Abstract Energy balance is defined as the equilibrium between energy consumed and expended. A substantial number of prospective epidemiological studies have been conducted to investigate the association of obesity and physical activity with risk of prostate cancer. The aim of this chapter is to provide an overall review and critical appraisal of the literature on these two purported risk factors and prostate cancer incidence overall, incidence of advanced and non-advanced disease, and prostate cancer mortality. Markers of general and central obesity have been associated with an increased risk of advanced and fatal disease, and a decreased risk of localized prostate cancer, but hints of bias were identified in this literature. The literature evidence is sparse and inconsistent for other adiposity indices and physical activity. Future prospective studies and large consortia with valid and direct assessment of the time-varying nature of body fatness and physical activity and with a focus on lethal prostate cancer are needed to draw firmer conclusions.

Keywords Relation BMI to Risk Prostate Cancer Severity • Relation BMI to Risk Prostate Cancer Fatality • Relation Physical Activity to Prostate Cancer Severity

---

N. Papadimitriou
Department of Hygiene and Epidemiology, University of Ioannina School of Medicine, University Campus, Ioannina 45110, Greece
e-mail: nicktzimas13@gmail.com

E. Critselis
Biomedical Research Foundation of the Academy of Athens, 4 Soranou Ephesiou Street, Athens 11527, Greece
e-mail: ecritselis@bioacademy.gr

K.K. Tsilidis (✉)
Department of Hygiene and Epidemiology, University of Ioannina School of Medicine, University Campus, Ioannina 45110, Greece

Department of Epidemiology and Biostatistics, Imperial College London, School of Public Health, London, UK
e-mail: ktsilidi@cc.uoi.gr

© Springer International Publishing AG 2018

E.A. Platz, N.A. Berger (eds.), *Energy Balance and Prostate Cancer*, Energy Balance and Cancer 14, DOI 10.1007/978-3-319-64940-5_1

Introduction

It is widely postulated that energy balance-related factors such as obesity and physical inactivity play an important role in the occurrence of several cancers. For prostate cancer, the literature investigating the role of obesity in prostate cancer incidence and mortality is extensive, while for physical inactivity the literature is less extensive. After reviewing the definition of energy balance, and the descriptive epidemiology of obesity, physical inactivity, and prostate cancer, in this chapter, we present the epidemiological evidence for obesity and physical activity in the etiology of prostate cancer incidence overall and by stage and grade, and mortality. We highlight the evidence for these associations with advanced disease and fatal prostate cancer, which are the most clinically important endpoints.

Definition of Energy Balance

Energy balance is defined as the equilibrium between energy consumed and expended. A sustained positive energy balance, when an individual consumes more energy than is needed for maintenance of body size, produces weight gain, which may be countered by increased energy expenditure through physical activity.

One of the most widely used anthropometric measures is body mass index (BMI). BMI is calculated as an individual's weight in kilograms divided by the square of height in meters. A higher BMI is indicative of increased body size [1]. The presence of adult obesity is defined as BMI larger than or equal to 30 kg/m^2 and is classified into the following subcategories: (a) Class 1: $30 \leq BMI < 35\ kg/m^2$; (b) Class 2: $35 \leq BMI < 40\ kg/m^2$; and, (c) Class 3: $BMI \geq 40\ kg/m^2$ [2]. A BMI of 25 to less than 30 kg/m^2 is classified as the overweight range. BMI less than 18.5 kg/m^2 is considered to be in the underweight range. BMI is a readily applicable and reliable surrogate measure of body size, but it does not measure body fat directly and it does not provide information about the distribution of body fat (i.e., abdominal vs. general obesity) [3, 4]. Waist circumference (WC) and waist to hip circumference ratio (WHR) are widely used as markers of abdominal (i.e., central) obesity. Abdominal obesity is linked to hyperinsulinemia and type II diabetes, and is hypothesized to be a stronger risk factor than general obesity for the development of several chronic, non-communicable diseases [5], although this hypothesis was not verified in a recent large pooled analysis [6].

Physical activity is defined as any movement that involves the use of skeletal muscles during occupational, household, and recreational activities. Based on its absolute and relative intensity, physical activity may be classified into sedentary, light, moderate (i.e., walking briskly, ballroom dancing, light gardening activities, etc.) and vigorous (i.e., jogging, intensive swimming, hiking uphill, etc.) activity [7]. Recently both the World Health Organization (WHO) and the American Cancer Society recommended that adults should engage in either at least 150 min of moderate or 75 min of vigorous aerobic physical activity each week [8, 9].

Descriptive Epidemiology of Obesity and Physical Inactivity

The worldwide prevalence of overweight and obesity is increasing and has achieved epidemic proportions particularly in developed countries [10]. In 2014, the prevalence of obesity worldwide was 11% in adult men and 15% in women [11]. During the period between 1975 and 2014, the global age-standardized mean BMI increased from 21.7 kg/m^2 to 24.2 kg/m^2 in men, an increase of 0.63 kg/m^2 per decade, and from 22.1 kg/m^2 to 24.4 kg/m^2 in women, an increase of 0.59 kg/m^2 per decade [12]. It is anticipated that by 2025, 18% of men and more than 20% of women will be obese [12]. The prevalence of obesity is more than two-fold higher in developed countries [11]. In particular, the highest prevalence was documented in the United States of American (USA), where more than 30% of the adult population is obese [12]. Since 2006, the rise in the prevalence of obesity appears to be curtailed in developed countries, but the corresponding rates are rising in developing countries [13].

Globally, 20% of men and 27% of women were unable to meet WHO recommendations for physical activity levels [11]. The prevalence of inadequate physical activity was highest in the WHO regions of America and East Mediterranean, while the lowest rates were observed in Africa and South-East Asia [11]. Physical inactivity rates were almost two-fold greater in high (33%) as compared to low-income countries (17%). Rising trends in physical inactivity are primarily attributed to urbanization and sedentary lifestyles, which have been readily adopted in high income countries [11, 14, 15]. Worldwide, approximately 1.6 million deaths in 2015 alone and 35 million lost disability adjusted life years are attributed to physical inactivity [16].

Epidemiology of Prostate Cancer

Incidence Rates

Prostate cancer is the second most commonly diagnosed cancer in men following lung cancer. It is estimated that 1.1 million men worldwide were diagnosed with prostate cancer in 2012, 70% of whom resided in economically developed countries [17]. The age-adjusted incidence rate of prostate cancer in developed countries is 69 cases per 100,000 person-years exceeding corresponding rates for lung and colorectal cancers [17]. There is large variability in the incidence rates of prostate cancer across the globe with highest rates (85–110 cases per 100,000) reported in Australia, New Zealand, North America and Europe, whereas the lowest incidence rates are observed in Asian populations (about 9 cases per 100,000) [17, 18]. The different trends in prostate cancer incidence may be partly attributed to differences in country-specific recommendations for the use of prostate-specific antigen (PSA) as a screening tool for detecting prostate cancer [19]. In countries such as the USA, Canada and Australia, where regular PSA screening was adopted early on in clinical practice, initial dramatic spikes in incidence rates of prostate cancer were observed [20–22]. Similar, albeit deduced, increases were observed in Western Europe, where regular PSA testing was adopted later [23]. Rates have since been declining in these countries, but continued increases of smaller magnitude in the incidence rates of prostate cancer during the past two decades have been observed in several Asian and Eastern European countries, where PSA testing is not widely used, suggesting changes in prostate cancer risk factors [20, 21, 24]. In addition, geographic differences in prostate cancer incidence rates were apparent prior to the introduction of PSA screening, further highlighting a potential role of environmental and lifestyle factors in the etiology of this disease.

Mortality Rates

Prostate cancer is the fifth most common cause of cancer death worldwide, corresponding to approximately 6.6% of all deaths in men [17]. Mortality rates are generally high in populations of African descent (19–29 deaths per 100,000), intermediate in the Americas and Oceania, and very low in Asia (2.9 per 100,000). During the past one or two decades, prostate cancer mortality rates have declined in many countries in men of all race/ethnicities, the reasons of which remain controversial [25]. However, it is noteworthy that most recently rising mortality rates have been reported in Russia, Belarus, and Bulgaria [17, 19, 21, 26, 27].

Heterogeneity of Prostate Cancer

Prostate cancer is a clinically heterogeneous disease ranging from microscopic, well-differentiated indolent tumors to aggressive disease; the latter comprises 10–20 % of all tumors and can lead to considerable morbidity and mortality [28]. This clinical heterogeneity may reflect the underlying heterogeneity and inconsistency of study results on putative risk factors, and may have implications for screening, treatment and prognosis. Efforts to understand risk factors for prostate cancer with a lethal phenotype are central to contemporary prostate cancer research.

Risk Factors

Despite the large amount of epidemiological research on prostate cancer etiology, the only well-established risk factors are age, race, family history, and low-penetrance genetic variants. The probability of developing prostate cancer increases from 0.3% in men aged younger than 49 years to 11.2% in those older than 70 years [29, 30]. Individuals of African descent are at highest risk of developing prostate cancer, followed by those of Caucasian and Asian descent. In particular, African-American men have 1.6 times higher incidence rates than Caucasian-Americans [31]. A positive family history of prostate cancer in a first degree relative puts men at an approximately two-fold increased risk of developing prostate cancer [29]. During the last decade, genome-wide association studies have identified more than 100 independent low-penetrance genetic loci associated with risk of prostate cancer, which combined explain more than one third of the disease variability [32, 33].

Epidemiological Evidence of an Association Between Obesity and Prostate Cancer

Overview

If this association is causal, it may be important for public health, because obesity and prostate cancer affect substantial proportions of men. However, reported associations could also be a product of residual confounding or several biases as shown in prior empirical research in the field of cancer epidemiology [34–38]. We recently conducted two umbrella reviews to evaluate the strength of the evidence and assess the extent of potential biases in the field of diet, nutrition, obesity, physical activity and risk of several cancers [39, 40]. We systematically identified all published systematic reviews or meta-analyses of prospective studies in this field and applied several criteria to assess evidence strength and validity. Data from 46 meta-analyses on the association between seven somatometric factors (i.e., BMI, weight, WC, WHR, weight gain, BMI at age 18–21, and birth weight) and risk of eight different prostate cancer endpoints were retrieved, a summary of which is presented in Table 1.1. The associations were categorized into five evidence judgments: strong, highly suggestive, suggestive, weak, and not significant evidence.

While none of these associations presented strong evidence (Table 1.1), statistically significant positive associations were observed for BMI and risk of advanced or fatal prostate cancer, the majority of which were graded with suggestive evidence. Similar associations in magnitude and direction were observed for weight, WC and WHR with risk of advanced or fatal disease, but the evidence judgments were in general weaker compared to associations for BMI. Statistically significant inverse associations between BMI and risk of low-grade or localized prostate cancer were observed, but these associations were graded with suggestive or weak evidence. None of the associations between the other measures of the adiposity and risk the other prostate cancer endpoints, including total prostate cancer, was statistically significant (Table 1.1). All of these associations are described in more detail in the following sections.

Table 1.1 Associations between adiposity indices and risk of prostate cancer (unless otherwise specified) in published meta-analyses[a]

Author, year	Risk factor	Contrast	Outcome	Studies	Sample size Cohort/Cases	Summary random effects RR	95% CI	*P*-value	I^2	Egger's P-value[b]	Evidence grading[c]
WCRF, 2014	BMI	Per 5 kg/m²	PrCa (inc & mort)	45	4,271,317/91,206	1.00	0.98, 1.03	0.75	67	0.59	Not significant
WCRF, 2014	BMI	per 5 kg/m²	PrCa	39	3,798,746/88,632	1.00	0.97, 1.03	0.92	70	0.45	Not significant
Renehan, 2008	BMI	Per 5 kg/m²	PrCa	26	3,027,773/69,740	1.03	0.99, 1.06	0.10	76	0.72	Not significant
WCRF, 2014	BMI	Per 5 kg/m²	Low-grade PrCa	4	293,630/9928	0.93	0.89, 0.97	5.1E-04	32	0.33	Suggestive
WCRF, 2014	BMI	Per 5 kg/m²	Non-advanced PrCa	14	1,142,902/25,887	0.95	0.92, 0.98	1.4E-03	40	0.48	Weak
Discaccati, 2012	BMI	Per 5 kg/m²	Localised PrCa	12	1,033,009/19,130	0.94	0.91, 0.97	4.6E-4	20	0.46	Suggestive
WCRF, 2014	BMI	Per 5 kg/m²	High-grade PrCa	6	306,596/3485	1.08	1.01, 1.15	0.02	13	0.98	Weak
WCRF, 2014	BMI	Per 5 kg/m²	Advanced PrCa	23	1,676,220/11,204	1.08	1.04, 1.12	2.4E-04	19	0.11	Suggestive
Discaccati, 2012	BMI	Per 5 kg/m²	Advanced PrCa	13	1,080,790/7067	1.09	1.02, 1.16	0.01	40	0.02	Weak
WCRF, 2014	BMI	Per 5 kg/m²	PrCa mort	12	1,580,914/9826	1.11	1.06, 1.17	1.5E-05	20	0.40	Suggestive
Cao, 2011	BMI	Per 5 kg/m²	PrCa mort	6	1,263,483/6817	1.15	1.06, 1.25	8.3E-4	59	0.30	Suggestive
WCRF, 2014	BMI	Highest—lowest	PrCa (inc & mort)	43	4,224,170/91,655	0.99	0.94, 1.04	0.64	37	0.83	Not significant

Zhang, 2015	BMI	Obese—normal	PrCa	14	2,342,066/73,851	1.00	0.95, 1.06	0.92	40	0.64	Not significant
WCRF, 2014	BMI	Highest—lowest	Advanced PrCa	21	1,591,046/10,210	1.14	1.04, 1.25	3.7E-03	13	0.46	Weak
WCRF, 2014	BMI	Highest—lowest	Fatal PrCa	21	1,591,046/8596	1.14	1.04, 1.25	3.7E-03	13	0.46	Weak
WCRF, 2014	BMI	Highest—lowest	PrCa mort	12	1,601,800/10,032	1.30	1.17, 1.44	1.8E-06	0	0.70	Suggestive
Zhang, 2015	BMI	Obese—normal	PrCa mort	10	2,339,669/14,179	1.24	1.15, 1.33	1.8E-08	0	0.03	Highly suggestive
WCRF, 2014	Weight	Per 5 kg	PrCa	14	807,552/26,176	1.01	1.00, 1.02	0.23	24	0.06	Not significant
WCRF, 2014	Weight	Per 5 kg	Non-advanced PrCa	5	433,176/15,655	0.99	0.97, 1.00	0.15	56	0.69	Not significant
WCRF, 2014	Weight	Per 5 kg	Advanced PrCa	5	433,176/3376	1.03	1.01, 1.06	2.6E-03	0	0.83	Weak
WCRF, 2014	Weight	Per 5 kg	PrCa mort	4	485,756/1180	1.09	1.04, 1.14	3.7E-04	16	0.98	Suggestive
WCRF, 2014	Weight	Highest—lowest	PrCa (inc & mort)	16	2,128,085/59,340	1.09	1.00, 1.18	0.05	76	0.23	Not significant
WCRF, 2014	Waist circum.	Per 10 cm	PrCa (inc & mort)	9	203,342/6624	1.00	0.97, 1.03	0.98	0	0.65	Not significant
MacInnis, 2006	Waist circum.	Per 10 cm	PrCA	4	56,699/1936	1.03	0.97, 1.09	0.34	0	0.44	Not significant

(continued)

Table 1.1 (continued)

Author, year	Risk factor	Contrast	Outcome	Studies	Sample size Cohort/Cases	Summary random effects RR	95% CI	*P*-value	I^2	Egger's P-value[b]	Evidence grading[c]
WCRF, 2014	Waist circum.	Per 10 cm	Non-advanced PrCa	4	182,460/2906	1.01	0.90, 1.12	0.87	71	0.42	Not significant
WCRF, 2014	Waist circum.	Per 10 cm	Advanced PrCa	4	182,460/1230	1.12	1.04, 1.21	4.0E-03	14	0.95	Weak
WCRF, 2014	Waist circum.	Highest—lowest	PrCa (inc & mort)	8	230,204/7428	0.99	0.91, 1.08	0.79	0	0.83	Not significant
WCRF, 2014	Waist circum.	Highest—lowest	Advanced PrCa	3	187,541/1427	1.25	1.05, 1.50	0.01	0	0.37	Weak
WCRF, 2014	Waist-to-hip	Per 0.1 units	PrCa (inc & mort)	5	183,283/5633	1.01	0.96, 1.06	0.73	0	0.35	Not significant
WCRF, 2014	Waist-to-hip	Per 0.1 units	Non-advanced PrCa	4	182,460/2906	0.99	0.90, 1.09	0.87	20	0.82	Not significant
WCRF, 2014	Waist-to-hip	Per 0.1 units	Advanced PrCa	4	182,460/1230	1.15	1.03, 1.28	0.01	0	0.30	Weak
WCRF, 2014	Waist-to-hip	Highest—lowest	PrCa (inc & mort)	5	214,728/6494	1.01	0.92, 1.10	0.90	0	0.14	Not significant
WCRF, 2014	Waist-to-hip	Highest—lowest	Advanced PrCa	3	187,541/1427	1.22	0.99, 1.50	0.06	0	0.03	Not significant
Keum, 2015	Weight gain	Per 5 kg	PrCA	4	102,109/6882	0.98	0.94, 1.02	0.23	51	0.67	Not significant
Keum, 2015	Weight gain	Per 5 kg	Localised PrCA	4	101,742/5404	0.96	0.92, 1.00	0.08	35	0.12	Not significant
Keum, 2015	Weight gain	Per 5 kg	Advanced PrCA	4	101,692/1094	1.04	0.99, 1.09	0.12	0	<0.01	Not significant
Keum, 2015	Weight gain	Highest—lowest	PrCA	8	426,104/19,377	0.98	0.91, 1.06	0.59	31	0.67	Not significant

WCRF, 2014	BMI (age 18-21)	Per 5 kg/m²	PrCa	7	465,132/14,815	0.99	0.93, 1.06	0.79	29	0.09	Not significant
WCRF, 2014	BMI (age 18-21)	Per 5 kg/m²	Non-advanced PrCa	4	397,318/10,158	1.00	0.86, 1.16	0.99	71	0.09	Not significant
WCRF, 2014	BMI (age 18-21)	Per 5 kg/m²	Advanced PrCa	5	445,099/11,388	1.04	0.86, 1.25	0.70	71	0.73	Not significant
WCRF, 2014	BMI (age 18-21)	Per 5 kg/m²	PrCa mort	3	323,878/729	1.13	0.93, 1.37	0.21	0	0.52	Not significant
WCRF, 2014	BMI (age 18-21)	Highest—lowest	PrCa (inc & mort)	8	492,297/15,152	0.98	0.91, 1.07	0.72	36	0.06	Not significant
WCRF, 2014	Birth weight	Per 500 g	PrCa	7	177,548/2695	1.03	0.99, 1.08	0.18	0	0.13	Not significant
WCRF, 2014	Birth weight	Per 500 g	Advanced PrCa	2	40,821/246	1.09	0.97, 1.22	0.13	0	NA	Not significant
WCRF, 2014	Birth weight	Per 500 g	PrCa mort	2	3,316/902	1.09	0.96, 1.25	0.18	0	NA	Not significant
WCRF, 2014	Birth weight	Highest—lowest	PrCa (inc & mort)	5	64,843/1559	1.18	0.97, 1.44	0.09	64	0.09	Not significant

Abbreviations: *WCRF* World Cancer Research Fund, *BMI* body mass index, *CI* confidence interval, *inc* incidence, *mort* mortality, *circum* circumference, *PrCA* prostate cancer, *RR* relative risk

[a]A selection of published meta-analyses of only prospective studies are shown using data from two published relevant umbrella reviews [39, 40]

[b]*P*-value from the Egger's regression asymmetry test

[c]For more details, please see the following references [39, 40]

BMI and Risk of Total Prostate Cancer

BMI was not associated with risk of total prostate cancer in a comprehensive meta-analysis of 39 prospective cohorts published in 2014 (Table 1.1) by the World Cancer Research Fund (WCRF) Continuous Update Project (CUP) [41]. The risk for developing total prostate cancer was 1.00 (95% CI: 0.97–1.03) for every 5 kg/m^2 higher BMI. Large between-study heterogeneity was observed, as denoted by an I^2 value of 70%. Similar findings were reported by another five meta-analyses that included fewer prospective studies [42–45]. In agreement, three recent large Mendelian randomization studies did not find evidence of a causal effect between BMI and risk of total prostate cancer [46–48]. Several studies have explored whether screening PSA tests influence the association of BMI with risk of total prostate cancer, but none of the studies identified a statistically significant interaction [49–53]. Some evidence of a non-linear association was observed in the report by WCRF-CUP and the meta-analysis by Hu and colleagues [41, 42]. Specifically, an inverse J-shaped relationship was suggested with a peak in prostate cancer risk for BMI equal to approximately 25 kg/m^2 and a significant reduction from that point on, which was also reported in a recent large cohort study in the UK [54].

BMI and Risk of Prostate Cancer by Disease Severity

The association between body size and incidence of advanced or aggressive and non-advanced or non-aggressive prostate cancer is complex [41–43, 55, 56]. Elevated BMI has been associated with an increased risk of high-grade and advanced prostate cancer, whereas inverse associations have been observed for low-grade and localized disease (Table 1.1). More specifically, a meta-analysis of 23 cohorts showed an 8% (95% CI: 1.04–1.12) increase in the risk of advanced prostate cancer for each 5 kg/m^2 higher BMI, whereas a meta-analysis of 12 cohorts showed an inverse association for localized disease (RR: 0.94; 95% CI: 0.91–0.97) [41].

The different associations of obesity by prostate cancer severity have been attributed in part to biology and part to detection biases associated with obesity [38]. Studies have shown that obese men have lower circulating PSA concentrations [57–59], which could produce a lower likelihood of having localized disease detected by screening compared to normal weight men. In addition, obesity may make the performance of a digital-rectal examination more challenging due to excess perirectal fat [60]. Obese men have also larger prostates, which further reduces the likelihood of finding an occult prostate cancer by biopsy [61]. All of the latter factors could lead to a reduced probability of detection of early-stage cancers, but they could also contribute to elevated incidence of advanced disease in obese men, because their cancers may grow undetected for a long time. However, some studies conducted before the PSA era [62] observed a positive association between obesity and prostate cancer mortality, which means that detection bias cannot fully explain the link between obesity and aggressive prostate cancer.

The extent to which the literature on body size and prostate cancer is affected by detection or other biases or confounding is difficult to prove definitively. In two published critical appraisals of the literature, we probed whether there is evidence for bias using an array of statistical tests and sensitivity analyses [39, 40]. The majority of the associations between body size and risk of aggressive and non-aggressive prostate cancer were graded by suggestive or weak evidence. No association was graded with strong evidence.

To further address whether bias may explain all or part of the association between obesity and advanced and non-advanced prostate cancer, we reviewed two large Mendelian randomization studies. Mendelian randomization is a statistical technique that uses polymorphisms in genes strongly associated with the exposure and associated with the outcome only via the exposure to estimate causal effects. These studies found little evidence of a substantial causal effect of BMI on prostate cancer endpoints [47, 48]. The risk estimate for aggressive prostate cancer (N: 4450 cases) produced by the GAME-ON consortium was 1.11 (95% CI: 0.85–1.44) [47], and the estimate for advanced disease (N: 4325 cases) from the PRACTICAL consortium was 1.01 (95% CI: 0.97–1.05) both per one standard deviation higher adult BMI [48]. Similar very weak associations were observed in PRACTICAL for localized (N: 12,975; RR: 0.98; 95% CI: 0.96–1.00), low-grade (N: 8784; RR: 0.97; 95% CI: 0.94–1.00) and high-grade disease (N: 8230; RR: 1.00; 95% CI: 0.98–1.01) per one standard deviation higher adult BMI. The associations for localized and low-grade disease were borderline statistically significant [48]. However, the genetic risk scores explained only a small amount of the variance (1.46% in PRACTICAL) in BMI. In addition, Mendelian randomization estimates have a causal interpretation only if the assumptions of the method hold. No evidence of assumption violation was detected in the Mendelian randomization studies [47, 48], although some of the assumptions are not easily testable. Further research in this area is warranted to better address these limitations.

BMI and Risk of Fatal Prostate Cancer

Four meta-analyses have examined the association between BMI and prostate cancer mortality [41, 43, 63, 64]. A 5 kg/m^2 higher BMI was associated with an 11% (95% CI: 1.06–1.17) increased risk of prostate cancer mortality in a meta-analysis of 12 cohorts (Table 1.1) [41]. Another meta-analysis of 15 cohorts observed an RR of 1.33 (95% CI: 1.22–1.45) comparing obese to normal weight men [63]. This positive association may be due in part to delayed prostate cancer diagnosis in obese versus normal weight men, but it could be also causal as studies have shown that obesity is associated with higher concentrations of insulin and inflammatory cytokines and lower concentrations of adiponectin and testosterone, all of which may be factors that influence prostate cancer progression [38, 65]. The Mendelian randomization study from the PRACTICAL consortium did not observe a statistically significant causal effect per standard deviation in BMI and prostate cancer mortality (OR: 1.00; 95% CI: 0.96–1.04), but this study only included 1483 prostate cancer deaths [48].

Other Measures of Adiposity and Risk of Prostate Cancer

The association between measures of adiposity other than BMI and risk of prostate cancer has been assessed in fewer studies. A meta-analysis of 14 prospective studies observed that weight was not associated with risk of total prostate cancer (Table 1.1), but a statistically significant association was observed for advanced (N: 5 studies; OR per 5 kg higher weight: 1.03; 95% CI: 1.01–1.06) and fatal disease (N: 4 studies; OR: 1.09; 95% CI: 1.04–1.14) [41], which were judged with weak and suggestive evidence in our umbrella reviews, respectively [39, 40].

WC and WHR in mid- and later-adulthood have been associated with advanced disease, but not generally with risk of total prostate cancer incidence or other prostate cancer endpoints (Table 1.1). Meta-analyses of four studies yielded a 12% (95% CI: 1.04–1.21) and 15% (95% CI: 1.03–1.28) increase in risk of advanced prostate cancer per 10 cm and 0.1 units higher WC and WHR, respectively [41], which were both judged with weak evidence [39, 40]. WHR was not associated with risk of total or aggressive prostate cancer in the Mendelian randomization study performed by the GAME-ON consortium [47].

The role of body size in childhood and early adulthood has also been studied. In the meta-analysis conducted by WCRF, BMI in early adulthood (18–21 years) was not associated with prostate cancer incidence or mortality (Table 1.1) [41], but in general few studies have investigated these hypotheses. The Health Professionals Follow-up Study found that high BMI at age 21 was inversely associated with risk of total, advanced and fatal prostate cancer [66]. It is possible that obesity in childhood and adolescence impacts sex hormone concentrations during periods of prostate growth and development that may be important for later prostate cancer risk. However, when the Mendelian randomization study in the GAME-ON consortium investigated whether childhood BMI was associated with total or aggressive prostate cancer, null associations were observed [47].

The meta-analysis conducted by WCRF did not report statistically significant associations between birth weight and risk of any prostate cancer endpoint [41], but a positive association was observed between the genetic risk score for birth weight and aggressive prostate cancer (OR: 1.63 per standard deviation increase in birth weight; 95% CI: 1.03, 2.57) in the GAME-ON Mendelian randomization study [47].

A few prospective cohort studies have examined adult weight change, which may be a better metric of the dynamic nature of adiposity during adulthood that is when obesity becomes central and has more metabolic effects, and the risk of prostate cancer. Two meta-analyses observed null associations for most prostate cancer endpoints (Table 1.1) [67, 68]. The only exception was a statistically significant positive association observed for fatal disease per 5 kg weight gain (RR: 1.15; 95% CI: 1.08–1.23) in a meta-analysis of only two prospective studies [67].

Epidemiological Evidence for an Association Between Physical Activity and Prostate Cancer

Physical Activity and Risk of Total Prostate Cancer

Physical activity has not been consistently associated with total prostate cancer incidence. We recently critically appraised this evidence using data from four published meta-analyses of prospective cohort studies (Table 1.2) that investigated whether total, occupational or recreational physical activity was associated with risk of prostate cancer [39]. Total physical activity was not associated with risk of prostate cancer incidence in a meta-analysis of ten prospective studies published in 2014 comparing men in the highest versus the lowest physical activity quartile (RR: 0.97; 95% CI: 0.90–1.04) [41]. Another meta-analysis published in 2011 identified 24 prospective studies, and estimated a weak but statistically significant summary RR of 0.94 (95% CI: 0.91–0.98), which was attenuated when only high-quality prospective studies were retained (N: 19 studies; RR: 0.96; 95% CI: 0.92–1.00) [69].

High occupational physical activity was associated with a 13% (RR: 0.87; 95% CI: 0.80–0.95) decreased risk of total prostate cancer incidence in a meta-analysis of 13 prospective studies (Table 1.1) [41], which was judged with weak evidence in our published umbrella review [39]. No statistically significant associations were observed for recreational physical activity and risk of total prostate cancer in the published meta-analyses [41, 69, 70]. However, a recent pooled analysis of 12 prospective studies in the USA and Europe reported a weak but statistically significant increased risk of total prostate cancer comparing men with high (90th percentile) versus low (10th percentile) levels of leisure-time physical activity (HR: 1.04; 95% CI: 1.01–1.07) [71]. This finding might be due to detection bias as there is no known biological rationale to explain this association and it has been hypothesized that physically active men are more likely than inactive men to receive digital rectal examinations and/or PSA screening [72].

Physical Activity and Risk of Prostate Cancer by Disease Severity

No statistically significant associations have been reported in published meta-analyses for total, occupational, or recreational physical activity with risk of localized or advanced prostate cancer (Table 1.2) [41, 69]. Leisure-time physical activity was associated with a higher risk of non-advanced disease (HR [90th vs. 10th

Table 1.2 Associations between physical activity indices and risk of prostate cancer (unless otherwise specified) in published meta-analyses[a]

Author, year	Risk factor	Contrast	Outcome	Studies	Sample size Cohort/ Cases	Summary random effects RR	95% CI	*P*-value	I^2	Egger's P-value[b]	Evidence grading[c]
WCRF, 2014	Total PA	Highest—lowest	PrCa (inc & mort)	10	500,121/22,354	0.97	0.90, 1.04	0.38	34	1.00	Not significant
WCRF, 2014	Occupational PA	Highest—lowest	PrCa (inc & mort)	13	3,861,201/101,304	0.87	0.80, 0.95	1.6E-03	28	0.24	Weak
WCRF, 2014	Recreational PA	Highest—lowest	Localised PrCa	3	176,145/2522	0.93	0.77, 1.13	0.46	45	0.04	Not significant
WCRF, 2014	Recreational PA	Highest—lowest	Advanced PrCa	6	522,052/21,064	0.93	0.73, 1.18	0.53	75	0.36	Not significant
WCRF, 2014	Recreational PA	Highest—lowest	Fatal PrCa	5	402,766/19,634	0.89	0.76, 1.05	0.18	0	0.49	Not significant

Abbreviations: *WCRF* World Cancer Research Fund, *CI* confidence interval, *inc* incidence, *mort* mortality, *PrCA* prostate cancer, *RR* relative risk

[a]A selection of published meta-analyses of only prospective studies are shown using data from two published relevant umbrella reviews [39, 40]

[b]*P*-value from the Egger's regression asymmetry test

[c]For more details, please see the following references [39, 40]

percentile]: 1.08; 95% CI: 1.03–1.12), but not with advanced prostate cancer (HR: 0.99; 95% CI, 0.88–1.10) in the recent pooled analysis of 12 prospective studies [71], which implies that results for total and non-advanced prostate cancer are probably influenced by detection bias. Recreational physical activity was not associated with prostate cancer mortality in a meta-analysis of five prospective studies (Table 1.2; RR [highest vs. lowest quartile]: 0.89; 95% CI: 0.76–1.05) [41].

Discussion and Directions for Future Research

The existing epidemiological literature on the relationship of correlates of energy balance—body size and physical activity—with risk of prostate cancer was summarized in this review. From a public health perspective, the potential identification of obesity and physical inactivity as risk factors for prostate cancer, especially for aggressive and fatal disease, is of paramount importance due to the high incidence of the disease and the high prevalence and modifiable nature of the exposures. Overall, the association of body size and physical activity with prostate cancer has been extensively studied. Meta-analyses of prospective studies have shown that high BMI is associated with a decreased risk of localized prostate cancer and an increased risk of advanced and fatal disease [39–41]. The magnitude of the observed associations was modest, ranging up to 10% of risk decrease or increase per 5 kg/m^2 higher BMI, respectively. It is generally difficult to distinguish such modest relative risks from potential chance or bias, and there is evidence that these results may be attributed, in part, to detection biases associated with obesity [38], although it is impossible to prove the definitive presence or the exact source of biases in epidemiological research. To diminish the probability of detection bias in obese men, it has been suggested that BMI-adjusted PSA cut-points should be used and more biopsy cores should be obtained in obese men who tend to have larger prostates [38], but studies are warranted to test this hypothesis.

The notable biological heterogeneity of prostate cancer adds further uncertainty in the determination of prostate cancer risk factors, and future research should focus in identifying more valid and accurate markers of this biological heterogeneity than stage and grade of the disease. Until then, prostate cancer death remains the most robust and clinically relevant outcome and future prospective studies and large consortia should focus on this endpoint, as approximately only one in four published studies in the field of obesity and prostate cancer have included fatal prostate cancer as an outcome (Table 1.1). In the absence of data from randomized controlled trials examining the effects of weight loss on prostate cancer endpoints, Mendelian randomization analyses might prove useful in determining whether an observed association is likely to be causal. Two large Mendelian randomization studies have been published, but found little evidence of a substantial causal effect of BMI on the different prostate cancer endpoints [47, 48]. Only one of these studies investigated risk of fatal prostate cancer, but included only 1483 deaths and was likely underpowered for this outcome [48].

Fewer prospective studies have investigated the association between other indices of adiposity, including markers of central obesity, body size in childhood and early adulthood and weight change, with risk of prostate cancer. The existing observational evidence supports a potential positive association between markers of central adiposity and risk of advanced prostate cancer, but again this evidence is not robust and the evidence is sparse for other adiposity indices [39–41]. Large prospective studies should be conducted in the future to investigate these associations, as they may prove useful in explaining part of the underlying heterogeneity of the observed associations between adiposity and prostate cancer and may also improve our understanding of the potential mechanisms involved in these associations.

Physical activity is not robustly associated with risk of prostate cancer [39–41]. The different sources of physical activity (i.e. total, occupational, recreational) and the wide variability and potential measurement error in the methods of its assessment add complexity. Further research, in the form of randomized controlled trials and epidemiological studies is necessary to understand whether the hypothesized benefits of exercise on prostate cancer are real. In the near future, new large prospective studies and bio-banks are expected to provide more valid estimates of the associations of obesity and physical activity with risk of prostate cancer endpoints using direct measurements of body fat (e.g. bioelectrical impedance analysis and DXA) and motion (e.g. accelerometry) in hundreds of thousands of participants [73, 74].

Conclusions

Markers of general and central obesity have been associated with an increased risk of advanced and fatal disease, and a decreased risk of localized prostate cancer, but hints of bias are present in this literature. The literature evidence is sparse and inconsistent for other adiposity indices and physical activity. Future prospective studies and large consortia with valid and direct assessment of the time-varying nature of body fatness and physical activity and with a focus on lethal prostate cancer are needed to draw firmer conclusions.

Funding NP and KKT were supported by the World Cancer Research Fund International Regular Grant Programme (WCRF 2014/1180 to KKT).

References

1. Centers for Disease Control and Prevention. Defining adult overweight and obesity [cited 2016 29 Nov]. Available from: https://www.cdc.gov/obesity/adult/defining.html.
2. Obesity: preventing and managing the global epidemic. Report of a WHO consultation. World Health Organ Tech Rep Ser. 2000;894(i-xii):1–253.
3. Garn SM, Leonard WR, Hawthorne VM. Three limitations of the body mass index. Am J Clin Nutr. 1986;44(6):996–7.

4. Gallagher D, Visser M, Sepulveda D, Pierson RN, Harris T, Heymsfield SB. How useful is body mass index for comparison of body fatness across age, sex, and ethnic groups? Am J Epidemiol. 1996;143(3):228–39.
5. Pischon T, Boeing H, Hoffmann K, Bergmann M, Schulze MB, Overvad K, et al. General and abdominal adiposity and risk of death in Europe. N Engl J Med. 2008;359(20):2105–20.
6. Emerging Risk Factors Collaboration, Wormser D, Kaptoge S, Di Angelantonio E, Wood AM, Pennells L, et al. Separate and combined associations of body-mass index and abdominal adiposity with cardiovascular disease: collaborative analysis of 58 prospective studies. Lancet. 2011;377(9771):1085–95.
7. World Cancer Research Fund/American Institute for Cancer Research. Food, nutrition, physical activity, and the prevention of cancer: a global perspective. Washington DC: AIRC; 2007.
8. World Health Organisation. Global Recommendations on Physical Activity for Health. WHO Guidelines Approved by the Guidelines Review Committee. Geneva. 2010.
9. Kushi LH, Doyle C, McCullough M, Rock CL, Demark-Wahnefried W, Bandera EV, et al. American Cancer Society guidelines on nutrition and physical activity for cancer prevention: reducing the risk of cancer with healthy food choices and physical activity. CA Cancer J Clin. 2012;62(1):30–67.
10. Swinburn BA, Sacks G, Hall KD, McPherson K, Finegood DT, Moodie ML, et al. The global obesity pandemic: shaped by global drivers and local environments. Lancet. 2011;378(9793):804–14.
11. World Health Organisation. Global status report on noncommunicable diseases 2014. Geneva: World Health Organisation; 2015.
12. NCD Risk Factor Collaboration. Trends in adult body-mass index in 200 countries from 1975 to 2014: a pooled analysis of 1698 population-based measurement studies with 19.2 million participants. Lancet. 2016;387(10,026):1377–96.
13. Ng M, Fleming T, Robinson M, Thomson B, Graetz N, Margono C, et al. Global, regional, and national prevalence of overweight and obesity in children and adults during 1980–2013: a systematic analysis for the Global Burden of Disease Study 2013. Lancet. 2014;384(9945):766–81.
14. Pratt M, Sarmiento OL, Montes F, Ogilvie D, Marcus BH, Perez LG, et al. The implications of megatrends in information and communication technology and transportation for changes in global physical activity. Lancet. 2012;380(9838):282–93.
15. Bauman AE, Reis RS, Sallis JF, Wells JC, Loos RJ, Martin BW, et al. Correlates of physical activity: why are some people physically active and others not? Lancet. 2012;380(9838):258–71.
16. GBD Risk Factors Collaborators. Global, regional, and national comparative risk assessment of 79 behavioural, environmental and occupational, and metabolic risks or clusters of risks, 1990–2015: a systematic analysis for the Global Burden of Disease Study 2015. Lancet. 2016;388(10,053):1659–724.
17. Ferlay J, Soerjomataram I, Dikshit R, Eser S, Mathers C, Rebelo M, et al. Cancer incidence and mortality worldwide: sources, methods and major patterns in GLOBOCAN 2012. Int J Cancer. 2015;136(5):E359–86.
18. Torre LA, Bray F, Siegel RL, Ferlay J, Lortet-Tieulent J, Jemal A. Global cancer statistics, 2012. CA Cancer J Clin. 2015;65(2):87–108.
19. Ferlay J, Steliarova-Foucher E, Lortet-Tieulent J, Rosso S, Coebergh JW, Comber H, et al. Cancer incidence and mortality patterns in Europe: estimates for 40 countries in 2012. Eur J Cancer. 2013;49(6):1374–403.
20. Feletto E, Bang A, Cole-Clark D, Chalasani V, Rasiah K, Smith DP. An examination of prostate cancer trends in Australia, England, Canada and USA: Is the Australian death rate too high? World J Urol. 2015;33(11):1677–87.
21. Wong MC, Goggins WB, Wang HH, Fung FD, Leung C, Wong SY, et al. Global incidence and mortality for prostate cancer: analysis of temporal patterns and trends in 36 countries. Eur Urol. 2016;
22. Kvale R, Auvinen A, Adami HO, Klint A, Hernes E, Moller B, et al. Interpreting trends in prostate cancer incidence and mortality in the five Nordic countries. J Natl Cancer Inst. 2007;99(24):1881–7.

23. Torre LA, Siegel RL, Ward EM, Jemal A. Global cancer incidence and mortality rates and trends—an update. Cancer Epidemiol Biomark Prev. 2016;25(1):16–27.
24. Ito K. Prostate cancer in Asian men. Nat Rev. Urol. 2014;11(4):197–212.
25. Ferlay J, Soerjomataram I, Ervik M, Dikshit R, Eser S, Mathers C, et al. GLOBOCAN 2012 v1.0, cancer incidence and mortality worldwide: IARC CancerBase No. 11 [Internet]. International Agency for Research on Cancer: Lyon, France; 2013. Available from: http://globocan.iarc.fr, accessed on 16 September 2015
26. Hashim D, Boffetta P, La Vecchia C, Rota M, Bertuccio P, Malvezzi M, et al. The global decrease in cancer mortality: trends and disparities. Ann Oncol. 2016;27(5):926–33.
27. Center MM, Jemal A, Lortet-Tieulent J, Ward E, Ferlay J, Brawley O, et al. International variation in prostate cancer incidence and mortality rates. Eur Urol. 2012;61(6):1079–92.
28. Siegel R, Naishadham D, Jemal A. Cancer statistics, 2013. CA Cancer J Clin. 2013;63(1):11–30.
29. Bayne CE, Jarrett TW. Cancer of the prostate: incidence in the USA. In: Mydlo JH, Godec CJ, editors. Prostate cancer science and clinical practice. 2nd ed. London: Academic; 2015. p. 119–25.
30. Platz EA, Giovannucci E. Prostate cancer. In: Schottenfeld D, Fraumeni Jr JF, editors. Cancer epidemiology and prevention. 3rd ed. New York: Oxford University Press; 2006. p. 1128–50.
31. Brawley OW. Trends in prostate cancer in the United States. J Natl Cancer Inst Monogr. 2012;2012(45):152–6.
32. Al Olama AA, Kote-Jarai Z, Berndt SI, Conti DV, Schumacher F, Han Y, et al. A meta-analysis of 87,040 individuals identifies 23 new susceptibility loci for prostate cancer. Nat Genet. 2014;46(10):1103–9.
33. Eeles R, Goh C, Castro E, Bancroft E, Guy M, Al Olama AA, et al. The genetic epidemiology of prostate cancer and its clinical implications. Nat Rev Urol. 2014;11(1):18–31.
34. Ioannidis JP. Why most published research findings are false. PLoS Med. 2005;2(8):e124.
35. Tsilidis KK, Kasimis JC, Lopez DS, Ntzani EE, Ioannidis JP. Type 2 diabetes and cancer: umbrella review of meta-analyses of observational studies. BMJ. 2015;350:g7607.
36. Tsilidis KK, Papatheodorou SI, Evangelou E, Ioannidis JP. Evaluation of excess statistical significance in meta-analyses of 98 biomarker associations with cancer risk. J Natl Cancer Inst. 2012;104(24):1867–78.
37. Schoenfeld JD, Ioannidis JP. Is everything we eat associated with cancer? A systematic cookbook review. Am J Clin Nutr. 2013;97(1):127–34.
38. Allott EH, Masko EM, Freedland SJ. Obesity and prostate cancer: weighing the evidence. Eur Urol. 2013;63(5):800–9.
39. Markozannes G, Tzoulaki I, Karli D, Evangelou E, Ntzani E, Gunter MJ, et al. Diet, body size, physical activity and risk of prostate cancer: an umbrella review of the evidence. Eur J Cancer. 2016;69:61–9.
40. Kyrgiou M, Kalliala I, Markozannes G, Gunter MJ, Paraskevaidis E, Gabra H, et al. Adiposity and cancer at major anatomical sites: an umbrella review of the literature. BMJ. 2017;356:j477.
41. World Cancer Research Fund/American Institute for Cancer Research. Continuous Update Project Report. Diet, nutrition, physical activity, and prostate cancer. 2014.
42. Hu MB, Liu SH, Jiang HW, Bai PD, Ding Q. Obesity affects the biopsy-mediated detection of prostate cancer, particularly high-grade prostate cancer: a dose-response meta-analysis of 29,464 patients. PLoS One. 2014;9(9):e106677.
43. Zhang X, Zhou G, Sun B, Zhao G, Liu D, Sun J, et al. Impact of obesity upon prostate cancer-associated mortality: A meta-analysis of 17 cohort studies. Oncol Lett. 2015;9(3):1307–12.
44. Renehan AG, Tyson M, Egger M, Heller RF, Zwahlen M. Body-mass index and incidence of cancer: a systematic review and meta-analysis of prospective observational studies. Lancet. 2008;371(9612):569–78.
45. Bergstrom A, Pisani P, Tenet V, Wolk A, Adami HO. Overweight as an avoidable cause of cancer in Europe. Int J Cancer. 2001;91(3):421–30.
46. Benn M, Tybjaerg-Hansen A, Smith GD, Nordestgaard BG. High body mass index and cancer risk-a Mendelian randomisation study. Eur J Epidemiol. 2016;31(9):879–92.

47. Gao C, Patel CJ, Michailidou K, Peters U, Gong J, Schildkraut J, et al. Mendelian randomization study of adiposity-related traits and risk of breast, ovarian, prostate, lung and colorectal cancer. Int J Epidemiol. 2016;45(3):896–908.
48. Davies NM, Gaunt TR, Lewis SJ, Holly J, Donovan JL, Hamdy FC, et al. The effects of height and BMI on prostate cancer incidence and mortality: a Mendelian randomization study in 20,848 cases and 20,214 controls from the PRACTICAL consortium. Cancer Causes Control. 2015;26(11):1603–16.
49. Giovannucci E, Liu Y, Platz EA, Stampfer MJ, Willett WC. Risk factors for prostate cancer incidence and progression in the health professionals follow-up study. Int J Cancer. 2007;121(7):1571–8.
50. Hernandez BY, Park SY, Wilkens LR, Henderson BE, Kolonel LN. Relationship of body mass, height, and weight gain to prostate cancer risk in the multiethnic cohort. Cancer Epidemiol Biomark Prev. 2009;18(9):2413–21.
51. Littman AJ, White E, Kristal AR. Anthropometrics and prostate cancer risk. Am J Epidemiol. 2007;165(11):1271–9.
52. Rodriguez C, Freedland SJ, Deka A, Jacobs EJ, McCullough ML, Patel AV, et al. Body mass index, weight change, and risk of prostate cancer in the Cancer Prevention Study II Nutrition Cohort. Cancer Epidemiol Biomark Prev. 2007;16(1):63–9.
53. Wright ME, Chang SC, Schatzkin A, Albanes D, Kipnis V, Mouw T, et al. Prospective study of adiposity and weight change in relation to prostate cancer incidence and mortality. Cancer. 2007;109(4):675–84.
54. Bhaskaran K, Douglas I, Forbes H, dos Santos-Silva I, Leon DA, Smeeth L. Body-mass index and risk of 22 specific cancers: a population-based cohort study of 5.24 million UK adults. Lancet. 2014;384(9945):755–65.
55. Discacciati A, Orsini N, Wolk A. Body mass index and incidence of localized and advanced prostate cancer—a dose-response meta-analysis of prospective studies. Ann Oncol. 2012;23(7):1665–71.
56. MacInnis RJ, English DR. Body size and composition and prostate cancer risk: systematic review and meta-regression analysis. Cancer Causes Control. 2006;17(8):989–1003.
57. Baillargeon J, Pollock BH, Kristal AR, Bradshaw P, Hernandez J, Basler J, et al. The association of body mass index and prostate-specific antigen in a population-based study. Cancer. 2005;103(5):1092–5.
58. Grubb RL 3rd, Black A, Izmirlian G, Hickey TP, Pinsky PF, Mabie JE, et al. Serum prostate-specific antigen hemodilution among obese men undergoing screening in the prostate, lung, colorectal, and ovarian cancer screening trial. Cancer Epidemiol Biomark Prev. 2009;18(3):748–51.
59. Hekal IA, Ibrahiem EI. Obesity-PSA relationship: a new formula. Prostate Cancer Prostatic Dis. 2010;13(2):186–90.
60. Chu DI, De Nunzio C, Gerber L, Thomas JA 2nd, Calloway EE, Albisinni S, et al. Predictive value of digital rectal examination for prostate cancer detection is modified by obesity. Prostate Cancer Prostatic Dis. 2011;14(4):346–53.
61. Freedland SJ, Platz EA, Presti JC Jr, Aronson WJ, Amling CL, Kane CJ, et al. Obesity, serum prostate specific antigen and prostate size: implications for prostate cancer detection. J Urol. 2006;175(2):500–4. discussion 4
62. Rodriguez C, Patel AV, Calle EE, Jacobs EJ, Chao A, Thun MJ. Body mass index, height, and prostate cancer mortality in two large cohorts of adult men in the United States. Cancer Epidemiol Biomark Prev. 2001;10(4):345–53.
63. Zhong S, Yan X, Wu Y, Zhang X, Chen L, Tang J, et al. Body mass index and mortality in prostate cancer patients: a dose-response meta-analysis. Prostate Cancer Prostatic Dis. 2016;19(2):122–31.
64. Cao Y, Ma J. Body mass index, prostate cancer-specific mortality, and biochemical recurrence: a systematic review and meta-analysis. Cancer Prev Res (Phila). 2011;4(4):486–501.

65. Wilson KM, Giovannucci EL, Mucci LA. Lifestyle and dietary factors in the prevention of lethal prostate cancer. Asian J Androl. 2012;14(3):365–74.
66. Moller E, Wilson KM, Batista JL, Mucci LA, Balter K, Giovannucci E. Body size across the life course and prostate cancer in the Health Professionals Follow-up Study. Int J Cancer. 2016;138(4):853–65.
67. Chen Q, Chen T, Shi W, Zhang T, Zhang W, Jin Z, et al. Adult weight gain and risk of prostate cancer: a dose-response meta-analysis of observational studies. Int J Cancer. 2016;138(4):866–74.
68. Keum N, Greenwood DC, Lee DH, Kim R, Aune D, Ju W, et al. Adult weight gain and adiposity-related cancers: a dose-response meta-analysis of prospective observational studies. J Natl Cancer Inst. 2015;107(2):djv088.
69. Liu Y, Hu F, Li D, Wang F, Zhu L, Chen W, et al. Does physical activity reduce the risk of prostate cancer? A systematic review and meta-analysis. Eur Urol. 2011;60(5):1029–44.
70. Liu L, Shi Y, Li T, Qin Q, Yin J, Pang S, et al. Leisure time physical activity and cancer risk: evaluation of the WHO's recommendation based on 126 high-quality epidemiological studies. Br J Sports Med. 2016;50(6):372–8.
71. Moore SC, Lee IM, Weiderpass E, Campbell PT, Sampson JN, Kitahara CM, et al. Association of leisure-time physical activity with risk of 26 types of cancer in 1.44 million adults. JAMA Intern Med. 2016;176(6):816–25.
72. Moore SC, Peters TM, Ahn J, Park Y, Schatzkin A, Albanes D, et al. Physical activity in relation to total, advanced, and fatal prostate cancer. Cancer Epidemiol Biomark Prev. 2008;17(9):2458–66.
73. German National Cohort C. The German National Cohort: aims, study design and organization. Eur J Epidemiol. 2014;29(5):371–82.
74. Sudlow C, Gallacher J, Allen N, Beral V, Burton P, Danesh J, et al. UK biobank: an open access resource for identifying the causes of a wide range of complex diseases of middle and old age. PLoS Med. 2015;12(3):e1001779.

Chapter 2
Racial/Ethnic Differences in the Association Between Energy Balance and Prostate Cancer

David S. Lopez

Abstract Population-based studies now generally support a positive association between correlates of energy imbalance and prostate cancer risk. However, despite the fact that prostate cancer shows notable racial/ethnic disparities, and the fact that modifiable and non-modifiable risk factors for prostate cancer show racial/ethnic variation, little work has been done to investigate whether the association between energy balance and prostate cancer differs by race/ethnicity. This chapter reviews the still evolving literature, including on lifestyle risk factors that are correlated with energy balance, with a focus on risk of advanced and fatal prostate cancer in different racial and ethnic groups. The majority of studies on energy balance and prostate cancer have been conducted in non-Hispanic white men, including from North America, Europe, and Australia. Very few studies on this topic have been conducted among minority populations, and of those studies that included minority populations, the sample sizes were so small that meaningful conclusions could not be derived. Some studies adjusted for race/ethnicity, but findings from these analyses do not inform whether the association between energy imbalance and prostate differs by race/ethnicity. Adequately powered studies seeking to document similarities and differences among racial/ethnic groups in energy-balance related risk factors for prostate cancer, especially lethal disease, are needed to be able to tailoring interventions to subpopulations. Standard definitions of race, ethnicity, and more generally ancestry, must be developed for such research in population-based studies, to make the comparison among study findings more valid and reliable. More work is also needed to understand the biological pathways that may underlie any racial/ethnic differences in the association between energy balance and prostate cancer: testosterone remains a possible explanatory mechanism.

Keywords Prostate cancer • Race • Ethnicity disparities • Risk • Obesity • Physical inactivity • Diet

---

D.S. Lopez, DrPH, MPH, MS (✉)
Division of Epidemiology, Human Genetics and Environmental Sciences, University of Texas School of Public Health, 1200 Pressler Street, suite E-629, Houston, TX 77030, USA

Division of Urology, University of Texas-Medical School at Houston, Houston, TX 77030, USA
e-mail: David.S.Lopez@uth.tmc.edu

© Springer International Publishing AG 2018

E.A. Platz, N.A. Berger (eds.), *Energy Balance and Prostate Cancer*, Energy Balance and Cancer 14, DOI 10.1007/978-3-319-64940-5_2

In the last ten years, the investigation of the role of energy balance, especially the imbalance between excessive energy intake relative to energy expenditure, in prostate cancer has increased substantially. Population-based studies now generally support a positive association between correlates of energy imbalance and prostate cancer risk. However, despite the fact that prostate cancer shows notable racial/ethnic disparities, and the fact that modifiable and non-modifiable risk factors for prostate cancer show racial/ethnic variation (Fig. 2.1), little work has been done to investigate whether the association between energy balance and prostate cancer differs by race/ethnicity. This chapter reviews the still evolving literature, including on lifestyle risk factors that are correlated with energy balance, with a focus on risk of advanced and fatal prostate cancer in different racial and ethnic groups. In addition, we will focus thoroughly in one biological mechanism, i.e. testosterone, as the

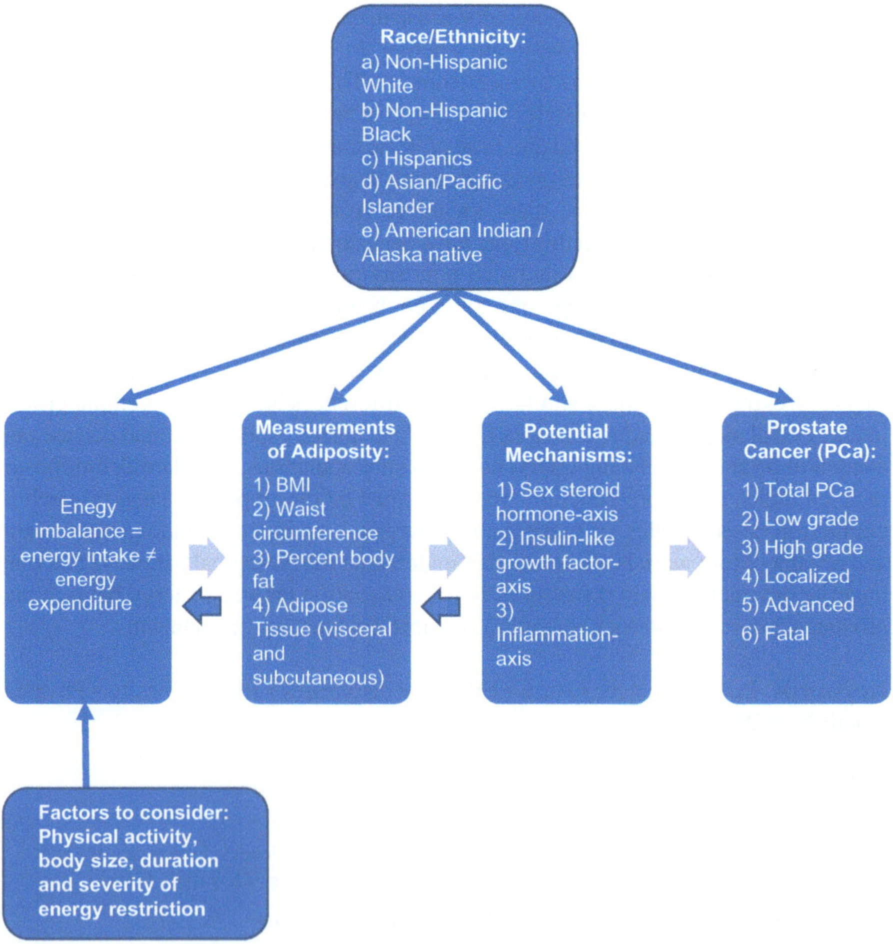

Fig. 2.1 Impact of race and ethnicity in the association of energy imbalance and natural history of prostate cancer

interplay among energy imbalance (specifically obesity), testosterone, and prostate cancer by race and ethnicity has begun to receive attention.

Race and Ethnicity: Description and Its Use in Research

The inclusion of race and ethnicity in research, especially in the investigation of energy balance and prostate cancer, is a growing and evolving field. Therefore, before we discuss the impact of race of race and ethnicity in the association of energy balance and prostate cancer, it is important to understand the implications of using race and ethnicity in research. We will (1) describe the different racial and ethnic groups in the United States (US); (2) report the use of race/ethnicity in epidemiological studies and its implications; and (3) understand the historical low participation of minority populations (other than non-Hispanic White) in randomized clinical trials, and the ongoing efforts to increase these numbers [1, 2].

Characterization of Race and Ethnicity in the US

The US Census Bureau collects race and ethnicity information following the US Office of Management and Budget's guidelines and this information is based on self-identification [3]. The racial groups included in the Census questionnaire generally reflect a social definition of race recognized in the US and not an attempt to define race biologically, anthropologically, or genetically. The Census uses five racial groups and one ethnic group: White, Black/African-American, American Indian/Alaska Native, Asian, and Native Hawaiian/other Pacific Islander, and the Hispanic/Latino ethnic group. People may self-identify with more than one race group, and also people who identify their origin as Hispanic/Latino may be of any race [3, 4].

- **White**—A person having origins in any of the original peoples of Europe, the Middle East, or North Africa.
- **Black or African American**—A person having origins in any of the Black racial groups of Africa.
- **American Indian/Alaska Native**—A person having origins in any of the original peoples of North and South America (including Central America) and who maintains tribal affiliation or community attachment.
- **Asian**—A person having origins in any of the original peoples of the Far East, Southeast Asia, or the Indian subcontinent including, for example, Cambodia, China, India, Japan, Korea, Malaysia, Pakistan, the Philippine Islands, Thailand, and Vietnam.
- **Native Hawaiian/Other Pacific Islander**—A person having origins in any of the original peoples of Hawaii, Guam, Samoa, or other Pacific Islands.

- **Hispanic/Latino ethnicity**—A person having origins from Mexico, Puerto Rico, Cuba, or Spanish Origin (any country from South America). Hispanics/ Latino ethnicity may be of any other race mentioned above.

From 2000 to 2010, more than half of the growth in the total US population was due to the increase in the Hispanic population. Hispanic population grew by 43% increasing from 35.3 million in 2000 to 50.5 million in 2010 [4]. The White population grew 5.7% (211.4–223.5 million), Black/African American population grew 12.3% (34.6–38.9 million), American Indian/Alaska Native grew 18.4% (2.4–2.9 million), Asian population grew 43.3% (10.2–14.6 million), and Native Hawaiian/ Other Pacific Islander population grew 35.4% (398,835–540,013). From this information and compared to the White population, the percent increased almost double in all the other racial and ethnic groups from 2000 to 2010.

Use of Race and Ethnicity in Epidemiological Studies

In parallel to the growth of the minority population, the use of race and ethnicity in research has increased over the past five decades [5, 6]. Yet, there is still confusion regarding the meaning of the terms. In a comprehensive review of 1198 articles, researchers determined how current investigators address the use of race and ethnicity as scientific variables in epidemiologic and public health studies [7]. These articles were published from 1996 to 1999 in two well-established and peer-reviewed journals that focused on publishing research of public health importance, the *American Journal of Epidemiology* and the *American Journal of Public Health*. One of the main findings in this review was the wide diversity of terms used to characterize the variables of race and ethnicity and the categories used to describe these variables. Because race and ethnicity is self-reported, researchers have no standard methodology to know how and when to use race and ethnicity terms/variables in randomized trials, epidemiologic studies, or research in general. Therefore, research findings from studies using race and ethnicity as a variable should be interpreted with caution to avoid generalizations as this variable is self-reported and there is no standard methodology among researchers for its use.

Participation of Race and Ethnicity in Randomized Clinical Trials and Observational Studies

Several studies have shown that minority populations are underrepresented in clinical trials and biobanking [8, 9], yet little is known about the reasons for their low participation and reasons may differ among different for each racial and ethnic group [1, 8, 10]. For instance, Scott et al. [9] in the Retrovirus Epidemiology Donor Studies (REDS-I/-II) demonstrated repository participation rates were lower among

Table 2.1 Prostate cancer incidence and mortality rates by race and ethnicity, United States, 2008–2012

Non-Hispanic White	Non-Hispanic Black	Asian/Pacific Islander	American Indian/Alaska native	Hispanic
		INCIDENCE		
123.0	208.7	67.8	90.5	112.1
		MORTALITY		
19.9	47.2	9.4	20.2	17.8

Adapted from Siegel RL et al. [12]
Rates are per 100,000 population and age adjusted to the 2000 US standard population. Nonwhite and nonblack race categories are not mutually exclusive of Hispanic origin
Data based on Indian Health Service Contract Health Service Delivery Areas (CHSDA) counties. Incidence rates exclude data from Kansas

African-Americans and Hispanics than among non-Hispanic Whites. A number of studies has suggested that minority populations are less likely to participate in clinical trials and biobanking because they have concerns related to sharing of genetic data and lack of credibility and trust in research institutions [1, 11]. Although there is a great effort to include minority populations in clinical trials, there are still few studies with very small numbers of minority study participants, including those investigating energy balance and prostate cancer or modifiable factors strongly correlated with energy balance. This information provides understanding about the few randomized trials found different racial and ethnic groups. Although the evaluation of associations separately among racial and ethnic groups in observational studies has increased, the sample sizes by race/ethnicity are, in general, small and therefore drawing race/ethnicity-specific inferences to inform population-specific recommendations has been difficult.

Prostate Cancer Incidence and Mortality Rates: Race and Ethnicity

Prostate cancer is the most common cancer diagnosed in men from any racial and ethnic group in the U.S. [12]. Furthermore, prostate cancer is the second most common cause of death among US men from any racial and ethnic group, with the exception in Asian/Pacific Islander men. Yet, one of the interesting characteristics of prostate cancer is that its incidence and mortality rates vary significantly by race and ethnicity (Table 2.1) [12, 13]. Non-Hispanic Black men have both the highest incidence and mortality rates of prostate cancer. They are followed by non-Hispanic White men with the second highest incidence rate, and subsequently by Hispanics, American Indian/Alaska Native, and lastly by Asian/Pacific Islander men. However, mortality rates are the second highest among American Indian/Alaska Native men, followed by non-Hispanic Whites, Hispanics, and again lastly by Asian/Pacific Islanders. Therefore, it is interesting to note that one group is consistent with having both the highest incidence and mortality rates (non-Hispanic Black men) and another one with having both the lowest incidence and mortality rates (Asian/Pacific Islander men).

Worldwide, reported prostate cancer incidence rates vary more than 25-fold and mortality rates vary more than 10-fold [14]. This cancer is the second most common type in men globally [15, 16]. With an estimated 307,000 deaths in 2012, prostate cancer is the fifth leading cause of death from cancer in men [16]. The highest incidence rates of prostate cancer are observed in Australia/New Zealand and North America (annual rates standardized to the world age standard: 111.6 and 97.2 per 100,000 men, respectively); however, these high rates have been attributed mainly to the widespread practice of prostate-specific antigen testing and subsequent biopsy in those regions. When the mortality rates of prostate cancer are stratified by race and ethnicity, mortality is highest predominantly in black populations (annual rates standardized to the world age standard: Caribbean, 29 per 100,000 men; sub-Saharan Africa, 19–24 per 100,000 men), intermediate among men from the Americas and Oceania, and the lowest among Asian men (2.9 per 100,000 men) [16].

The future of prostate cancer is and will remain as a significant public health concern. It is estimated that in just over a decade, prostate cancer will overtake lung cancer as the most common form of cancer in men around the globe [17, 18]. Therefore, racial/ethnic disparities in prostate cancer are expected to increase in parallel.

Modifiable and Non-Modifiable Risk Factors for Prostate Cancer: Race and Ethnicity

Race (black or African ancestry), older age and family history of prostate cancer are the only well-established risk factors for prostate cancer [19, 20]. Unfortunately, these factors are non-modifiable, and although they are important to identify high-risk groups to develop and target specific interventions, men have no control over them. While not established risk factors, epidemiological studies suggest associations between modifiable factors and prostate cancer, primarily advanced and fatal prostate cancer cases, suggesting that they may have an effect on the progression of the disease rather than initiation of disease [20–22]. A list of these modifiable factors include total fat intake, saturated fat, low physical activity and body size (total and distribution of adiposity) [17, 20, 22]. Interestingly, several of these modifiable factors are aspects of or strongly linked to energy balance. Of these energy-related factors, body size (total and distribution of adiposity) is considered one the most valid and reliable measure of health exposure related to energy balance [23]. Therefore, a substantial number of studies have focused on body size to make inferences about energy balance. Race and ethnicity have been shown to play an independent role in any of these modifiable and non-modifiable factors, including stage and grade of prostate cancer (Fig. 2.1).

Energy Balance and Prostate Cancer: By Race and Ethnicity

Experimental studies have shown the plausibility of the role of energy imbalance (excessive energy intake in relation to energy expenditure) in the development and progression of prostate cancer. A number of experimental studies in mouse and rat models have confirmed that energy restriction reduced the development of tumors and they have explored the beneficial effects of energy restriction in models of carcinogenesis [24–26]. However, in population-based studies, for obvious ethical reasons it will be difficult to investigate the long-term effect of energy restriction on prostate cancer. Therefore, the evidence of the role of energy imbalance in advanced and fatal prostate cancer is obtained largely from observational studies investigating the effect of modifiable factors strongly correlated with energy balance on the natural history of prostate cancer [17, 21, 27–30]. Although there is a clear racial and ethnic disparity in prostate cancer and evidence that energy imbalance influences prostate cancer carcinogenesis as shown in experimental, migrant, ecological, and observational studies [21], it is surprising there are still few studies that have investigated the full impact of race and ethnicity in that association. This lack of study makes the generalizability of findings from previous studies to minority populations uncertain. Studies investigating the association between energy intake itself and prostate cancer are difficult to perform because of inaccuracies in methods of measuring caloric intake in large observational studies. Yet, the importance of addressing racial/ethnic disparities in prostate cancer that might result from differences in energy intake may be suggested based on a study that quantified the energy imbalance gap responsible for the US adult obesity epidemic among racial and ethnic groups [31]. Fallah-Fini et al. 2014 [31] concluded that no racial and ethnic group showed a negative or zero energy imbalance gap, suggesting that the obesity epidemic continues to worsen, albeit at a slower rate. In the past decade the epidemic has slowed down for non-Hispanic Whites, is starting to slow for non-Hispanic Blacks, but continues to accelerate among Mexican-Americans, suggesting that future interventions addressing energy imbalance should be tailored to minority population's needs.

Energy Balance and Prostate Cancer in Randomized Trials and Observational Studies: Race and Ethnicity

Randomized Controlled Trials (RCTs) of Lifestyle Interventions (Diet and Physical Activity), Lycopene, and Selenium and Prostate Cancer

In general, participation of minority populations in RCTs is very limited, including those investigating the interplay of energy imbalance, prostate cancer and race and ethnicity. A number of RCTs have been conducted investigating the association of lifestyle interventions (diet and physical activity), nutrients (selenium and lycopene) with all stages of prostate cancer. Some of these RCTs have included a few participants from different racial ethnic groups.

Lifestyle Interventions (Diet, Physical Activity): Race/Ethnicity

In a systematic review of randomized controlled trials of the influence of lifestyle interventions on breast and prostate cancer outcomes published between 1980 and 2010 [32], only one [33] trial (n = 84 participants) reported on a possibly relevant outcome. That trial reported that a 12-month lifestyle intervention (vegan diet, supplements, aerobic exercise, stress management techniques) produced declines in prostate specific antigen (PSA) level, but did not investigate whether the intervention reduced the rate of progression. That trial and two other RCTs [34, 35] identified by the systematic review, investigated the effect of lifestyle interventions on secondary outcomes, such as fat intake (calories from fat), among prostate cancer patients. In general, the systematic review concluded that the strength of evidence for effects on these secondary outcomes was insufficient. The two main racial groups included in these three RCTs were White and Black men. Yet, it is important to note that in the three studies more than 85% of the study participants were White. Therefore, there was insufficient information to derive a conclusion among Black men.

Lycopene: Race/Ethnicity

A body of literature supports that tomatoes, tomato-based products, and blood lycopene levels may be inversely associated with prostate cancer [36]. A recent double-blind, randomized, placebo-controlled trial of 105 African-American men reported higher lycopene levels in prostate tissue after comparing the lycopene intervention (30 mg/day of lycopene) groups vs placebo group for 21-days (0.446 ± 0.53 vs 0.593 ± 0.472; P = 0.005) [37]. A 6-month repeat biopsy randomized trial among men with high-grade prostatic intraepithelial neoplasia investigating a lycopene-rich tomato extract reported that no treatment effects on PSA, insulin-like growth factor proteins, or on prostate tissue markers of proliferation were apparent [38]. This latter trial included 58 men and only 6 African-American men were included in the intervention group and 9 in the placebo group.

Selenium: Race/Ethnicity

Two large randomized controlled trials have been conducted on the association between selenium intake and prostate cancer [39, 40]. However, the independent results from these RCTs are inconsistent. The Nutritional Prevention Cancer (NPC) [40] trial, which included prostate cancer as a secondary outcome, showed a reduced risk for prostate cancer for those men with low selenium status at the beginning of the trial. However, no race and ethnicity information was included in the trial. In the second trial, the large SELECT trial [39], selenium did not affect prostate cancer incidence (hazard ratio = 1.04; 99% CI = 0.87–1.24). The authors of this large trial indicated that racial and ethnic groups were recruited for generalizability, however, no racial/ethnic-specific analyses were conducted (White, n = 27,569 [79%]; African American, n = 4314 [12%]; Hispanic, n = 2294 [6.6%]; Asian, n = 420 [1.2%]; Native American, n = 99 [0.28%]; and Pacific Islander, n = 39 [0.11%]).

Prospective Cohort Studies, Case-Control and Other Study Designs on Energy Intake, Total Fat Intake, Saturated Fat and Body Size: Race and Ethnicity

Prospective Cohort Studies: Race and Ethnicity

In a 2016 meta-analysis of three prospective studies, the pooled analyses showed that men exposed to early-life energy restriction (ranging from 220 to 800 kcal/day) had a higher prostate cancer risk than those not exposed (Relative Risk [RR] = 1.16; 95% CI = 1.03–1.30) [41]. The endpoint for two of these studies was prostate cancer risk [42, 43] and was prostate cancer mortality for the third one [44]. Only one of the three studies reported a statistically significant association for energy restriction (prostate cancer risk, RR = 1.5; 95 CI = 1.01–1.31) [43]. The racial background for each study population was White: Dirx et al. included men from the Netherlands, Keinan-Boker et al. from Israel, and Koupil et al. from Leningrad-USSR. However, it is important to note that the findings from these studies should interpreted with caution because the range of energy restriction was severe and obtained from adolescent men during World War II or places/cities with economic depression or famine. It is unclear whether the findings from this meta-analysis can be generalized to other racial and ethnic groups.

A 2002 meta-analysis of epidemiologic studies reported that among prospective cohort studies (n = 4), the summary RR for the association between higher energy intake and total prostate cancer was 1.0 (95% CI = 0.8–1.2) [21]. None of the included prospective studies reported a significant association of high-energy intake with risk of prostate cancer independent of other factors. Three of these studies [45–47] included European white men, while Severson et al. [48] was conducted among Hawaiian men with Japanese ancestry.

A 2004 meta-analysis focused mainly on the relationship between total or saturated fat intake and prostate cancer [49], and consisting of four prospective studies [46–48, 50] (case-control studies will be discussed the section below), reported no association for total fat intake (summary RR = 1.00, 95% CI = 0.86–1.16). Two of the four studies were conducted among white European [46, 47], while the other two were conducted in the US, but one of studies had approximately 95% of White men [50] and the second study had mainly men with Japanese ancestry [48]. Similar findings were reported with saturated fat (summary RR = 1.00; 95% CI = 0.87–1.16); this analysis included an additional cohort study of Belgian men [51].

Subsequent cohort studies have also investigated total and saturated fat intake and prostate cancer risk. The Multiethnic Cohort Study found no significant associations with overall prostate cancer risk or risk of non-localized or high-grade prostate cancer [52]. The Multiethnic Cohort Study (n = 82,483) is composed of White (25.6%), African-American (13.0%), Native Hawaiian (7.1%), Japanese American (30.4%), and Latino (24.0%) men. Similar associations remained even after stratifying by race and ethnicity ($P_{trend} \geq 0.05$). Neuhouser et al. [53], in a prospective study with 11 years of follow-up and a total population of 12,000 participants (White 92%, Black 3.7%, Hispanics 1.6%), reported that total and saturated fat were not associated with total, non-aggressive, or aggressive prostate cancer. Race was not associated with any fat measures in relation to prostate cancer risk. A prospective study of 10,564 men conducted in Sweden reported no association between fat intake and risk of total or advanced prostate cancer [54]. A European prospective study of 142,520 men found no association between total fat intake (% of total energy) or saturated fat (% of total energy) intake with localized, high-grade, or advanced prostate cancer [55]. In a cohort analysis in the Prostate Cancer Prevention Trial [56], in general, energy, total fat, and saturated fat were not statistically significantly associated with risk of either high- or low-grade cancer in both the percent energy models and the total energy models. The study population was mainly composed of White men (93.2%), followed by African-American (4.4%), Asian/Pacific Islander (0.3%), and Hispanic (1.9%) men. In the US National Institutes of Health (NIH)-AARP Diet and Health Study, which included 288,268 men with an average follow-up of 9 years [57] saturated fat intake was associated with an increased risk of advanced prostate cancer. More than 90% of this cohort was white; the cohort included <3% each non-Hispanic black, Hispanic and other race/ethnicity men.

One of the latest and most comprehensive dose-response meta-analyses, which included 13 prospective studies, investigated the relationship between total fat intake (28.35 g increment/day; RR = 0.99, 95% CI = 0.98–1.01, n = 13 studies) and saturated fat intake (RR = 1.00, 95% CI = 1.00–1.00, n = 9 studies) and risk for prostate cancer reported no significant associations [58]. Similar findings were reported for total fat intake (RR = 1.02, 95% CI = 0.96–1.08; n = 5 studies) and saturated fat (RR = 0.96, 95% CI: 0.84–1.11; n = 6) and advanced stage of prostate cancer. The main conclusion from this meta-analysis of prospective studies was that there is little evidence from published cohort studies to support the statement that total fat or saturated fat increases the risk for prostate cancer or advanced stage disease. The majority of the included studies were conducted in American or European countries. American studies adjusted for race and others for race and ethnicity [52, 53, 56, 57, 59]. With the exception of Park et al. [52] conducted in the Multiethnic Cohort Study the studies included too few men from diverse racial and ethnic groups to conduct independent analyses.

Case-Control Studies: Race and Ethnicity

One of the first systematic reviews and meta-analyses on energy intake and prostate cancer, which used 14 case-control studies (population- and hospital-based) [21], reported the odds of prostate cancer was 30% higher (odds ratio $[OR]_{summary} = 1.3$, 95% CI = 1.1–1.4) in the top compared with the bottom quintile of energy intake. However, the findings from the included studies had significant heterogeneity, therefore, results should be interpreted with caution. Four case-control studies from this meta-analysis evaluated advanced disease, and suggested a higher risk with higher energy intake ($OR_{summary} = 1.6$, 95% CI = 1.2–2.0). Four of these case-control studies were conducted in European countries (Sweden, England, Spain, Serbia) [60–63], nine in North or South American countries [64–72] (two in USA, one Uruguay, six Canada), and one in Japan [73]. Eight studies showed direct associations, specifically two of the European (Vlajinac et al. [63] in Serbia and Andersson et al. [60] in Sweden) and six of the North or South American (three in Canada [64, 69, 70], one Uruguay [65], two in USA [68, 72]) studies. While these studies were conducted in several different countries on four continents, these studies do not shed light on whether the association of energy intake and prostate cancer differs by race/ethnicity.

Dennis et al. [49] investigated a source of energy intake—total fat and saturated fat—with prostate cancer in eight population-based case-control studies. Associations for intake of total fat ($OR_{summary} = 1.20$, 95% CI = 1.11–1.30) and saturated fat ($OR_{summary} = 1.19$, 95% CI = 0.87–1.16) were statistically significant. However, the heterogeneity in findings among the studies was large making it difficult to provide a definitive conclusion. Five of these population-based case-control studies were conducted in American countries (US [72, 74, 75] and Canada [67, 70]), two in Europe (England [61] and Sweden [76]) and one in Asia (China [77]). One study conducted in the US specifically investigated associations of total fat and saturated fat intakes with prostate cancer among different racial and ethnic groups: Whittemore et al. [76] reported that saturated fat intake was more strongly positively associated with prostate cancer among Asian-Americans than among blacks and whites. While not directly informing whether this association is similar among racial/ethnic groups, a case-control study among Japanese, Caucasian, Hawaiian, Filipino, and Chinese men reported a positive association between fat intake and prostate cancer in older men (highest vs lowest quartile: OR = 1.7, 95% CI = 1.0–2.8) after adjusting for race/ethnicity [77].

Other Study Designs: Race and Ethnicity

In a population based study of 2212 black (~50%) and white men with prostate cancer called the North Carolina-Louisiana Prostate Cancer Project (PCaP), Arab et al. [78] investigated the association between adherence with lifestyle recommendations (low fat, physical activity, etc.) from the World Cancer Research Fund (WCRF) and the odds of high aggressive (versus low/intermediate aggressive) prostate cancer in both white and black men. In men from both racial groups, lower total energy intake (≤125 kcal/100 g per day) was possibly associated with a lower risk of aggressive prostate cancer.

Also in the PCaP, Allott et al. [79] investigated the association of total fat and saturated fat intakes with aggressive prostate cancer. The associations of high total fat intake and high saturated fat intake with high aggressive prostate cancer were stronger in white (OR = 1.84, 95% CI = 1.13–2.98, OR = 1.96, 95% CI = 1.23–3.12, respectively) than in black (OR = 1.19, 95% CI = 0.77–1.83, OR = 1.25, 95% CI = 0.81–1.93, respectively) men.

Body Size and Weight Change and Prostate Cancer: By Race and Ethnicity

Obesity and weight change are among the most valid and reliable health exposures related to energy balance [23]. Emerging evidence supports a link between obesity and weight change and an elevated incidence of advanced and fatal prostate cancer [80–82]. Here, we will review whether these links differ by race and ethnicity.

The prevalence of obesity is higher in some racial/ethnic minority groups [83, 84]. Given the well-documented racial and ethnic differences in the morbidity and mortality of prostate cancer (described above), it has been suggested that that racial/ethnic differences in the prevalence of overweight and obesity may, in part, underlie racial/ethnic disparities in the risk of cancer [85].

Discacciati et al. [82] conducted a dose-response, meta-analyses of prospective studies that investigated the association of body mass index (BMI) with localized (n = 12 studies) and advanced prostate cancer (n = 13 studies). Focusing on the findings for advanced prostate cancer, which is the most clinically relevant endpoint, there was a linear direct relationship for BMI (RR = 1.09, 95% CI = 1.02–1.16 for every 5 kg/m [2] increase, P_{trend} = 0.001). Six studies were conducted in the US, three in Sweden, one in The Netherlands, one in Australia, one in Japan, and one in several European countries (the multi-center EPIC study: Italy, Spain, United Kingdom, Netherlands, Greece, Germany, Sweden and Denmark). Only two (in Australia [86] and in the US [87]) out of these 13 studies reported independent, positive significant associations (RR = 1.51, 95% CI = 1.14–2.01 and RR = 1.19, 95% CI = 1.03–1.38, respectively). The US [87] study consisted of mainly of white men (>95%).

A 2016 dose-response meta-analyses of observational studies (case-control and cohort) addressed weight gain and prostate cancer [81]. Focusing on the findings for high-risk (at least one of the following criteria at diagnosis: T3/T4, N1 or M1; Gleason score 8–10; or serum PSA ≥ 20 ng/mL; n = 5 studies: 1 case-control, 4 cohort studies) and fatal prostate cancer (prostate cancer-specific death during follow-up; n = 3: 1 case-control, 2 cohort studies) for clinical relevance, investigators reported a positive association for adult weight gain with high risk prostate cancer (per 5-kg increase: RR = 1.02, 95% CI = 1.00–1.04) and with fatal prostate cancer (RR = 1.12, 95% CI = 1.05–1.19). For the outcome of high-risk prostate cancer, studies were from Sweden (one case-control), Australia (one cohort [88]), and the US (three cohort [89–91]). With the exception of the Australian [88] study (RR = 1.37, 95% CI = 1.02–1.83), none reported a significant association for high-risk prostate cancer when comparing the highest versus lowest categories of adult weight gain. The studies that investigated fatal prostate cancer (n = 3) included studies from Sweden (one case-control [92]), Australian (one cohort [88]), and US (one cohort [90]). The only study that observed a statistically significant association was the Australian cohort study (RR = 1.84; 95% CI = 1.09–3.09) [88]. Of the studies included in the meta-analysis [81], only one evaluated this association within racial/ethnic groups. In the Multiethnic Cohort study (n = 82,483), which is composed of white (25.6%), African-American (13.0%), Native Hawaiian (7.1%), Japanese American (30.4%), and Latino (24.0%) participants, Hernandez et al. [91] compared a weight gain of 40 lb to <10 lb and reported that the trends for the risk of advanced prostate cancer were not statistically significant in any racial and ethnic group (white, $P_{trend} = 0.43$; African-American, $P_{trend} = 0.54$; Japanese, $P_{trend} = 0.29$; Latino, $P_{trend} = 0.96$). Similar results were found for high-grade prostate cancer, except possibly for a positive association among Latino men (RR = 1.53, 95% CI = 0.97–2.36, $P_{trend} = 0.02$). The other two studies conducted in the US [90, 93], adjusted for race but did not separately report on race-specific associations.

Biological Mechanism: Testosterone: Race and Ethnicity

Three mechanisms have been consistently suggested to underlie, in part, the association between energy balance and prostate cancer, insulin-like growth factor (IGF) [93], inflammation [28], and sex steroid hormones [27, 29, 94, 95]. In other instances, studies have expanded by investigating the interplay among these three mechanisms [28, 93, 96, 97]. However, to provide a more concise message in this chapter on the impact of race/ethnicity on the association between energy balance and prostate cancer, we will focus on one mediating mechanism, testosterone. To provide insight about these links, first we briefly review the historical and controversial relationship between endogenous and exogenous testosterone and prostate cancer. Then, we describe the well-known bidirectional relationship between endogenous and exogenous testosterone and obesity, and the influence of replacement testosterone in hypogonadism on adiposity. Understanding the testosterone-adiposity relationship is important to interpreting the emerging evidence supporting a link between obesity and an elevated incidence of advanced and fatal prostate cancer [80–82]. Finally, we review the evidence of racial variation in testosterone levels.

Endogenous and Exogenous Testosterone and Prostate Cancer

Circa 1941, Charles Huggins asserted that testosterone plays a role in the risk of prostate cancer [98]. Later, other studies suggested a positive association between testosterone and prostate cancer and that the role of androgens in prostate cancer is notable since estimates indicated that 80–90% of prostate cancers is dependent on circulating androgens for growth [94, 95, 99]. Furthermore, androgen deprivation, directly or through administration of luteinizing hormone-releasing hormone agonists, is a highly successful mainstay of anti-prostate cancer therapy [100]. However, modern evidence does not seem to support the contention that higher circulating levels of testosterone or the use of testosterone replacement therapy for hypogonadism increases the risk of prostate cancer [101–110]. Despite this wealth of evidence, very little research has been conducted on whether race and ethnicity influence the association of circulating testosterone or use of testosterone therapy and risk of prostate cancer.

Bidirectional Relationship Between Low Levels of Testosterone and Obesity
The inverse relationship between low levels of testosterone and body fatness (measured by BMI ≥ 30 kg/m [2], waist circumference ≥102 cm, percent body fat ≥25%, or increased adipose tissue), has been shown to be consistent in cross-sectional studies [111–113], prospective cohort studies [114–116], and two systematic reviews and meta-analyses (MacDonald et al. [117]: 19 observational studies, n = 15,060 participants; Brand et al. [118]: 20 observational studies, n = 8094 participants). Interestingly, this relationship has been shown to be bidirectional; that is, low levels of testosterone increase the risk of body fatness, and body fatness increases the risk of low levels of testosterone [119–122].

Treatment of Low Levels of Testosterone with Testosterone Therapy and Its Beneficial Effects on Measures of Adiposity and Lean Mass
In response to the prevalence of low testosterone resulting from the aging of the male population and of the obesity epidemic, the treatment of low testosterone with testosterone therapy has increased dramatically in the last decade from 0.81% in 2001 to 2.9% in 2011 [123, 124].

Traish [125] reported in a narrative review that testosterone therapy increased lean body mass and reduced fat mass in all 28 intervention studies spanning treatment periods of 3–36 months. In the same article, 20 intervention studies reported reduced waist circumference over a similar range of treatment periods, and out of these 20 intervention studies, 10 reported reduced BMI and greater weight loss; the remaining studies did not report on these outcomes. In 2015, Neto et al. [126] conducted a systematic review and meta-analysis of eight randomized placebo-controlled trials of testosterone replacement in men over 60 years old with serum testosterone ≤550 ng/mL and reported a significant increase in lean mass and decrease in fat mass.

A comprehensive meta-analyses of 32 observational studies (i.e., studies other than randomized controlled trials) of a total of 4513 patients by Corona et al. [127] reported testosterone therapy was associated with weight loss, reduced BMI, increased lean mass, and reduced fat mass. Compared with published randomized controlled trials of testosterone therapy and change in body composition, per these authors, participants in the observational studies [121, 128–132] were younger and had lower testosterone levels [121, 130, 132, 133].

Variation in Testosterone Levels by Race and Ethnicity

In a population-based cross-sectional study in the third National Health and Nutrition and Examination Survey (NHANES III), Rohrmann et al. found that total testosterone concentration was highest in Mexican-American (MA) compared with non-Hispanic black (NHB) and white (NHW) men, and total estradiol and sex hormone binding globulin (SHBG) concentrations were highest in NHB compared with NHW and MA men [134]. Subsequently, Lopez et al. [135] extended the analysis in a nationally-representative sample to US adolescent males (12–19 years old), which is the time of prostate maturation. This latter study reported that adolescent Mexican-Americans had higher total and free testosterone than NHB, but Mexican-Americans had the lowest total and free estradiol and SHBG than NHW and NHB adolescents. Other studies have also found similar testosterone concentrations between young NHW and NHB men. However, previous studies have reported differences in circulating testosterone concentration between black and white men [136–139]. A meta-analysis reported that black men had modestly higher free testosterone (2.5–4.9% higher) than white men, but black and white men did not differ on total testosterone [140].

Another cross-sectional study looking at trends in the NHANES 1988–1991 and 1999–2004 reported no decline in testosterone levels among NHW, NHB and MA men after taking into account body fatness [141]. However, the Massachusetts Male Aging Study reported that testosterone declined among men followed from 1987–1989 to 2002–2004, even after adjustment for BMI and other factors, yet no racial/ethnic specific results were provided [142].

Summary and Future Directions

While the association of energy imbalance and its correlated lifestyle factors with prostate cancer, especially aggressive disease, shows growing consistency whether these same associations are similar or different among racial and ethnic groups remains understudied. The majority of studies on energy balance and prostate cancer have been conducted in non-Hispanic white men, including from North America, Europe, and Australia. Very few studies on this topic have been conducted among minority populations, and of those studies that included minority populations, the sample sizes were so small that meaningful conclusions could not be derived. Some studies adjusted for race/ethnicity, but findings from these analyses do not inform whether the association between energy imbalance and prostate differs by race/ethnicity.

With the growing attention to tailoring interventions to subpopulations, research documenting similarities and differences among racial/ethnic groups and among even more understudied populations not discussed here in risk factors for cancer, including prostate cancer, is needed [143]. Standard definitions of race, ethnicity, and more generally ancestry, must be developed for such research in population-based studies, to make the comparison among study findings more valid and reliable. Future studies must be adequately powered to investigate the association between energy balance and prostate cancer, especially lethal disease within population subgroups to provide a definitive conclusion. More work is also needed to understand the biological pathways that may underlie any racial/ethnic differences in the association between energy balance and prostate cancer: testosterone remains a possible explanatory mechanism.

References

1. Wallington SF, Luta G, Noone AM, et al. Assessing the awareness of and willingness to participate in cancer clinical trials among immigrant Latinos. J Community Health. 2012;37(2):335–43.
2. Brooks SE, Muller CY, Robinson W, et al. Increasing minority enrollment onto clinical trials: practical strategies and challenges emerge from the NRG oncology accrual workshop. J Oncol Pract. 2015;11(6):486–90.
3. Ennis SR, Rios-Vargas M, Albert NG. US Census Bureau. The Hispanic population: 2010. 2011;C2010BR-04.
4. US Census Bureau. Overview of race and Hispanic origin: 2010. http://Www.census.gov/prod/cen2010/briefs/c2010br-02.pdf.
5. Drevdahl D, Taylor JY, Phillips DA. Race and ethnicity as variables in nursing research, 1952–2000. Nurs Res. 2001;50(5):305–13.
6. Ahdieh L, Hahn RA. Use of the terms 'race', 'ethnicity', and 'national origins': A review of articles in the American Journal of Public Health, 1980–1989. Ethn Health. 1996;1(1):95–8.
7. Comstock RD, Castillo EM, Lindsay SP. Four-year review of the use of race and ethnicity in epidemiologic and public health research. Am J Epidemiol. 2004;159(6):611–9.
8. Ramirez AG, Wildes K, Talavera G, Napoles-Springer A, Gallion K, Perez-Stable EJ. Clinical trials attitudes and practices of Latino physicians. Contemp Clin Trials. 2008;29(4):482–92.
9. Scott EA, Schlumpf KS, Mathew SM, et al. Biospecimen repositories: are blood donors willing to participate? Transfusion. 2010;50(9):1943–50.
10. Lopez DS, Fernandez ME, Cano MA, et al. Association of acculturation, nativity, and years living in the United States with biobanking among individuals of Mexican descent. Cancer Epidemiol Biomarkers Prev. 2014;23(3):402–8.
11. Rivera-Goba MV, Dominguez DC, Stoll P, Grady C, Ramos C, Mican JM. Exploring decision-making of HIV-infected Hispanics and African Americans participating in clinical trials. J Assoc Nurses AIDS Care. 2011;22(4):295–306.
12. Siegel RL, Miller KD, Jemal A. Cancer statistics, 2016. CA Cancer J Clin. 2016;66(1):7–30.
13. Siegel RL, Fedewa SA, Miller KD, et al. Cancer statistics for Hispanics/Latinos, 2015. CA Cancer J Clin. 2015;65(6):457–80.
14. Wong MC, Goggins WB, Wang HH, et al. Global incidence and mortality for prostate cancer: analysis of temporal patterns and trends in 36 countries. Eur Urol. 2016;70:862–74.
15. Gelband H, Jha P, Sankaranarayanan R, Horton S. Disease control priorities: cancer, vol. 3. 3rd ed. Washington, DC: World Bank; 2015. doi:10.1596/978-1-4648-0349-9. license: Creative commons attribution CC BY 3.0 IGO.
16. World Health Organization. GLOBOCAN cancer fact sheets: prostate cancer in 2012. http://Globocan.iarc.fr/old/FactSheets/cancers/prostate-new.asp [10/5/2016 11:14:18 AM] 2015.
17. World Cancer Research Fund International/American Institute for Cancer Research. Continuous update project report: diet, nutrition, physical activity, and prostate cancer. 2014. Available at: www.wcrf.org/sites/default/files/prostate-cancer-2014-report.pdf

18. Quick Stats. Age-adjusted death rates for top five causes of cancer death, by race/Hispanic ethnicity—United States, 2014. MMWR Morb Mortal Wkly Rep. 2016;65:989. doi:10.15585/mmwr.mm6536a10.
19. Crawford ED. Epidemiology of prostate cancer. Urology. 2003;62(6 Suppl 1):3–12.
20. Giovannucci E, Liu Y, Platz EA, Stampfer MJ, Willett WC. Risk factors for prostate cancer incidence and progression in the health professionals follow-up study. Int J Cancer. 2007;121(7):1571–8.
21. Platz EA. Energy imbalance and prostate cancer. J Nutr. 2002;132(11 Suppl):3471S–81S.
22. Wilson KM, Giovannucci EL, Mucci LA. Lifestyle and dietary factors in the prevention of lethal prostate cancer. Asian J Androl. 2012;14(3):365–74.
23. Doyle C. Obesity and cancer: Epidemiology in racial/ethnic minorities. In: Berger NA, editor. Cancer and energy balance, epidemiology and overview. New York: Springer; 2010. p. 45.
24. Mukherjee P, Sotnikov AV, Mangian HJ, Zhou JR, Visek WJ, Clinton SK. Energy intake and prostate tumor growth, angiogenesis, and vascular endothelial growth factor expression. J Natl Cancer Inst. 1999;91(6):512–23.
25. Zhu Z, Haegele AD, Thompson HJ. Effect of caloric restriction on pre-malignant and malignant stages of mammary carcinogenesis. Carcinogenesis. 1997;18(5):1007–12.
26. Thompson HJ, Jiang W, Zhu Z. Mechanisms by which energy restriction inhibits carcinogenesis. Adv Exp Med Biol. 1999;470:77–84.
27. Key TJ, Allen NE, Verkasalo PK, Banks E. Energy balance and cancer: the role of sex hormones. Proc Nutr Soc. 2001;60(1):81–9.
28. Wang H, Ye J. Regulation of energy balance by inflammation: common theme in physiology and pathology. Rev Endocr Metab Disord. 2015;16(1):47–54.
29. Hursting SD, Digiovanni J, Dannenberg AJ, et al. Obesity, energy balance, and cancer: new opportunities for prevention. Cancer Prev Res (Phila). 2012;5(11):1260–72.
30. Saxton JM. Diet, physical activity and energy balance and their impact on breast and prostate cancers. Nutr Res Rev. 2006;19(2):197–215.
31. Fallah-Fini S, Rahmandad H, Huang TT, Bures RM, Glass TA. Modeling US adult obesity trends: a system dynamics model for estimating energy imbalance gap. Am J Public Health. 2014;104(7):1230–9.
32. Sumano E, Ha C, Korownyk C, Vandermeer B, Dryden DM. Lifestylee interventions for four conditions: Type 2 diabetes, metabolic syndrome, breast cancer and prostate cancer [Internet]. Rockville, MD: Agency for Healthcare Research and Quality (US); 2011 May 26. Available from http://www.ncbi.nlm.nih.gov/books/NBK254022/
33. Ornish D, Weidner G, Fair WR, et al. Intensive lifestyle changes may affect the progression of prostate cancer. J Urol. 2005;174(3):1065–9. discussion 1069–70
34. Morey MC, Snyder DC, Sloane R, et al. Effects of home-based diet and exercise on functional outcomes among older, overweight long-term cancer survivors: RENEW: a randomized controlled trial. JAMA. 2009;301(18):1883–91.
35. Demark-Wahnefried W, Clipp EC, Morey MC, et al. Lifestyle intervention development study to improve physical function in older adults with cancer: outcomes from project LEAD. J Clin Oncol. 2006;24(21):3465–73.
36. Giovannucci E. Tomatoes, tomato-based products, lycopene, and cancer: review of the epidemiologic literature. J Natl Cancer Inst. 1999;91(4):317–31.
37. van Breemen RB, Sharifi R, Viana M, et al. Antioxidant effects of lycopene in African American men with prostate cancer or benign prostate hyperplasia: a randomized, controlled trial. Cancer Prev Res (Phila). 2011;4(5):711–8.
38. Gann PH, Deaton RJ, Rueter EE, et al. A phase II randomized trial of lycopene-rich tomato extract among men with high-grade prostatic intraepithelial neoplasia. Nutr Cancer. 2015;67(7):1104–12.
39. Lippman SM, Klein EA, Goodman PJ, et al. Effect of selenium and vitamin E on risk of prostate cancer and other cancers: the selenium and vitamin E cancer prevention trial (SELECT). JAMA. 2009;301(1):39–51.

40. Duffield-Lillico AJ, Dalkin BL, Reid ME, et al. Selenium supplementation, baseline plasma selenium status and incidence of prostate cancer: an analysis of the complete treatment period of the nutritional prevention of cancer trial. BJU Int. 2003;91(7):608–12.
41. Elands RJ, Simons CC, Dongen M, et al. A systematic literature review and meta-regression analysis on early-life energy restriction and cancer risk in humans. PLoS One. 2016;11(9):e0158003.
42. Dirx MJ, Zeegers MP, Dagnelie PC, van den Bogaard T, van den Brandt PA. Energy restriction and the risk of spontaneous mammary tumors in mice: a meta-analysis. Int J Cancer. 2003;106(5):766–70.
43. Keinan-Boker L, Vin-Raviv N, Liphshitz I, Linn S, Barchana M. Cancer incidence in Israeli Jewish survivors of world war II. J Natl Cancer Inst. 2009;101(21):1489–500.
44. Koupil I, Plavinskaja S, Parfenova N, Shestov DB, Danziger PD, Vagero D. Cancer mortality in women and men who survived the siege of Leningrad (1941–1944). Int J Cancer. 2009;124(6):1416–21.
45. Chan JM, Pietinen P, Virtanen M, et al. Diet and prostate cancer risk in a cohort of smokers, with a specific focus on calcium and phosphorus (Finland). Cancer Causes Control. 2000;11(9):859–67.
46. Schuurman AG, van den Brandt PA, Dorant E, Brants HA, Goldbohm RA. Association of energy and fat intake with prostate carcinoma risk: results from the Netherlands Cohort Study. Cancer. 1999;86(6):1019–27.
47. Veierod MB, Laake P, Thelle DS. Dietary fat intake and risk of prostate cancer: a prospective study of 25,708 Norwegian men. Int J Cancer. 1997;73(5):634–8.
48. Severson RK, Nomura AM, Grove JS, Stemmermann GN. A prospective study of demographics, diet, and prostate cancer among men of Japanese ancestry in Hawaii. Cancer Res. 1989;49(7):1857–60.
49. Dennis LK, Snetselaar LG, Smith BJ, Stewart RE, Robbins ME. Problems with the assessment of dietary fat in prostate cancer studies. Am J Epidemiol. 2004;160(5):436–44.
50. Giovannucci E, Rimm EB, Colditz GA, et al. A prospective study of dietary fat and risk of prostate cancer. J Natl Cancer Inst. 1993;85(19):1571–9.
51. Staessen L, De Bacquer D, De Henauw S, De Backer G, Van Peteghem C. Relation between fat intake and mortality: an ecological analysis in Belgium. Eur J Cancer Prev. 1997;6(4):374–81.
52. Park SY, Murphy SP, Wilkens LR, Henderson BE, Kolonel LN. Fat and meat intake and prostate cancer risk: the multiethnic cohort study. Int J Cancer. 2007;121(6):1339–45.
53. Neuhouser ML, Barnett MJ, Kristal AR, et al. (N-6) PUFA increase and dairy foods decrease prostate cancer risk in heavy smokers. J Nutr. 2007;137(7):1821–7.
54. Wallstrom P, Bjartell A, Gullberg B, Olsson H, Wirfalt E. A prospective study on dietary fat and incidence of prostate cancer (Malmo, Sweden). Cancer Causes Control. 2007;18(10):1107–21.
55. Crowe FL, Key TJ, Appleby PN, et al. Dietary fat intake and risk of prostate cancer in the European prospective investigation into cancer and nutrition. Am J Clin Nutr. 2008;87(5):1405–13.
56. Kristal AR, Arnold KB, Neuhouser ML, et al. Diet, supplement use, and prostate cancer risk: results from the prostate cancer prevention trial. Am J Epidemiol. 2010;172(5):566–77.
57. Pelser C, Mondul AM, Hollenbeck AR, Park Y. Dietary fat, fatty acids, and risk of prostate cancer in the NIH-AARP diet and health study. Cancer Epidemiol Biomarkers Prev. 2013;22(4):697–707.
58. Xu C, Han FF, Zeng XT, Liu TZ, Li S, Gao ZY. Fat intake is not linked to prostate cancer: a systematic review and dose-response meta-analysis. PLoS One. 2015;10(7):e0131747.
59. Agalliu I, Kirsh VA, Kreiger N, Soskolne CL, Rohan TE. Oxidative balance score and risk of prostate cancer: results from a case-cohort study. Cancer Epidemiol. 2011;35(4):353–61.
60. Andersson SO, Wolk A, Bergstrom R, et al. Energy, nutrient intake and prostate cancer risk: a population-based case-control study in Sweden. Int J Cancer. 1996;68(6):716–22.

61. Key TJ, Silcocks PB, Davey GK, Appleby PN, Bishop DT. A case-control study of diet and prostate cancer. Br J Cancer. 1997;76(5):678–87.
62. Ramon JM, Bou R, Romea S, et al. Dietary fat intake and prostate cancer risk: a case-control study in Spain. Cancer Causes Control. 2000;11(8):679–85.
63. Vlajinac HD, Marinkovic JM, Ilic MD, Kocev NI. Diet and prostate cancer: a case-control study. Eur J Cancer. 1997;33(1):101–7.
64. Bairati I, Larouche R, Meyer F, Moore L, Fradet Y. Lifetime occupational physical activity and incidental prostate cancer (Canada). Cancer Causes Control. 2000;11(8):759–64.
65. Deneo-Pellegrini H, De Stefani E, Ronco A, Mendilaharsu M. Foods, nutrients and prostate cancer: a case-control study in Uruguay. Br J Cancer. 1999;80(3–4):591–7.
66. Fincham SM, Hill GB, Hanson J, Wijayasinghe C. Epidemiology of prostatic cancer: a case-control study. Prostate. 1990;17(3):189–206.
67. Ghadirian P, Lacroix A, Maisonneuve P, et al. Nutritional factors and prostate cancer: a case-control study of French Canadians in Montreal, Canada. Cancer Causes Control. 1996;7(4):428–36.
68. Hayes RB, Ziegler RG, Gridley G, et al. Dietary factors and risks for prostate cancer among blacks and whites in the United States. Cancer Epidemiol Biomarkers Prev. 1999;8(1):25–34.
69. Meyer F, Bairati I, Fradet Y, Moore L. Dietary energy and nutrients in relation to preclinical prostate cancer. Nutr Cancer. 1997;29(2):120–6.
70. Rohan TE, Howe GR, Burch JD, Jain M. Dietary factors and risk of prostate cancer: a case-control study in Ontario, Canada. Cancer Causes Control. 1995;6(2):145–54.
71. Villeneuve PJ, Johnson KC, Kreiger N, Mao Y. Risk factors for prostate cancer: results from the Canadian national enhanced cancer surveillance system. The Canadian cancer registries epidemiology research group. Cancer Causes Control. 1999;10(5):355–67.
72. West DW, Slattery ML, Robison LM, French TK, Mahoney AW. Adult dietary intake and prostate cancer risk in Utah: a case-control study with special emphasis on aggressive tumors. Cancer Causes Control. 1991;2(2):85–94.
73. Oishi K, Okada K, Yoshida O, et al. A case-control study of prostatic cancer with reference to dietary habits. Prostate. 1988;12(2):179–90.
74. Whittemore AS, Kolonel LN, Wu AH, et al. Prostate cancer in relation to diet, physical activity, and body size in blacks, whites, and Asians in the United States and Canada. J Natl Cancer Inst. 1995;87(9):652–61.
75. Kolonel LN, Yoshizawa CN, Hankin JH. Diet and prostatic cancer: a case-control study in Hawaii. Am J Epidemiol. 1988;127(5):999–1012.
76. Andersson SO, Baron J, Wolk A, Lindgren C, Bergstrom R, Adami HO. Early life risk factors for prostate cancer: a population-based case-control study in Sweden. Cancer Epidemiol Biomarkers Prev. 1995;4(3):187–92.
77. Lee MM, Wang RT, Hsing AW, Gu FL, Wang T, Spitz M. Case-control study of diet and prostate cancer in China. Cancer Causes Control. 1998;9(6):545–52.
78. Arab L, Su J, Steck SE, et al. Adherence to world cancer research fund/American institute for cancer research lifestyle recommendations reduces prostate cancer aggressiveness among African and Caucasian Americans. Nutr Cancer. 2013;65(5):633–43.
79. Allott EH, Arab L, Su LJ, et al. Saturated fat intake and prostate cancer aggressiveness: results from the population-based North Carolina-Louisiana prostate cancer project. Prostate Cancer Prostatic Dis. 2017;20:48–54.
80. Allott EH, Masko EM, Freedland SJ. Obesity and prostate cancer: weighing the evidence. Eur Urol. 2013;63(5):800–9.
81. Chen Q, Chen T, Shi W, et al. Adult weight gain and risk of prostate cancer: a dose-response meta-analysis of observational studies. Int J Cancer. 2016;138(4):866–74.
82. Discacciati A, Orsini N, Wolk A. Body mass index and incidence of localized and advanced prostate cancer—a dose-response meta-analysis of prospective studies. Ann Oncol. 2012;23(7):1665–71.

83. Flegal KM, Carroll MD, Ogden CL, Curtin LR. Prevalence and trends in obesity among US adults, 1999–2008. JAMA. 2010;303(3):235–41.
84. Flegal KM, Carroll MD, Kit BK, Ogden CL. Prevalence of obesity and trends in the distribution of body mass index among US adults, 1999–2010. JAMA. 2012;307(5):491–7.
85. Calle EE, Kaaks R. Overweight, obesity and cancer: epidemiological evidence and proposed mechanisms. Nat Rev Cancer. 2004;4(8):579–91.
86. MacInnis RJ, English DR, Gertig DM, Hopper JL, Giles GG. Body size and composition and prostate cancer risk. Cancer Epidemiol Biomarkers Prev. 2003;12(12):1417–21.
87. Rodriguez C, Freedland SJ, Deka A, et al. Body mass index, weight change, and risk of prostate cancer in the Cancer Prevention Study II Nutrition Cohort. Cancer Epidemiol Biomarkers Prev. 2007;16(1):63–9.
88. Bassett JK, Severi G, Baglietto L, et al. Weight change and prostate cancer incidence and mortality. Int J Cancer. 2012;131(7):1711–9.
89. Hernandez BY, Park SY, Wilkens LR, Henderson BE, Kolonel LN. Relationship of body mass, height, and weight gain to prostate cancer risk in the multiethnic cohort. Cancer Epidemiol Biomarkers Prev. 2009;18(9):2413–21.
90. Wright ME, Chang SC, Schatzkin A, et al. Prospective study of adiposity and weight change in relation to prostate cancer incidence and mortality. Cancer. 2007;109(4):675–84.
91. Littman AJ, White E, Kristal AR. Anthropometrics and prostate cancer risk. Am J Epidemiol. 2007;165(11):1271–9.
92. Moller E, Adami HO, Mucci LA, et al. Lifetime body size and prostate cancer risk in a population-based case-control study in Sweden. Cancer Causes Control. 2013;24(12):2143–55.
93. Kaaks R, Lukanova A. Energy balance and cancer: the role of insulin and insulin-like growth factor-I. Proc Nutr Soc. 2001;60(1):91–106.
94. Platz EA, Rimm EB, Willett WC, Kantoff PW, Giovannucci E. Racial variation in prostate cancer incidence and in hormonal system markers among male health professionals. J Natl Cancer Inst. 2000;92(24):2009–17.
95. Platz EA, Giovannucci E. The epidemiology of sex steroid hormones and their signaling and metabolic pathways in the etiology of prostate cancer. J Steroid Biochem Mol Biol. 2004;92(4):237–53.
96. Tsilidis KK, Rohrmann S, McGlynn KA, et al. Association between endogenous sex steroid hormones and inflammatory biomarkers in US men. Andrology. 2013;1(6):919–28.
97. Baillargeon J, Al Snih S, Raji MA, et al. Hypogonadism and the risk of rheumatic autoimmune disease. Clin Rheumatol. 2016;35(12):2983–7.
98. Huggins C, Hodges C. Studies on prostate cancer. I. The effect of castration, of estrogen and of androgen injection on serum phosphatases in metastatic carcinoma of the prostate. Cancer Res. 1941;1:293.
99. Heinlein CA, Chang C. Androgen receptor in prostate cancer. Endocr Rev. 2004;25(2):276–308.
100. Kawakami J, Cowan JE, Elkin EP, et al. Androgen-deprivation therapy as primary treatment for localized prostate cancer: data from Cancer of the Prostate Strategic Urologic Research Endeavor (CaPSURE). Cancer. 2006;106(8):1708–14.
101. Endogenous Hormones and Prostate Cancer Collaborative Group, Roddam AW, Allen NE, Appleby P, Key TJ. Endogenous sex hormones and prostate cancer: a collaborative analysis of 18 prospective studies. J Natl Cancer Inst. 2008;100(3):170–83.
102. Klap J, Schmid M, Loughlin KR. The relationship between total testosterone levels and prostate cancer: a review of the continuing controversy. J Urol. 2015;193(2):403–13.
103. Morgentaler A. Controversies and advances with testosterone therapy: a 40-year perspective. Urology. 2016;89:27–32.
104. Morgentaler A. Goodbye androgen hypothesis, hello saturation model. Eur Urol. 2012;62(5):765–7.
105. Morgentaler A, Traish AM. Shifting the paradigm of testosterone and prostate cancer: the saturation model and the limits of androgen-dependent growth. Eur Urol. 2009;55(2):310–20.

106. Morgentaler A, Conners WP. Testosterone therapy in men with prostate cancer: literature review, clinical experience, and recommendations. Asian J Androl. 2015;17(2):206–11.
107. Baillargeon J, Kuo YF, Fang X, Shahinian VB. Long-term exposure to testosterone therapy and the risk of high grade prostate cancer. J Urol. 2015;194(6):1612–6.
108. Calof OM, Singh AB, Lee ML, et al. Adverse events associated with testosterone replacement in middle-aged and older men: a meta-analysis of randomized, placebo-controlled trials. J Gerontol A Biol Sci Med Sci. 2005;60(11):1451–7.
109. Cui Y, Zong H, Yan H, Zhang Y. The effect of testosterone replacement therapy on prostate cancer: a systematic review and meta-analysis. Prostate Cancer Prostatic Dis. 2014;17(2):132–43.
110. Schenk JM, Till C, Hsing AW, et al. Serum androgens and prostate cancer risk: results from the placebo arm of the Prostate Cancer Prevention Trial. Cancer Causes Control. 2016;27(2):175–82.
111. Rohrmann S, Shiels MS, Lopez DS, et al. Body fatness and sex steroid hormone concentrations in US men: results from NHANES III. Cancer Causes Control. 2011;22(8):1141–51.
112. Abate N, Haffner SM, Garg A, Peshock RM, Grundy SM. Sex steroid hormones, upper body obesity, and insulin resistance. J Clin Endocrinol Metab. 2002;87(10):4522–7.
113. Couillard C, Gagnon J, Bergeron J, et al. Contribution of body fatness and adipose tissue distribution to the age variation in plasma steroid hormone concentrations in men: the HERITAGE family study. J Clin Endocrinol Metab. 2000;85(3):1026–31.
114. Gapstur SM, Gann PH, Kopp P, Colangelo L, Longcope C, Liu K. Serum androgen concentrations in young men: a longitudinal analysis of associations with age, obesity, and race. The CARDIA male hormone study. Cancer Epidemiol Biomarkers Prev. 2002;11(10 Pt 1):1041–7.
115. Derby CA, Zilber S, Brambilla D, Morales KH, McKinlay JB. Body mass index, waist circumference and waist to hip ratio and change in sex steroid hormones: The Massachusetts Male Ageing Study. Clin Endocrinol (Oxf). 2006;65(1):125–31.
116. Travison TG, Araujo AB, Kupelian V, O'Donnell AB, McKinlay JB. The relative contributions of aging, health, and lifestyle factors to serum testosterone decline in men. J Clin Endocrinol Metab. 2007;92(2):549–55.
117. MacDonald AA, Herbison GP, Showell M, Farquhar CM. The impact of body mass index on semen parameters and reproductive hormones in human males: a systematic review with meta-analysis. Hum Reprod Update. 2010;16(3):293–311.
118. Brand JS, Rovers MM, Yeap BB, et al. Testosterone, sex hormone-binding globulin and the metabolic syndrome in men: an individual participant data meta-analysis of observational studies. PLoS One. 2014;9(7):e100409.
119. Lamm S, Chidakel A, Bansal R. Obesity and hypogonadism. Urol Clin North Am. 2016;43(2):239–45.
120. Kelly DM, Jones TH. Testosterone and obesity. Obes Rev. 2015;16(7):581–606.
121. Saad F, Haider A, Doros G, Traish A. Long-term treatment of hypogonadal men with testosterone produces substantial and sustained weight loss. Obesity (Silver Spring). 2013;21(10):1975–81.
122. Mammi C, Calanchini M, Antelmi A, et al. Androgens and adipose tissue in males: a complex and reciprocal interplay. Int J Endocrinol. 2012;2012:789653.
123. Baillargeon J, Urban RJ, Ottenbacher KJ, Pierson KS, Goodwin JS. Trends in androgen prescribing in the United States, 2001–2011. JAMA Intern Med. 2013;173(15):1465–6.
124. Layton JB, Li D, Meier CR, et al. Testosterone lab testing and initiation in the United Kingdom and the United States, 2000–2011. J Clin Endocrinol Metab. 2014;99(3):835–42.
125. Traish AM. Testosterone and weight loss: The evidence. Curr Opin Endocrinol Diabetes Obes. 2014;21(5):313–22.
126. Neto WK, Gama EF, Rocha LY, et al. Effects of testosterone on lean mass gain in elderly men: systematic review with meta-analysis of controlled and randomized studies. Age (Dordr). 2015;37(1):9742. doi:10.1007/s11357-014-9742-0.

127. Corona G, Giagulli VA, Maseroli E, et al. Testosterone supplementation and body composition: results from a meta-analysis of observational studies. J Endocrinol Invest. 2016;39:967–81.
128. Schwarz ER, Willix RD Jr. Impact of a physician-supervised exercise-nutrition program with testosterone substitution in partial androgen-deficient middle-aged obese men. J Geriatr Cardiol. 2011;8(4):201–6.
129. Tirabassi G, Delli Muti N, Corona G, Maggi M, Balercia G. Androgen receptor gene CAG repeat polymorphism regulates the metabolic effects of testosterone replacement therapy in male postsurgical hypogonadotropic hypogonadism. Int J Endocrinol. 2013;2013:816740.
130. Zitzmann M, Mattern A, Hanisch J, Gooren L, Jones H, Maggi M. IPASS: A study on the tolerability and effectiveness of injectable testosterone undecanoate for the treatment of male hypogonadism in a worldwide sample of 1,438 men. J Sex Med. 2013;10(2):579–88.
131. Yassin A, Doros G. Testosterone therapy in hypogonadal men results in sustained and clinically meaningful weight loss. Clin Obes. 2013;3(3–4):73–83.
132. Yassin DJ, Doros G, Hammerer PG, Yassin AA. Long-term testosterone treatment in elderly men with hypogonadism and erectile dysfunction reduces obesity parameters and improves metabolic syndrome and health-related quality of life. J Sex Med. 2014;11(6):1567–76.
133. Permpongkosol S, Tantirangsee N, Ratana-olarn K. Treatment of 161 men with symptomatic late onset hypogonadism with long-acting parenteral testosterone undecanoate: effects on body composition, lipids, and psychosexual complaints. J Sex Med. 2010;7(11):3765–74.
134. Rohrmann S, Nelson WG, Rifai N, et al. Serum estrogen, but not testosterone, levels differ between black and white men in a nationally representative sample of Americans. J Clin Endocrinol Metab. 2007;92(7):2519–25.
135. Lopez DS, Peskoe SB, Joshu CE, et al. Racial/ethnic differences in serum sex steroid hormone concentrations in US adolescent males. Cancer Causes Control. 2013;24(4):817–26.
136. Winters SJ, Brufsky A, Weissfeld J, Trump DL, Dyky MA, Hadeed V. Testosterone, sex hormone-binding globulin, and body composition in young adult African American and Caucasian men. Metabolism. 2001;50(10):1242–7.
137. Ellis L, Nyborg H. Racial/ethnic variations in male testosterone levels: a probable contributor to group differences in health. Steroids. 1992;57(2):72–5.
138. Ross R, Bernstein L, Judd H, Hanisch R, Pike M, Henderson B. Serum testosterone levels in healthy young black and white men. J Natl Cancer Inst. 1986;76(1):45–8.
139. Orwoll E, Lambert LC, Marshall LM, et al. Testosterone and estradiol among older men. J Clin Endocrinol Metab. 2006;91(4):1336–44.
140. Richard A, Rohrmann S, Zhang L, et al. Racial variation in sex steroid hormone concentration in black and white men: a meta-analysis. Andrology. 2014;2(3):428–35.
141. Nyante SJ, Graubard BI, Li Y, et al. Trends in sex hormone concentrations in US males: 1988–1991 to 1999–2004. Int J Androl. 2012;35(3):456–66.
142. Travison TG, Araujo AB, O'Donnell AB, Kupelian V, McKinlay JB. A population-level decline in serum testosterone levels in American men. J Clin Endocrinol Metab. 2007;92(1):196–202.
143. Martin DN, Lam TK, Brignole K, et al. Recommendations for cancer epidemiologic research in understudied populations and implications for future needs. Cancer Epidemiol Biomarkers Prev. 2016;25(4):573–80.

Chapter 3
Consequence of Energy Imbalance in Prostate Cancer and Comorbidities

Jeannette M. Schenk and Jonathan L. Wright

Abstract Obesity and prostate cancer are two of the most common conditions in older men and there is strong evidence that obesity influences the risk, aggressiveness and outcomes of men with prostate cancer. In addition, several comorbidities are observed with obesity, including diabetes mellitus, hypertension, hypercholesterolemia and cardiovascular disease. Separate study of these diagnoses has also identified associations with prostate cancer risk and outcomes. Whether the underlying obesity, the comorbid conditions, or both are responsible for the observed interactions with prostate cancer is not fully understood. Further, pharmacologic treatment of these comorbidities may influence prostate cancer, either by reducing the direct effect of the comorbidity, or independently through additional pharmacologic mechanisms. In this chapter, we review the relationship between common obesity related comorbidities and prostate cancer risk, progression and mortality. We also describe, when available, data on the medications used to treat these comorbidities and the influence these therapies may have on prostate cancer.

Keywords Prostate cancer • Obesity • Comorbidity • Diabetes mellitus • Metabolic syndrome • Hypercholesterolemia • Hypertension • Prostate cancer-specific mortality • Heart disease

---

J.M. Schenk, PhD, RD
Cancer Prevention Program, Fred Hutchinson Cancer Research Center,
1100 Fairview Ave N., M4-B402, Seattle, WA 98109-1024, USA
e-mail: jschenk@fredhutch.org

J.L. Wright, MD, MS, FACS (✉)
Department of Urology, University of Washington,
1959 NE Pacific Street, Box 356510, Seattle, WA 98195, USA

Epidemiology Program, Fred Hutchinson Cancer Research Center,
1100 Fariview Ave N., M4-A402, Seattle, WA 98109-1024, USA
e-mail: jlwright@uw.edu

© Springer International Publishing AG 2018
E.A. Platz, N.A. Berger (eds.), *Energy Balance and Prostate Cancer*, Energy Balance and Cancer 14, DOI 10.1007/978-3-319-64940-5_3

General Overview of Obesity and Prostate CancerRisk/ Incidence, Progression, Mortality

Obesity prevalence in the U.S. has risen dramatically over the past 20 years. Presently, more than one-third of adults are obese (body mass index (BMI) ≥30 kg/m²) and among older men, approximately 40% are obese [1]. Obesity is linked with an increase in cancer-specific mortality and an estimated 14% of cancer deaths in U.S. men are due to obesity [2]. The associations of obesity with prostate cancer risk are complex. Pooled/meta-analyses from prospective studies report no overall association of obesity with total PCa risk [3–7]; however, there is growing evidence that associations of obesity with PCa differ for aggressive and nonaggressive PCa. Numerous studies report that obesity is associated with a decreased risk of non-aggressive (low-grade and/or local stage) disease and an increased risk of aggressive (high-grade and/or advanced stage) disease [3–5, 7]. Furthermore, there is strong and consistent evidence for a positive association between obesity and PCa progression and PCa-specific mortality (PCSM) [1, 2, 8–21]. As shown in Table 3.1, obesity is associated with a 20–160% elevation in PCa-specific mortality. Pooled/meta analyses report that for every five-point increase in BMI, there is a corresponding 20% increase in PCSM (95% CI 0.99–1.46) and conclude that "cumulative data is compelling for a strong positive association between obesity and fatal prostate cancer" [23]. A 2011 Institute of Medicine Workshop on Obesity and Cancer Report noted: "evidence is building that obesity and weight gain are risk factors for poor outcome in prostate cancer" [24].

The mechanisms underlying the obesity-PCa progression relationship are unknown. However, a number of metabolic changes that occur in obese men may be responsible, including (1) impaired glucose regulation and insulin resistance; (2) altered adipokines (e.g., leptin and adiponectin); (3) sex hormones; and (4) chronic inflammation, among other potential etiologies. It is well recognized that several morbidities are associated with obesity, such that obesity is one of the leading causes of preventable disease and disability in the United States. Obese patients are at higher risk of having diabetes mellitus, hypertension, hypercholesterolemia and cardiovascular disease (Fig. 3.1) [25].

Table 3.1 Studies of obesity and PCa-specific mortality

	No.	Hazard ratios (95% Confidence intervals)			
Study, year	patients	BMI ≤ 25	BMI 26–29	BMI ≥ 30	P trend
Andersson (1997) [21]	2368	1.00 (ref)	1.3 (1.0–1.7)[a]	1.4 (1.1–1.8)[a]	0.04
Calle (2003) [1]	3314	1.00 (ref)	1.1 (1.0–1.2)	1.2 (1.1–1.4)	<0.001
Wright (2007) [2]	9.986	1.00 (ref)	1.3 (0.9–1.8)	1.5 (0.9–2.3)	0.02
Efstathiou (2007) [13]	945	1.00 (ref)	1.5 (1.0–2.3)	1.6 (1.0–2.7)	–[b]
Gong (2007) [8]	752	1.00 (ref)	1.1 (0.6–2.3)	2.6 (1.2–5.9)	0.03
Ma (2008) [22]	2456	1.00 (ref)	1.3 (1.0–1.6)	2.0 (1.2–3.2)	<0.001

[a]BMI (kg/m²) quartiles used
[b]p Trend not provided

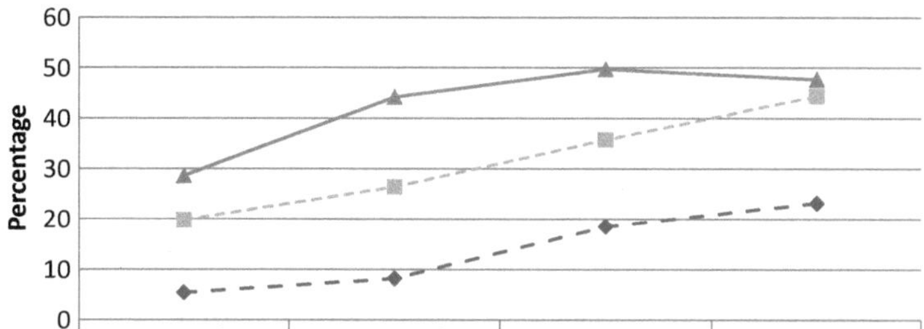

	Normal	Overweight	Obese	Morbid Obesity
Diabetes Mellitus	5.4	8.2	18.5	23.2
Hypertension	19.8	26.4	35.7	44.4
Dyslipidemia	28.6	44.2	49.7	47.7

Fig. 3.1 Comorbid conditions by obesity level, US 2007–2010 (Plotted from data in Saydah et al. [25])

Obesity is also associated with several other cardiovascular comorbid conditions in addition to hypertension, including coronary artery disease, heart failure, and arrhythmias. Interestingly, these diagnoses have also been associated with prostate cancer risk and outcomes. Whether it is obesity driving the relationship with prostate cancer, or if there is a separate effect of the comorbid condition is not fully understood, but there has been a great deal of research on the potential mechanisms underlying the links between the comorbidities and prostate cancer. Further, pharmacologic treatment of these conditions may impact the effects of the comorbidities on prostate cancer, either through reduction in the direct effect of the comorbidity, or separately through additional pharmacologic mechanisms.

In this chapter, we review the relationship between common obesity related comorbidities and prostate cancer. We review the literature, where available, for the association between these comorbidities and prostate cancer risk, progression and mortality. If applicable, we also describe the data on medications used to treat these comorbidities and the influence these medications may have on prostate cancer.

Metabolic Syndrome and Prostate Cancer Risk

Metabolic syndrome (MetS) is as a cluster of several metabolic abnormalities associated with increased risk of cardiovascular disease and diabetes. Components include hypertension, glucose intolerance, obesity, hypertriglyceridemia, and low high density lipoprotein cholesterol, with insulin resistance as the underlying hallmark feature (Table 3.2) [29].

The prevalence of MetS among US adults in the 2000–2003 National Health and Nutrition Examination Survey was 34% overall [30]. However, among older men the prevalence was much higher, with 41% of men age 40–59 years and 52% of men

Table 3.2 Definitions of metabolic syndrome

	NCEP ATP III (2005) [26]	WHO (1998) [27]	IDF (2005) [28]
Criteria requirements	Any three of the five criteria below	Insulin resistance or diabetes PLUS two of the five criteria below	Central obesity PLUS two of the four criteria below
Obesity	Waist circumference: >40 inches (M), >35 inches (F)	Waist/hip ratio: >0.90 (M), >0.85 (F); or BMI > 30 kg/m^2	Central obesity (Waist circumference: ≥94 cm (M), ≥80 cm (F))
Insulin resistance/ Hyperglycemia	Fasting glucose ≥100 mg/dl or Rx	IGT, IFG, T2DM or other evidence of IR	Fasting glucose ≥100 mg/dl
Dyslipidemia	TG ≥ 150 mg/dl or Rx	TG ≥ 150 mg/dl or HDL-C: <35 mg/dl (M), <39 mg/dl (F)	TG ≥ 150 mg/dl or Rx
Dyslipidemia (second, separate criteria)	HDL-C: <40 mg/dl (M), <50 mg/dl (F); or Rx		HDL-C: <40 mg/dl (M), <50 mg/dl (F); or Rx
Hypertension	>130 mm Hg systolic or >85 mm Hg diastolic or Rx	≥140/90 mm Hg	>130 mm Hg systolic or >85 mm Hg diastolic or Rx
Other criteria		Microalbuminuria	

Rx Pharmacologic treatment, *NCEP* National Cholesterol Education Program Adult Treatment Panel, *IDF* International Diabetes Federation
Impaired Fasting Glucose (IFG) defined as a fasting glucose level above a predetermined cutoff, commonly 100 milligrams per deciliter (mg/dl) or impaired glucose tolerance (IGT, defined as a glucose level above a predetermined cutoff, commonly 140 mg/dl, for 120 min after ingestion of 75 g of glucose load during an oral glucose tolerance test or other evidence of insulin resistance, such as an elevated homeostatic model assessment of insulin resistance (HOMA-IR) value

age 60 or older meeting the criteria for metabolic syndrome [30]. Over the past decade, a growing body of literature suggests that the metabolic syndrome may be involved in the pathogenesis and progression of prostate cancer.

Data on the association between metabolic syndrome and prostate cancer risk are conflicting. Several studies have reported significant positive associations between metabolic syndrome and prostate cancer risk. Two studies from northern Europe that found an increased risk for men with three metabolic syndrome components (RR = 1.56, 95% CI, 1.21–2.00) [31] and OR = 3.36, 95% CI 1.19–9.44) [32], and one study from Finland that reported an increased risk (RR = 1.94, 95% CI 1.06–3.53) among non-diabetic men with metabolic syndrome [33]. Three additional case-control studies reported an increased risk of prostate cancer among men with metabolic syndrome [34–36], two of which reported positive associations among African Americans (OR = 1.76, 95% CI = 1.1–2.88 [35] and OR = 1.71, 95% CI 0.97–3.01 [36]). In contrast, a number of studies reported an inverse relationship between metabolic syndrome and prostate cancer risk. In two large cohorts, men with three or more metabolic syndrome components had a significantly lower risk of total prostate cancer than men with less than three components (RR = 0.77, 95%

CI 0.60–0.98 [37] and OR = 0.69, 95% CI 0.58–0.82) [38]. In the REDUCE trial, men with one metabolic syndrome component had a lower risk of overall prostate cancer (OR = 0.87, 95% CI 0.76–0.99), although two or three to four components were not significantly related to prostate cancer risk [39]. In a large Swedish cohort, a composite score of five metabolic syndrome factors was associated with a 7% lower risk of overall prostate cancer (RR = 0.93, 95% CI = 0.89–0.97) [40]. In addition, several cohort studies have reported no significant associations between metabolic syndrome and overall prostate cancer risk [41–46]. It is likely that the inconsistencies in these associations may be due, at least in part, to differences in the populations studied, definitions of metabolic syndrome or methodologies used.

Three meta-analyses have also evaluated the association of metabolic syndrome with risk of prostate cancer; one of which reported a significant increased risk of overall prostate cancer (RR = 1.54, 95% CI 1.23–1.94) [3] and two reported no overall association [47, 48]. One meta-analysis also evaluated associations of metabolic syndrome with prostate cancer risk among by region, and reported that metabolic syndrome was associated with a reduced risk of total prostate cancer among studies conducted in U.S. (primarily white) populations (RR = 0.79, 95% CI: 0.69–0.91) [47].

Few prospective studies have examined the association of metabolic syndrome and prostate cancer severity defined by grade, stage, and/or aggressiveness. In a large Canadian cohort, metabolic syndrome was associated with a reduced risk of low-grade (RR = 0.69, 95% CI 0.52–0.82) and high-grade (RR = 0.75, 95% CI 0.60–0.94) prostate cancer [38]. Similar associations of metabolic syndrome and a reduced risk of low- and high-grade prostate cancer were reported in the REDUCE trial [39]. However, one case-control study among African Americans in the US reported a significant increased risk of organ confined prostate cancer among men with metabolic syndrome, compared to men without (OR = 1.82 95% CI 1.02–3.23), and no association with advanced prostate cancer [35]. Similarly, a case-control study from Italy reported metabolic syndrome was associated with a significant increased risk of low-grade (Gleason <7; OR = 1.48, 95% CI 1.48–3.17) and high-grade (Gleason ≥7; OR = 1.80, 95% CI 1.17–2.78) prostate cancer [34]. In addition, several cross-sectional studies of men undergoing biopsy or treatment of prostate cancer (radical prostatectomy) have reported positive associations for metabolic syndrome with the presence of higher grade/stage or more aggressive prostate cancer [49–55].

Lastly, four studies have also examined the association of metabolic syndrome with prostate cancer specific mortality, of which one reported an increased risk (RR = 1.86, 95% CI 1.59–2.19) [46], one reported a decreased risk (RR = 1.14, 95% CI = 1.01–1.28), and two reported no association [45, 56].

Diabetes Mellitus and Prostate Cancer Risk

Diabetes mellitus commonly co-exists with obesity, and there is a large body of epidemiologic evidence providing strong support for the notion that diabetes mellitus is associated with a decreased risk for prostate cancer. To date, three meta-analyses have reported a statistically significant inverse association of diabetes mellitus with risk of total prostate cancer [57–59]. The most recent of these analyses, which reviewed 45 studies (29 cohort and 16 case-control) of more than 132,000 total prostate cancer cases, reported a 15% lower risk of overall prostate cancer (95% CI 0.82–0.89) for type-2 diabetes mellitus compared to non-diabetics [57]. Although many studies did not indicate the type of diabetes mellitus, given that type-2 is far more common than type-1, the associations between diabetes mellitus and prostate cancer risk are generally interpreted in terms of type-2 [60].

The inverse association is fairly consistent across various ethnic groups within the US [61, 62]; although evidence is limited to two studies with sufficient numbers of minority participants. Data from populations outside of the US are less consistent with some studies reporting no association [63, 64] or positive associations [65, 66] between diabetes mellitus and prostate cancer. In addition, one meta-analysis reported the opposite association of diabetes mellitus with prostate cancer risk between western studies (RR = 0.81; 95% CI 0.76–0.85) and Asian studies (RR = 1.64; 95% CI 1.00–2.88) (p-interaction = 0.01) [57].

Many studies have also examined the association of diabetes mellitus and prostate cancer severity defined by grade, stage, and/or aggressiveness. Among studies reporting inverse associations between diabetes mellitus and total prostate cancer risk, most reported similar associations by prostate cancer grade, stage or aggressiveness [61, 62, 67–71]. One recent meta-analysis reported the risk of low-grade (RR = 0.74; 95% CI 0.64–0.86) and localized disease (RR = 0.72; 95% CI 0.67–0.76) was modestly stronger than for high grade (RR = 0.78; 95% CI 0.67–0.90) and advanced disease (RR = 0.85; 95% CI 0.75–0.97) [72]. In contrast, a small number of studies found no differences in associations between diabetes mellitus and prostate cancer aggressiveness. At least three large studies reported significant inverse associations for low-grade, localized or less-aggressive disease only [67, 73–75]. One study reported an increased risk for diabetes mellitus with early-stage disease (stage A), but inverse association for higher stage (stages B–D) disease [76], and one study reported a positive association between diabetes mellitus and risk of advanced prostate cancer [65]. Given the relatively small proportion of advanced tumors in many of the studies with screen-detected cases, additional epidemiologic studies are needed to more fully explore the association of diabetes mellitus with more advanced prostate cancer.

In contrast to the relatively consistent inverse associations reported between diabetes mellitus and risk of total and low-risk prostate cancer, multiple studies have reported that diabetes mellitus is associated with an *increased* risk of both all-cause and prostate cancer-specific mortality in men with prostate cancer. A recent meta-analysis of these data concluded that diabetes mellitus was associated with a 29% increase in risk of prostate cancer-specific mortality (RR = 1.29; 95% CI 1.22–1.38) and a 37% (RR = 1.37, 95% CI 1.29–1.45) increase in all-cause mortality [77]. Although individual findings are consistent across the majority of studies, many did not account for potentially important confounders such as prostate cancer characteristics (grade and stage), prostate specific antigen (PSA), prostate cancer treatment(s) or the possible impact of competing risks from other diabetes mellitus-related co-morbidities on the association of diabetes mellitus with prostate cancer-specific mortality. Few studies have evaluated the association of diabetes mellitus prostate cancer mortality among men without prostate cancer at baseline. In a study of almost 18,000 men in London, UK, with 40 years of follow-up, neither impaired glucose tolerance nor diabetes mellitus were associated with prostate cancer-specific mortality [78]. In a study of approximately 2000 male American Indians, diabetes mellitus was associated with an increased risk of prostate cancer mortality; however, among men without diabetes mellitus, a higher level of insulin resistance (measured by homeostasis model assessment to quantify insulin resistance (HOMA-IR)) was associated with a lower risk of prostate-cancer specific mortality [79].

Timing of Diabetes Mellitus and Prostate Cancer Risk

There is growing evidence to suggest that the association of diabetes mellitus with prostate cancer risk may differ by duration of diabetes mellitus. The early stage of type 2 diabetes mellitus is characterized by hyperinsulinemia, which is accompanied by increased levels of circulating insulin like growth factor 1 (IGF-1) and testosterone, and decreased levels of insulin-like growth factor binding protein 3 (IGF-BP3) and serum hormone binding globulin (SHBG) [80]. In contrast, as diabetes mellitus progresses, insulin levels decline and IGF-1 and testosterone levels decrease, and IGF-BP3 and SHBG levels increase [81, 82]. Numerous studies have reported data on duration of diabetes mellitus and risk of prostate cancer, the majority of which report stronger inverse associations of diabetes mellitus and prostate cancer risk with an increasing number of years elapsed since diabetes mellitus diagnosis [68–71, 76, 80]. Others have reported no meaningful differences [74, 75, 83] and two studies have reported positive associations of PCa risk with increasing duration of diabetes mellitus [84, 85]. Many of the studies reporting stronger inverse associations with increasing duration of diabetes mellitus have also reported a positive association between prostate cancer and recently diagnosed diabetes mellitus [63, 68, 70, 86], which is likely attributable to increased surveillance and health care utilization around the time of diabetes mellitus diagnosis. Larger studies have also examined associations of diabetes mellitus duration and different prostate cancer stage, grade or aggressiveness. All have reported similar associations between diabetes mellitus duration and prostate cancer severity [69, 71, 83]. Notably, few of the studies evaluating diabetes mellitus duration and prostate cancer risk directly assessed diabetes mellitus duration (as opposed to evaluating length of follow-up during the study) [68, 71, 74–76, 87], although the findings of these studies do not differ substantively from the overall literature.

Diabetes Mellitus Treatment and Prostate Cancer Risk and Outcomes

It is unknown whether the observed findings above between diabetes and prostate cancer are due to the diabetes, or due to the pharmacologic treatment of diabetes mellitus. Metformin is the most commonly used medication for diabetes mellitus and a great deal of interest exists on its potential anti-cancer properties. Metformin has several potential mechanisms that may influence cancer, including increased AMP-activated protein kinase (AMPK) activation, decreased hepatic gluconeogenesis (with resultant decrease in hyperinsulinemia), and improved insulin sensitivity [88, 89]. AMPK is activated in response to cellular stress [90] leading to a reduction of mammalian target of rapamycin (mTOR) activation, protein synthesis and cellular proliferation [91, 92]. Hyperglycemia and hyperinsulinemia have been associated with multiple malignancies [93–99]. As metformin use results in lower serum insulin levels [89, 93, 100, 101] the result may produce decreased downstream activation of these mitogenic pathways and potentially, a decrease in PCa growth (Fig. 3.2 [92]).

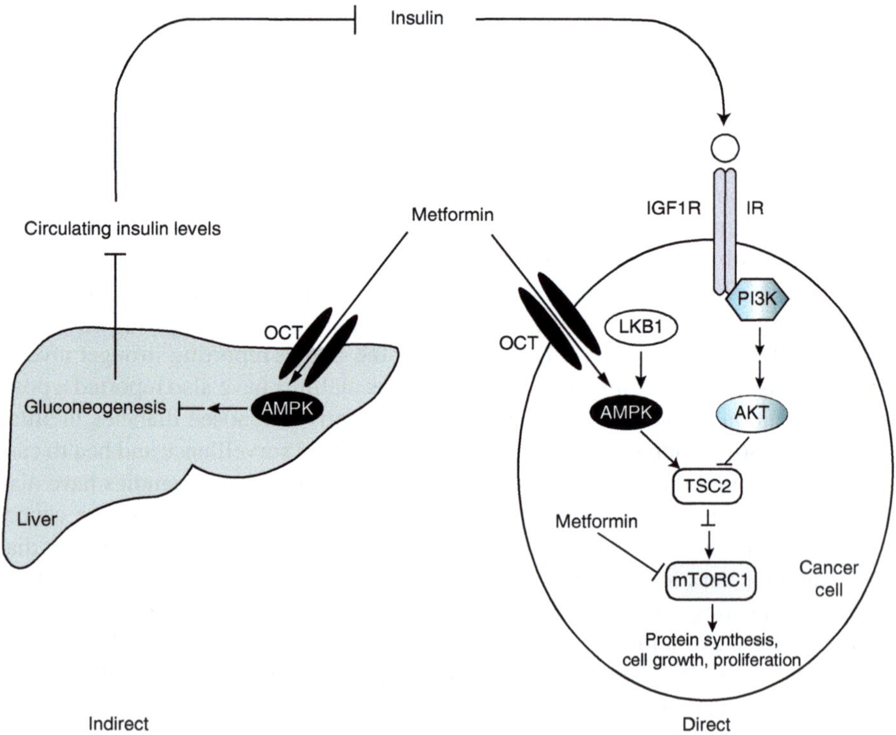

Fig. 3.2 Mechanism of action of metformin in cancer

Several studies of metformin and prostate cancer risk have been performed with some finding a reduction in prostate cancer risk [102–105] and others finding no effect [40, 106–109]. Two meta-analyses [110, 111] found no evidence for an effect of metformin on prostate cancer risk with similar odds ratios (OR 0.96, 95% CI 0.87–1.05; and OR 0.93, 95% CI 0.82–1.05, respectively). It should be noted that the main indication for metformin is the treatment of diabetes mellitus, so comparing metformin users to non-users may just be comparing diabetics to nondiabetics, which makes interpreting results for use of any diabetes medication difficult.

There are stronger data for an effect of metformin on prostate cancer outcomes, and several meta-analyses have been performed with evidence of metformin leading to a reduction in the risk of biochemical recurrence after primary therapy and also a reduction in both prostate cancer-specific and overall mortality [112–116]. In the meta analysis by Coyle et al., the reduction in risk of recurrence after primary treatment was seen following radiation therapy (HR 0.45, 95% CI 0.29–0.70) but not following radical prostatectomy (0.94, 0.77–1.15) [115].

Small clinical trials of metformin and prostate cancer outcomes have been completed and several studies are ongoing. One trial of 40 men starting ADT randomized men to either ADT alone or ADT in combination with metformin and a lifestyle intervention (diet and exercise) [117]. After 6 months, men in the intervention arm had significant improvements in weight, BMI, abdominal girth and blood pressure [117]. Metformin is being studied in various stages of prostate cancer (pre-prostatectomy, active surveillance, adjuvant for high risk localized disease, biochemical recurrence, at time of salvage radiation, castrate resistant prostate cancer, advanced hormone sensitive) (https://www.clinicaltrials.gov/).

Use of other medications for diabetes mellitus has also been studied with regards to prostate cancer. Several studies have investigated insulin and prostate cancer risk. A meta-analysis of 11 non-randomized studies from 2007 to 2013 and found that compared to use other glucose lowering agents, insulin was not associated with a reduction in risk of prostate cancer [118]. Sulfonylurea, which is an insulin-secretagogue, has also been studied with most showing no effect on prostate cancer risk compared to patients with diabetes mellitus taking metformin [119, 120], non-sulfonylurea therapy [121] or non-diabetes mellitus patients [122]. Recently, a study from Sweden found that those subjects with >1 year of diabetes mellitus and taking insulin/sulfonureas for >1 year had a reduction in the risk of prostate cancer compared to those not taking diabetes medications (OR 0.73, 95% CI 0.55–0.98) [40]. However, a study from the Finnish Randomized Study of Screening for Prostate Cancer found that use of sulphonylureas was associated with an increase in the risk of metastatic prostate cancer compared to other oral medications for diabetes mellitus (HR 2.04, 95% CI 1.11–3.77) [123]. Further research is needed to define the role of sulfonylurea and prostate cancer. Another class of diabetes medications, thiazolidinediones, are PPAR gamma ligands which can have anti-cancer properties and several preclinical studies have shown these agents to be active against prostate cancer cells [124]. Interestingly, higher levels of Peroxisome proliferator-activated receptor gamma (PPAR-γ)receptors have been identified on prostate cancer cells as opposed to benign prostate cells [125]. With prostate cancer, the data has suggested an increased risk [126, 127] or no effect [128, 129].

Hyperlipidemia and Prostate Cancer Risk

Hyperlipidemia is a well-established consequence of obesity, and there is growing evidence to suggest that men with hypercholesterolemia are at increased risk of high-grade or advanced prostate cancer. Several large prospective studies from various populations have reported that increasing cholesterol concentrations are associated with a greater risk of high-grade [130–134] and aggressive [135–137] prostate cancer. Two of these studies reported that the positive association between cholesterol level and high-risk prostate cancer was limited to overweight/obese men [133, 134]; although other studies have not reported differences in associations by obesity status [130, 131]. In an attempt to evaluate whether the use of cholesterol-lowering medications could explain associations between cholesterol concentrations and high-risk prostate cancer, three studies conducted analyses excluding men who reported use of these medications [130, 134, 136]. Associations were similar after excluding men who reported use of these medications, although no longer statistically significant in one study [130]. Few prospective studies have evaluated the relationship of cholesterol concentration with prostate cancer mortality. The majority report no association [45, 138]; however, one reported a significant increased risk for increasing total cholesterol concentrations [78].

The relationship between circulating cholesterol concentrations and total prostate cancer, however, is less clear. Initial studies of the association of cholesterol with risk of total prostate cancer, many of which were based on a small number of prostate cancer cases, reported no association [78, 139–142] or an inverse association [143, 144]. Since then, several prospective studies based on much larger sample sizes have confirmed findings from early studies [45, 130, 131, 133, 134, 145–148]; however, several recent studies have reported a significant increase in risk of total prostate cancer with increasing total cholesterol concentrations [132, 135–137].

Few prospective studies have evaluated associations of other lipids, such as high-density lipoprotein (HDL) and low-density lipoprotein (LDL), with risk of prostate cancer. Studies evaluating the relationship between HDL concentrations and risk of prostate cancer have been inconsistent. Some have reported a reduced risk of total prostate cancer [135, 148], while other report no association [45, 145] or an increased risk of total [132], high-risk [132] or low-risk [136] prostate cancer. Studies of the relationship between LDL concentrations and prostate cancer risk are also conflicting, with some studies reporting no association [45, 145, 148], and others reporting increased risks for total [132] and high-grade prostate cancer [132, 136]. The relationship of triglyceride concentrations with risk of prostate cancer has only been evaluated by three studies, all of which reported no association [45, 136, 147]. Only one study evaluated associations of apolipoproteins with risk of prostate cancer, and found a slight inverse association of apolipoprotein A-1 with risk of total cancer, but no association for apolipoprotein-B [148].

Hyperlipidemia Treatment and Prostate Cancer Risk

Statins use for high cholesterol has risen to almost 30% of US adults [149]. The potential mechanisms by which statins may reduce prostate cancer development and progression are multiple and can be divided into cholesterol-mediated pathways (e.g., reducing intra-tumor level of cholesterol precursor to androgens; altering cell membrane signaling) or non-cholesterol-mediated pathways (e.g., pro-apoptosis; lowering mevalonate levels and subsequent production of farnesyl and geranyl pyrophosphate which would block cellular proliferation and survival) (Fig. 3.3) [151].

Several studies have explored the relationship between statin use and primary prevention of incident prostate cancer. A meta analysis published in 2012 of 27 studies found that use of statins reduced incident prostate cancer (RR 0.93, 95% CI 0.87–0.99) and had a greater effect on reducing the risk of advanced prostate cancer (RR 0.80, 95% CI 0.70–0.98) [152]. Studies published since this meta analysis have been mixed with some showing a reduced risk of prostate cancer [153, 154] but several showing no protective effect [106, 155–158].

Tertiary prevention of prostate cancer recurrence and studies of prostate cancer specific mortality have also been performed. In a recent meta-analysis [159] of 22 studies of biochemical recurrence, use of statins was associated with a reduced risk of prostate cancer recurrence (HR 0.88, 95% CI 0.77–1.00). Interestingly, the effects were limited to treatment with radiation (HR 0.67, 95% CI 0.48–0.86; 7 studies)

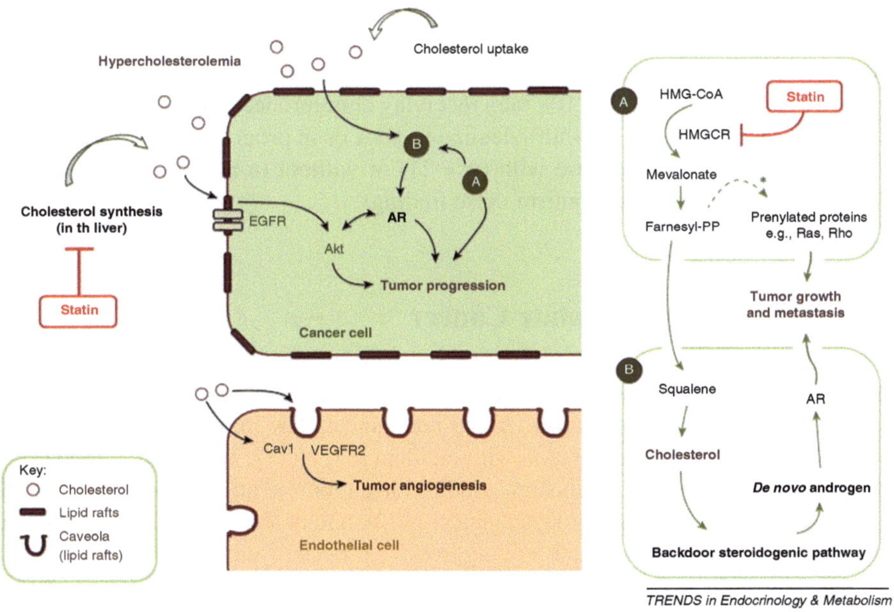

Fig. 3.3 Mechanism of action of statins in prostate cancer (from [150])

with no effect seen in those undergoing prostatectomy (HR 0.96, 95% CI 0.83–1.09). Whether statins (1) act as a radiosensitizer, or (2) if statins influence the effects of concomitant androgen deprivation therapy (ADT) use with radiation (ADT was used in 6 of 7 radiation studies with the proportion of men in those studies receiving ADT along with their radiation therapy ranging from 26 to 67%), or (3) if the statins association is due to unmeasured confounding is unknown. In a separate meta-analysis of mortality from 13 studies, use of statins reduced both overall (HR 0.56, 95% CI 0.38–0.83) and prostate cancer specific mortality (0.53, 95% CI 0.36–0.77) [160], with the effect observed for both pre and post-treatment use of statins.

An interesting interaction has recently been identified in steroid transport, statins and prostate cancer. The organic anion transporter, SLCO2B1, is involved in cellular uptake of several substrates, including steroid hormones such as dehydroepiandrosterone (DHEA) that prostate cancer cells can use as a precursor to dihydrotestosterone (DHT). Castrate resistant prostate cancer metastases have increased expression of SLCO genes compared to primary prostate cancer and genetic variants of SLCO transporters have been found to be associated with prostate cancer-specific mortality [161–163]. Statins are also a substrate for SLCO2B1 and act as a competitive inhibitor to DHEA for transport into prostate cancer cells [164]. In a study of 926 men starting ADT for advanced disease, use of statins (31% of cohort) had a longer time to progression compared to those not taking statins (adjusted HR 0.83, 95% CI 0.69–0.99) [164]. However, in castrate resistant disease, a common medication utilized is abiraterone, which is a CYP17A1 inhibitor that results in blocking all androgen production including DHEA. In this scenario, if adrenal DHEA is acting as an androgen source for prostate cancer cells in the setting of ADT, and abiraterone is blocking the production of DHEA, one would expect to not see a benefit to statin use if SLCO2B1 transport inhibition is the mechanism of statin effect on prostate cancer. In a study of 108 men receiving abiraterone, there was no difference in the percent experiencing >50% decline in PSA or in progression-free survival or overall survival between those with (n = 21) or without (n = 87) statin use [165]. Further study is needed to confirm these findings.

Hypertension and Prostate Cancer

Epidemiologic studies have reported inconsistent findings regarding the association of high blood pressure with risk of prostate cancer. The majority of studies have reported no significant association with incident [31, 32, 37, 166–170] or fatal [169, 171] prostate cancer, although some studies have reported an increased risk of total [32, 172, 173] or advanced prostate cancer [172], and at least one study reported an inverse association for total and non-aggressive prostate cancer [174].

Treatment for Hypertension and Prostate Cancer

Several classes of drugs are commonly used individually or in combination as pharmacological treatment for high blood pressure, including diuretics, beta-blockers (BBs), calcium channel (CC) blockers, angiotensin-converting enzyme (ACE) inhibitors, and angiotensin II-receptor (AR) blockers. Many of these medications have been shown to either suppress prostate cancer cell growth and proliferation, angiogenesis in vitro, and inhibit migration of PC-3 human prostate carcinoma in vivo [175]. Thus, numerous studies have evaluated the association of antihypertensive medication use with prostate cancer risk. For overall antihypertensive medication use, four large prospective studies found no evidence of an association with risk of prostate cancer [166, 172, 173, 176]. However, in one large population-based cohort, current use of any antihypertensive medication was associated with a slight decreased risk of total (RR = 0.90, 95% CI 0.83–0.98) and organ-confined low-grade prostate cancer (RR = 0.89, 95% CI 0.81–0.99) [177].

Studies on individual classes of antihypertensive medications and prostate cancer risk have also produced mixed results. Among studies evaluating the association of ACE inhibitor use and prostate cancer incidence, most have found no association [166, 167, 178–182], two found an inverse association [176, 177], although the inverse association was limited to one individual ACE inhibitor (captopril) in one study [176] and in the second one was no longer statistically significant after adjustment for other antihypertensive use [177], and two study reported a significant positive association for total prostate cancer only [183, 184]. A recent meta-analysis of the prospective studies found that use of ACE inhibitors or AR blockers was associated with a significant decreased risk of overall prostate cancer (RR = 0.88, 95% CI 0.80–0.97), [185] although two additional meta-analyses of data from clinical trials did not find an association with risk of prostate cancer for ACE inhibitor use [186, 187]. For calcium channel blockers, several large population-based cohort studies and a case-control study have reported no association with risk of total [167, 177, 183, 184, 188, 189], low-grade [177] or aggressive/fatal prostate cancer [177, 190]. Only one study reported a significant inverse association for CC blocker use with total prostate cancer risk (OR = 0.55; 95% CI, 0.31–0.97) [191]. The majority of studies evaluating the association of BB use and prostate cancer risk have also found no association [166, 167, 176, 177, 191]. However, in two observational studies, BB use was associated with lower overall prostate cancer risk (OR = 0.80; 95% CI, 0.70–1.0) [183], and in one was associated with a slight increased risk (OR = 1.16; 95% CI, 1.12–1.21) [184].

Heart Disease and Prostate Cancer Risk

An additional comorbidity that occurs with, or as a result of obesity, is heart disease. There are some data that a history of coronary artery disease (CAD) is associated with an increased risk of prostate cancer. In a secondary analysis of the REDUCE trial (a randomized controlled trial of dutasteride versus placebo for reducing the risk of prostate cancer in men with a prior negative biopsy), 9% of men had a history of CAD and this was associated with a 35% increased risk of prostate cancer in the multivariate model [192]. Men with CAD also were more likely to be obese, have diabetes mellitus, hypertension and hypercholesterolemia.

Treatment of Heart Disease and Prostate Cancer Risk

The cardiac glycosides (e.g., digoxin) are used in the treatment of congestive heart failure and cardiac arrhythmias. Cardiac glycosides also have been found to alter serum androgen levels [193, 194], inhibiting tumor growth and development, [195] and have inhibitory effects on prostate cancer cell lines [196–199]. In a study that screened a medication library for growth inhibition in prostate cancer cell lines, cardiac glycosides were among the most potent [199]. Although an analysis of the Health Professionals Follow-up Study found a significant reduction in the risk of prostate cancer for digoxin users (HR 0.76, 95% CI 0.60–0.95) [199], other studies have not shown a statistically significant reduction in prostate cancer risk [200, 201]. With regards to prostate cancer-specific mortality, the literature does not support a protective role for digoxin, with two of the studies showing non-significant increases in prostate cancer-specific mortality among users [202, 203]. Sotalol, a BB and potassium-channel inhibitor used for arrhythmias has commonly been studied along with glycosides, with one study finding a reduction in the risk of advanced prostate cancer associated with sotalol use [204].

Individuals with heart disease are often recommended to take aspirin daily to prevent to reduce the risk of vascular events (heart attack, stroke) [205]. There are several studies on aspirin use and cancer risk and mortality, with the strongest data present for colorectal cancer risk. The anti-cancer mechanisms for aspirin are hypothesized to include induction of apoptosis, reduced prostaglandin production with effects on angiogenesis, proliferation and host immunity [206, 207]. A meta analysis of the effects of aspirin on prostate cancer risk and mortality was published in 2014 [208]. Overall, use of aspirin was associated with a reduction in the incidence of total prostate cancer (OR 0.92, 95% CI 0.87–0.97) and advanced prostate cancer (OR 0.81, 95% CI 0.73–0.89). In a recent study with TMPRSS2:ERG fusion status available, aspirin users had a 37% reduction in the risk of TMPRSS2:ERG fusion positive tumors (95% CI 0.43–0.93) with dose effect present, whereas no association was seen with TMPRSS2:ERG fusion negative tumors and aspirin use (OR 0.99, 0.69–1.42) [209]. TMPRSS2:ERG fusion is the most common gene rearrangement in prostate cancer, present in approximately 50% of cases. As aspirin reduces the level of reactive oxygen species in a cell (which can create dsDNA breaks), use of aspirin may protect against DNA strand breaks required for TMPRSS2:ERG fusion. In a recent meta-analysis, use of aspirin was associated with a modest reduction in the risk of prostate cancer specific mortality (OR 0.86, 95% CI 0.78–0.96 for total prostate cancer; OR = 0.81, 95% CI 0.71–0.92 for advanced prostate cancer) [208].

Potential Biases of Associations of Obesity-Related Metabolic Conditions and Risk of Prostate Cancer

When considering the potential mechanisms that underlie the inverse association between comorbid conditions and prostate cancer, non-causal explanations should also be considered. Many obesity-related metabolic conditions have been associated with lower prostate-specific antigen (PSA) levels. For example, PSA has been shown to be lower in diabetics and lowest in individuals with a long duration of disease [62, 70, 210–215]. Similarly, obesity, which commonly coexists with diabetes, is believed to lowers PSA due to hemodilution [216–219]. Furthermore, some medications, such as statins and 5-alpha reductase inhibitors have been associated with lower PSA levels [220–222]. Because PSA drives biopsy recommendations and subsequent PCa detection in clinical practice, lower PSA in men with obesity-related medical conditions could lead to fewer biopsies and consequently to less diagnoses of cancer. Thus, it is possible that the observed associations between obesity-related metabolic conditions and prostate cancer risk are attributable, at least in part, to the effects of these conditions and/or their treatments on PSA values.

Conclusions

Obesity and prostate cancer are two common conditions in men over the age of 50 today and there appears to be a relationship between the two, with obesity potentially influencing the risk, aggressiveness and outcomes of men with prostate cancer. As our understanding of the mechanisms between these conditions grows, the appreciation of the complexity of the relationship and the likely contribution from multiple factors also increases. With obesity, a number of comorbid conditions also become more common. The observed associations between these diagnoses or their treatments and prostate cancer could be explained by confounding by the obesity:prostate cancer relationship. Or, these diagnoses and treatments may influence prostate cancer development and progression independent of obesity. Further research will help define the complex interplay. Until then, care of men at risk for, or with prostate cancer, should also include attention to weight management, glucose and lipid control, to promote both overall and prostate-cancer specific health.

References

1. Calle EE, Rodriguez C, Walker-Thurmond K, Thun MJ. Overweight, obesity, and mortality from cancer in a prospectively studied cohort of U.S. adults. N Engl J Med. 2003;348(17):1625–38. doi:10.1056/NEJMoa021423.
2. Wright ME, Chang SC, Schatzkin A, Albanes D, Kipnis V, Mouw T, Hurwitz P, Hollenbeck A, Leitzmann MF. Prospective study of adiposity and weight change in relation to prostate cancer incidence and mortality. Cancer. 2007;109(4):675–84. doi:10.1002/cncr.22443.

3. Hsing AW, Sakoda LC, Chua S Jr. Obesity, metabolic syndrome, and prostate cancer. Am J Clin Nutr. 2007;86(3):s843–57.
4. Allott EH, Masko EM, Freedland SJ. Obesity and prostate cancer: weighing the evidence. Eur Urol. 2013;63(5):800–9. doi:10.1016/j.eururo.2012.11.013.
5. MacInnis RJ, English DR. Body size and composition and prostate cancer risk: systematic review and meta-regression analysis. Cancer Causes Control. 2006;17(8):989–1003. doi:10.1007/s10552-006-0049-z.
6. Discacciati A, Orsini N, Wolk A. Body mass index and incidence of localized and advanced prostate cancer—a dose-response meta-analysis of prospective studies. Ann Oncol. 2012;23(7):1665–71. doi:10.1093/annonc/mdr603.
7. Zhang X, Zhou G, Sun B, Zhao G, Liu D, Sun J, Liu C, Guo H. Impact of obesity upon prostate cancer-associated mortality: a meta-analysis of 17 cohort studies. Oncol Lett. 2015;9(3):1307–12. doi:10.3892/ol.2014.2841.
8. Gong Z, Agalliu I, Lin DW, Stanford JL, Kristal AR. Obesity is associated with increased risks of prostate cancer metastasis and death after initial cancer diagnosis in middle-aged men. Cancer. 2007;109(6):1192–202. doi:10.1002/cncr.22534.
9. Snowdon DA, Phillips RL, Choi W. Diet, obesity, and risk of fatal prostate cancer. Am J Epidemiol. 1984;120(2):244–50.
10. Rodriguez C, Patel AV, Calle EE, Jacobs EJ, Chao A, Thun MJ. Body mass index, height, and prostate cancer mortality in two large cohorts of adult men in the United States. Cancer Epidemiol Biomark Prev. 2001;10(4):345–53.
11. Siddiqui SA, Inman BA, Sengupta S, Slezak JM, Bergstralh EJ, Leibovich BC, Zincke H, Blute ML. Obesity and survival after radical prostatectomy: a 10-year prospective cohort study. Cancer. 2006;107(3):521–9. doi:10.1002/cncr.22030.
12. Banez LL, Sun L, Trock BJ, Han M, Partin AW, Aronson WJ, Terris MK, Presti JC Jr, Kane CJ, Amling CL, Moul JW, Freedland SJ. Body mass index and prostate specific antigen as predictors of adverse pathology and biochemical recurrence after prostatectomy. J Urol. 2009;182(2):491–496. discussion 6–8. doi:10.1016/j.juro.2009.04.007.
13. Efstathiou JA, Bae K, Shipley WU, Hanks GE, Pilepich MV, Sandler HM, Smith MR. Obesity and mortality in men with locally advanced prostate cancer: analysis of RTOG 85-31. Cancer. 2007;110(12):2691–9. doi:10.1002/cncr.23093.
14. Freedland SJ, Grubb KA, Yiu SK, Humphreys EB, Nielsen ME, Mangold LA, Isaacs WB, Partin AW. Obesity and risk of biochemical progression following radical prostatectomy at a tertiary care referral center. J Urol. 2005;174(3):919–22. doi:10.1097/01.ju.0000169459.78982.d7.
15. Freedland SJ, Terris MK, Presti JC Jr, Amling CL, Kane CJ, Trock B, Aronson WJ. Search Database Study G. Obesity and biochemical outcome following radical prostatectomy for organ confined disease with negative surgical margins. J Urol. 2004;172(2):520–4. doi:10.1097/01.ju.0000135302.58378.ae.
16. Jayachandran J, Banez LL, Aronson WJ, Terris MK, Presti JC Jr, Amling CL, Kane CJ, Freedland SJ, Group SDS. Obesity as a predictor of adverse outcome across black and white race: results from the Shared Equal Access Regional Cancer Hospital (SEARCH) Database. Cancer. 2009;115(22):5263–71. doi:10.1002/cncr.24571.
17. Kane CJ, Im R, Amling CL, Presti JC Jr, Aronson WJ, Terris MK, Freedland SJ, Group SDS. Outcomes after radical prostatectomy among men who are candidates for active surveillance: results from the SEARCH database. Urology. 2010;76(3):695–700. doi:10.1016/j.urology.2009.12.073.
18. Major JM, Klonoff-Cohen HS, Pierce JP, Slymen DJ, Saltzstein SL, Macera CA, Mercola D, Kattan MW. Prostate cancer postoperative nomogram scores and obesity. PLoS One. 2011;6(2):e17382. doi:10.1371/journal.pone.0017382.
19. Strom SS, Wang X, Pettaway CA, Logothetis CJ, Yamamura Y, Do KA, Babaian RJ, Troncoso P. Obesity, weight gain, and risk of biochemical failure among prostate cancer patients following prostatectomy. Clin Cancer Res. 2005;11(19 Pt 1):6889–94. doi:10.1158/1078-0432.CCR-04-1977.

20. Calle EE, Kaaks R. Overweight, obesity and cancer: epidemiological evidence and proposed mechanisms. Nat Rev Cancer. 2004;4(8):579–91. doi:10.1038/nrc1408.
21. Andersson SO, Wolk A, Bergstrom R, Adami HO, Engholm G, Englund A, Nyren O. Body size and prostate cancer: a 20-year follow-up study among 135006 Swedish construction workers. J Natl Cancer Inst. 1997;89(5):385–9.
22. Ma J, Li H, Giovannucci E, Mucci L, Qiu W, Nguyen PL, Gaziano JM, Pollak M, Stampfer MJ. Prediagnostic body-mass index, plasma C-peptide concentration, and prostate cancer-specific mortality in men with prostate cancer: a long-term survival analysis. Lancet Oncol. 2008;9(11):1039–47. doi:10.1016/S1470-2045(08)70235-3.
23. Cao Y, Ma J. Body mass index, prostate cancer-specific mortality, and biochemical recurrence: a systematic review and meta-analysis. Cancer Prev Res (Phila). 2011;4(4):486–501. doi:10.1158/1940-6207.CAPR-10-0229.
24. Demark-Wahnefried W, Platz EA, Ligibel JA, Blair CK, Courneya KS, Meyerhardt JA, Ganz PA, Rock CL, Schmitz KH, Wadden T, Philip EJ, Wolfe B, Gapstur SM, Ballard-Barbash R, McTiernan A, Minasian L, Nebeling L, Goodwin PJ. The role of obesity in cancer survival and recurrence. Cancer Epidemiol Biomark Prev. 2012;21(8):1244–59. doi:10.1158/1055-9965.EPI-12-0485.
25. Saydah S, Bullard KM, Cheng Y, Ali MK, Gregg EW, Geiss L, Imperatore G. Trends in cardiovascular disease risk factors by obesity level in adults in the United States, NHANES 1999–2010. Obesity (Silver Spring). 2014;22(8):1888–95. doi:10.1002/oby.20761.
26. Grundy SM, Cleeman JI, Daniels SR, Donato KA, Eckel RH, Franklin BA, Gordon DJ, Krauss RM, Savage PJ, Smith SC Jr, Spertus JA, Costa F, American Heart A, National Heart L, Blood I. Diagnosis and management of the metabolic syndrome: an American Heart Association/National Heart, Lung, and Blood Institute Scientific Statement. Circulation. 2005;112(17):2735–52. doi:10.1161/CIRCULATIONAHA.105.169404.
27. Alberti KG, Zimmet PZ. Definition, diagnosis and classification of diabetes mellitus and its complications. Part 1: diagnosis and classification of diabetes mellitus provisional report of a WHO consultation. Diabet Med. 1998;15(7):539–53. doi:10.1002/(SICI)1096-9136(199807)15:7<539::AID-DIA668>3.0.CO;2-S.
28. Zimmet P, Magliano D, Matsuzawa Y, Alberti G, Shaw J. The metabolic syndrome: a global public health problem and a new definition. J Atheroscler Thromb. 2005;12(6):295–300.
29. Reaven GM. Banting lecture 1988. Role of insulin resistance in human disease. Diabetes. 1988;37(12):1595–607.
30. Ervin RB. Prevalence of metabolic syndrome among adults 20 years of age and over, by sex, age, race and ethnicity, and body mass index: United States, 2003–2006. Natl Health Stat Rep. 2009(13):1–7.
31. Lund Haheim L, Wisloff TF, Holme I, Nafstad P. Metabolic syndrome predicts prostate cancer in a cohort of middle-aged Norwegian men followed for 27 years. Am J Epidemiol. 2006;164(8):769–74. doi:10.1093/aje/kwj284.
32. Tuohimaa P, Tenkanen L, Syvala H, Lumme S, Hakulinen T, Dillner J, Hakama M. Interaction of factors related to the metabolic syndrome and vitamin D on risk of prostate cancer. Cancer Epidemiol Biomark Prev. 2007;16(2):302–7. doi:10.1158/1055-9965.EPI-06-0777.
33. Laukkanen JA, Laaksonen DE, Niskanen L, Pukkala E, Hakkarainen A, Salonen JT. Metabolic syndrome and the risk of prostate cancer in Finnish men: a population-based study. Cancer Epidemiol Biomark Prev. 2004;13(10):1646–50.
34. Pelucchi C, Serraino D, Negri E, Montella M, Dellanoce C, Talamini R, La Vecchia C. The metabolic syndrome and risk of prostate cancer in Italy. Ann Epidemiol. 2011;21(11):835–41. doi:10.1016/j.annepidem.2011.07.007.
35. Beebe-Dimmer JL, Dunn RL, Sarma AV, Montie JE, Cooney KA. Features of the metabolic syndrome and prostate cancer in African-American men. Cancer. 2007;109(5):875–81. doi:10.1002/cncr.22461.
36. Beebe-Dimmer JL, Nock NL, Neslund-Dudas C, Rundle A, Bock CH, Tang D, Jankowski M, Rybicki BA. Racial differences in risk of prostate cancer associated with metabolic syndrome. Urology. 2009;74(1):185–90. doi:10.1016/j.urology.2009.03.013.

37. Tande AJ, Platz EA, Folsom AR. The metabolic syndrome is associated with reduced risk of prostate cancer. Am J Epidemiol. 2006;164(11):1094–102. doi:10.1093/aje/kwj320.
38. Blanc-Lapierre A, Spence A, Karakiewicz PI, Aprikian A, Saad F, Parent ME. Metabolic syndrome and prostate cancer risk in a population-based case-control study in Montreal, Canada. BMC Public Health. 2015;15:913. doi:10.1186/s12889-015-2260-x.
39. Sourbeer KN, Howard LE, Andriole GL, Moreira DM, Castro-Santamaria R, Freedland SJ, Vidal AC. Metabolic syndrome-like components and prostate cancer risk: results from the Reduction by Dutasteride of Prostate Cancer Events (REDUCE) study. BJU Int. 2015;115(5):736–43. doi:10.1111/bju.12843.
40. Haggstrom C, Van Hemelrijck M, Zethelius B, Robinson D, Grundmark B, Holmberg L, Gudbjornsdottir S, Garmo H, Stattin P. Prospective study of Type 2 diabetes mellitus, anti-diabetic drugs and risk of prostate cancer. Int J Cancer. 2017;140(3):611–7. doi:10.1002/ijc.30480.
41. Lawrence YR, Morag O, Benderly M, Boyko V, Novikov I, Dicker AP, Goldbourt U, Behar S, Barchana M, Wolf I. Association between metabolic syndrome, diabetes mellitus and prostate cancer risk. Prostate Cancer Prostatic Dis. 2013;16(2):181–6. doi:10.1038/pcan.2012.54.
42. Wallner LP, Morgenstern H, McGree ME, Jacobson DJ, St Sauver JL, Jacobsen SJ, Sarma AV. The effects of metabolic conditions on prostate cancer incidence over 15 years of follow-up: results from the Olmsted County Study. BJU Int. 2011;107(6):929–35. doi:10.1111/j.1464-410X.2010.09703.x.
43. Russo A, Autelitano M, Bisanti L. Metabolic syndrome and cancer risk. Eur J Cancer. 2008;44(2):293–7. doi:10.1016/j.ejca.2007.11.005.
44. Inoue M, Noda M, Kurahashi N, Iwasaki M, Sasazuki S, Iso H, Tsugane S, Japan Public Health Center-based Prospective Study G. Impact of metabolic factors on subsequent cancer risk: results from a large-scale population-based cohort study in Japan. Eur J Cancer Prev. 2009;18(3):240–7. doi:10.1097/CEJ.0b013e3283240460.
45. Martin RM, Vatten L, Gunnell D, Romundstad P, Nilsen TI. Components of the metabolic syndrome and risk of prostate cancer: the HUNT 2 cohort, Norway. Cancer Causes Control. 2009;20(7):1181–92. doi:10.1007/s10552-009-9319-x.
46. Grundmark B, Garmo H, Loda M, Busch C, Holmberg L, Zethelius B. The metabolic syndrome and the risk of prostate cancer under competing risks of death from other causes. Cancer Epidemiol Biomark Prev. 2010;19(8):2088–96. doi:10.1158/1055-9965.EPI-10-0112.
47. Esposito K, Chiodini P, Colao A, Lenzi A, Giugliano D. Metabolic syndrome and risk of cancer: a systematic review and meta-analysis. Diabetes Care. 2012;35(11):2402–11. doi:10.2337/dc12-0336.
48. Xiang YZ, Xiong H, Cui ZL, Jiang SB, Xia QH, Zhao Y, Li GB, Jin XB. The association between metabolic syndrome and the risk of prostate cancer, high-grade prostate cancer, advanced prostate cancer, prostate cancer-specific mortality and biochemical recurrence. J Exp Clin Cancer Res. 2013;32:9. doi:10.1186/1756-9966-32-9.
49. De Nunzio C, Freedland SJ, Miano R, Trucchi A, Cantiani A, Carluccini A, Tubaro A. Metabolic syndrome is associated with high grade Gleason score when prostate cancer is diagnosed on biopsy. Prostate. 2011;71(14):1492–8. doi:10.1002/pros.21364.
50. De Nunzio C, Simone G, Brassetti A, Mastroianni R, Collura D, Muto G, Gallucci M, Tubaro A. Metabolic syndrome is associated with advanced prostate cancer in patients treated with radical retropubic prostatectomy: results from a multicentre prospective study. BMC Cancer. 2016;16:407. doi:10.1186/s12885-016-2442-7.
51. Morote J, Ropero J, Planas J, Bastaros JM, Delgado G, Placer J, Celma A, de Torres IM, Carles J, Reventos J, Doll A. Metabolic syndrome increases the risk of aggressive prostate cancer detection. BJU Int. 2013;111(7):1031–6. doi:10.1111/j.1464-410X.2012.11406.x.
52. Bhindi B, Locke J, Alibhai SM, Kulkarni GS, Margel DS, Hamilton RJ, Finelli A, Trachtenberg J, Zlotta AR, Toi A, Hersey KM, Evans A, van der Kwast TH, Fleshner NE. Dissecting the association between metabolic syndrome and prostate cancer risk: analysis of a large clinical cohort. Eur Urol. 2015;67(1):64–70. doi:10.1016/j.eururo.2014.01.040.

53. Bhindi B, Xie WY, Kulkarni GS, Hamilton RJ, Nesbitt M, Finelli A, Zlotta AR, Evans A, van der Kwast TH, Alibhai SM, Trachtenberg J, Fleshner NE. Influence of metabolic syndrome on prostate cancer stage, grade, and overall recurrence risk in men undergoing radical prostatectomy. Urology. 2016;93:77–85. doi:10.1016/j.urology.2016.01.041.
54. Kheterpal E, Sammon JD, Diaz M, Bhandari A, Trinh QD, Pokala N, Sharma P, Menon M, Agarwal PK. Effect of metabolic syndrome on pathologic features of prostate cancer. Urol Oncol. 2013;31(7):1054–9. doi:10.1016/j.urolonc.2011.12.012.
55. Macleod LC, Chery LJ, Hu EY, Zeliadt SB, Holt SK, Lin DW, Porter MP, Gore JL, Wright JL. Metabolic syndrome, dyslipidemia and prostate cancer recurrence after primary surgery or radiation in a veterans cohort. Prostate Cancer Prostatic Dis. 2015;18(2):190–5. doi:10.1038/pcan.2015.12.
56. Jaggers JR, Sui X, Hooker SP, LaMonte MJ, Matthews CE, Hand GA, Blair SN. Metabolic syndrome and risk of cancer mortality in men. Eur J Cancer. 2009;45(10):1831–8. doi:10.1016/j.ejca.2009.01.031.
57. Bansal D, Bhansali A, Kapil G, Undela K, Tiwari P. Type 2 diabetes and risk of prostate cancer: a meta-analysis of observational studies. Prostate Cancer Prostatic Dis. 2013;16(2):151–58. S1. doi:10.1038/pcan.2012.40.
58. Bonovas S, Filioussi K, Tsantes A. Diabetes mellitus and risk of prostate cancer: a meta-analysis. Diabetologia. 2004;47(6):1071–8. doi:10.1007/s00125-004-1415-6.
59. Kasper JS, Giovannucci E. A meta-analysis of diabetes mellitus and the risk of prostate cancer. Cancer Epidemiol Biomark Prev. 2006;15(11):2056–62. doi:10.1158/1055-9965.EPI-06-0410.
60. Cowie CC, Rust KF, Byrd-Holt DD, Eberhardt MS, Flegal KM, Engelgau MM, Saydah SH, Williams DE, Geiss LS, Gregg EW. Prevalence of diabetes and impaired fasting glucose in adults in the U.S. population: National Health And Nutrition Examination Survey 1999–2002. Diabetes Care. 2006;29(6):1263–8. doi:10.2337/dc06-0062.
61. Calton BA, Chang SC, Wright ME, Kipnis V, Lawson K, Thompson FE, Subar AF, Mouw T, Campbell DS, Hurwitz P, Hollenbeck A, Schatzkin A, Leitzmann MF. History of diabetes mellitus and subsequent prostate cancer risk in the NIH-AARP Diet and Health Study. Cancer Causes Control. 2007;18(5):493–503. doi:10.1007/s10552-007-0126-y.
62. Waters KM, Henderson BE, Stram DO, Wan P, Kolonel LN, Haiman CA. Association of diabetes with prostate cancer risk in the multiethnic cohort. Am J Epidemiol. 2009;169(8):937–45. doi:10.1093/aje/kwp003.
63. Adami HO, McLaughlin J, Ekbom A, Berne C, Silverman D, Hacker D, Persson I. Cancer risk in patients with diabetes mellitus. Cancer Causes Control. 1991;2(5):307–14.
64. Tavani A, Gallus S, Bertuzzi M, Dal Maso L, Zucchetto A, Negri E, Franceschi S, Ramazzotti V, Montella M, La Vecchia C. Diabetes mellitus and the risk of prostate cancer in Italy. Eur Urol. 2005;47(3):313–317.; discussion 7. doi:10.1016/j.eururo.2004.10.027.
65. Li Q, Kuriyama S, Kakizaki M, Yan H, Sone T, Nagai M, Sugawara Y, Ohmori-Matsuda K, Hozawa A, Nishino Y, Tsuji I. History of diabetes mellitus and the risk of prostate cancer: The Ohsaki Cohort Study. Cancer Causes Control. 2010;21(7):1025–32. doi:10.1007/s10552-010-9530-9.
66. Rousseau MC, Parent ME, Pollak MN, Siemiatycki J. Diabetes mellitus and cancer risk in a population-based case-control study among men from Montreal, Canada. Int J Cancer. 2006;118(8):2105–9. doi:10.1002/ijc.21600.
67. Gong Z, Neuhouser ML, Goodman PJ, Albanes D, Chi C, Hsing AW, Lippman SM, Platz EA, Pollak MN, Thompson IM, Kristal AR. Obesity, diabetes, and risk of prostate cancer: results from the prostate cancer prevention trial. Cancer Epidemiol Biomark Prev. 2006;15(10):1977–83. doi:10.1158/1055-9965.EPI-06-0477.
68. Rodriguez C, Patel AV, Mondul AM, Jacobs EJ, Thun MJ, Calle EE. Diabetes and risk of prostate cancer in a prospective cohort of US men. Am J Epidemiol. 2005;161(2):147–52. doi:10.1093/aje/kwh334.

69. Kasper JS, Liu Y, Giovannucci E. Diabetes mellitus and risk of prostate cancer in the health professionals follow-up study. Int J Cancer. 2009;124(6):1398–403. doi:10.1002/ijc.24044.
70. Giovannucci E, Rimm EB, Stampfer MJ, Colditz GA, Willett WC. Diabetes mellitus and risk of prostate cancer (United States). Cancer Causes Control. 1998;9(1):3–9.
71. Fall K, Garmo H, Gudbjornsdottir S, Stattin P, Zethelius B. Diabetes mellitus and prostate cancer risk; a nationwide case-control study within PCBaSe Sweden. Cancer Epidemiol Biomark Prev. 2013;22(6):1102–9. doi:10.1158/1055-9965.EPI-12-1046.
72. Xu H, Jiang HW, Ding GX, Zhang H, Zhang LM, Mao SH, Ding Q. Diabetes mellitus and prostate cancer risk of different grade or stage: a systematic review and meta-analysis. Diabetes Res Clin Pract. 2013;99(3):241–9. doi:10.1016/j.diabres.2012.12.003.
73. Leitzmann MF, Ahn J, Albanes D, Hsing AW, Schatzkin A, Chang SC, Huang WY, Weiss JM, Danforth KN, Grubb RL 3rd, Andriole GL, Prostate LC. Ovarian Trial Project T. Diabetes mellitus and prostate cancer risk in the Prostate, Lung, Colorectal, and Ovarian Cancer Screening Trial. Cancer Causes Control. 2008;19(10):1267–76. doi:10.1007/s10552-008-9198-6.
74. Tsilidis KK, Allen NE, Appleby PN, Rohrmann S, Nothlings U, Arriola L, Gunter MJ, Chajes V, Rinaldi S, Romieu I, Murphy N, Riboli E, Tzoulaki I, Kaaks R, Lukanova A, Boeing H, Pischon T, Dahm CC, Overvad K, Quiros JR, Fonseca-Nunes A, Molina-Montes E, Gavrila Chervase D, Ardanaz E, Khaw KT, Wareham NJ, Roswall N, Tjonneland A, Lagiou P, Trichopoulos D, Trichopoulou A, Palli D, Pala V, Tumino R, Vineis P, Bueno-de-Mesquita HB, Malm J, Orho-Melander M, Johansson M, Stattin P, Travis RC, Key TJ. Diabetes mellitus and risk of prostate cancer in the European Prospective Investigation into Cancer and Nutrition. Int J Cancer. 2015;136(2):372–81. doi:10.1002/ijc.28989.
75. Turner EL, Lane JA, Donovan JL, Davis MJ, Metcalfe C, Neal DE, Hamdy FC, Martin RM. Association of diabetes mellitus with prostate cancer: nested case-control study (Prostate testing for cancer and treatment study). Int J Cancer. 2011;128(2):440–6. doi:10.1002/ijc.25360.
76. Zhu K, Lee IM, Sesso HD, Buring JE, Levine RS, Gaziano JM. History of diabetes mellitus and risk of prostate cancer in physicians. Am J Epidemiol. 2004;159(10):978–82.
77. Lee J, Giovannucci E, Jeon JY. Diabetes and mortality in patients with prostate cancer: a meta-analysis. Springerplus. 2016;5(1):1548. doi:10.1186/s40064-016-3233-y.
78. Batty GD, Kivimaki M, Clarke R, Davey Smith G, Shipley MJ. Modifiable risk factors for prostate cancer mortality in London: forty years of follow-up in the Whitehall study. Cancer Causes Control. 2011;22(2):311–8. doi:10.1007/s10552-010-9691-6.
79. Best LG, Garcia-Esquinas E, Yeh JL, Yeh F, Zhang Y, Lee ET, Howard BV, Farley JH, Welty TK, Rhoades DA, Rhoades ER, Umans JG, Navas-Acien A. Association of diabetes and cancer mortality in American Indians: the Strong Heart Study. Cancer Causes Control. 2015;26(11):1551–60. doi:10.1007/s10552-015-0648-7.
80. Baradaran N, Ahmadi H, Salem S, Lotfi M, Jahani Y, Baradaran N, Mehrsai AR, Pourmand G. The protective effect of diabetes mellitus against prostate cancer: role of sex hormones. Prostate. 2009;69(16):1744–50. doi:10.1002/pros.21023.
81. Giovannucci E, Michaud D. The role of obesity and related metabolic disturbances in cancers of the colon, prostate, and pancreas. Gastroenterology. 2007;132(6):2208–25. doi:10.1053/j.gastro.2007.03.050.
82. Weir GC, Bonner-Weir S. Five stages of evolving beta-cell dysfunction during progression to diabetes. Diabetes. 2004;53(Suppl 3):S16–21.
83. Wu C, Moreira DM, Gerber L, Rittmaster RS, Andriole GL, Freedland SJ. Diabetes and prostate cancer risk in the REDUCE trial. Prostate Cancer Prostatic Dis. 2011;14(4):326–31. doi:10.1038/pcan.2011.28.
84. Will JC, Vinicor F, Calle EE. Is diabetes mellitus associated with prostate cancer incidence and survival? Epidemiology. 1999;10(3):313–8.
85. Tseng CH. Diabetes and risk of prostate cancer: a study using the National Health Insurance. Diabetes Care. 2011;34(3):616–21. doi:10.2337/dc10-1640.
86. Tavani A, Gallus S, Bosetti C, Tzonou A, Lagiou P, Negri E, Trichopoulos D, La Vecchia C. Diabetes and the risk of prostate cancer. Eur J Cancer Prev. 2002;11(2):125–8.

87. Atchison EA, Gridley G, Carreon JD, Leitzmann MF, McGlynn KA. Risk of cancer in a large cohort of U.S. veterans with diabetes. Int J Cancer. 2011;128(3):635–43. doi:10.1002/ijc.25362.
88. Joshua AM, Zannella VE, Downes MR, Bowes B, Hersey K, Koritzinsky M, Schwab M, Hofmann U, Evans A, van der Kwast T, Trachtenberg J, Finelli A, Fleshner N, Sweet J, Pollak M. A pilot 'window of opportunity' neoadjuvant study of metformin in localised prostate cancer. Prostate Cancer Prostatic Dis. 2014;17(3):252–8. doi:10.1038/pcan.2014.20.
89. Pernicova I, Korbonits M. Metformin—mode of action and clinical implications for diabetes and cancer. Nat Rev Endocrinol. 2014;10(3):143–56. doi:10.1038/nrendo.2013.256.
90. Hardie DG. Minireview: the AMP-activated protein kinase cascade: the key sensor of cellular energy status. Endocrinology. 2003;144(12):5179–83. doi:10.1210/en.2003-0982.
91. Hadad SM, Fleming S, Thompson AM. Targeting AMPK: a new therapeutic opportunity in breast cancer. Crit Rev Oncol Hematol. 2008;67(1):1–7. doi:10.1016/j.critrevonc.2008.01.007.
92. Dowling RJ, Niraula S, Stambolic V, Goodwin PJ. Metformin in cancer: translational challenges. J Mol Endocrinol. 2012;48(3):R31–43. doi:10.1530/JME-12-0007.
93. Pollak M. Insulin and insulin-like growth factor signalling in neoplasia. Nat Rev Cancer. 2008;8(12):915–28. doi:10.1038/nrc2536.
94. Pollak MN. Investigating metformin for cancer prevention and treatment: the end of the beginning. Cancer Discov. 2012;2(9):778–90. doi:10.1158/2159-8290.CD-12-0263.
95. Belfiore A. The role of insulin receptor isoforms and hybrid insulin/IGF-I receptors in human cancer. Curr Pharm Des. 2007;13(7):671–86.
96. Wright JL, Plymate SR, Porter MP, Gore JL, Lin DW, Hu E, Zeliadt SB. Hyperglycemia and prostate cancer recurrence in men treated for localized prostate cancer. Prostate Cancer Prostatic Dis. 2013;16(2):204–8. doi:10.1038/pcan.2013.5.
97. Goodwin PJ, Ennis M, Pritchard KI, Trudeau ME, Koo J, Madarnas Y, Hartwick W, Hoffman B, Hood N. Fasting insulin and outcome in early-stage breast cancer: results of a prospective cohort study. J Clin Oncol. 2002;20(1):42–51. doi:10.1200/JCO.2002.20.1.42.
98. Hammarsten J, Hogstedt B. Hyperinsulinaemia: a prospective risk factor for lethal clinical prostate cancer. Eur J Cancer. 2005;41(18):2887–95. doi:10.1016/j.ejca.2005.09.003.
99. Heni M, Hennenlotter J, Scharpf M, Lutz SZ, Schwentner C, Todenhofer T, Schilling D, Kuhs U, Gerber V, Machicao F, Staiger H, Haring HU, Stenzl A. Insulin receptor isoforms A and B as well as insulin receptor substrates-1 and -2 are differentially expressed in prostate cancer. PLoS One. 2012;7(12):e50953. doi:10.1371/journal.pone.0050953.
100. Anwar MA, Kheir WA, Eid S, Fares J, Liu X, Eid AH, Eid AA. Colorectal and prostate cancer risk in diabetes: metformin, an actor behind the scene. J Cancer. 2014;5(9):736–44. doi:10.7150/jca.9726.
101. Bailey CJ, Turner RC. Metformin. N Engl J Med. 1996;334(9):574–9. doi:10.1056/NEJM199602293340906.
102. Wright JL, Stanford JL. Metformin use and prostate cancer in Caucasian men: results from a population-based case-control study. Cancer Causes Control. 2009;20(9):1617–22. doi:10.1007/s10552-009-9407-y.
103. Murtola TJ, Tammela TL, Lahtela J, Auvinen A. Antidiabetic medication and prostate cancer risk: a population-based case-control study. Am J Epidemiol. 2008;168(8):925–31. doi:10.1093/aje/kwn190.
104. Preston MA, Riis AH, Ehrenstein V, Breau RH, Batista JL, Olumi AF, Mucci LA, Adami HO, Sorensen HT. Metformin use and prostate cancer risk. Eur Urol. 2014;66(6):1012–20. doi:10.1016/j.eururo.2014.04.027.
105. Evans JM, Donnelly LA, Emslie-Smith AM, Alessi DR, Morris AD. Metformin and reduced risk of cancer in diabetic patients. BMJ. 2005;330(7503):1304–5. doi:10.1136/bmj.38415.708634.F7.
106. Nordstrom T, Clements M, Karlsson R, Adolfsson J, Gronberg H. The risk of prostate cancer for men on aspirin, statin or antidiabetic medications. Eur J Cancer. 2015;51(6):725–33. doi:10.1016/j.ejca.2015.02.003.

107. Feng T, Sun X, Howard LE, Vidal AC, Gaines AR, Moreira DM, Castro-Santamaria R, Andriole GL, Freedland SJ. Metformin use and risk of prostate cancer: results from the REDUCE study. Cancer Prev Res (Phila). 2015;8(11):1055–60. doi:10.1158/1940-6207.CAPR-15-0141.
108. Azoulay L, Dell'Aniello S, Gagnon B, Pollak M, Suissa S. Metformin and the incidence of prostate cancer in patients with type 2 diabetes. Cancer Epidemiol Biomark Prev. 2011;20(2):337–44. doi:10.1158/1055-9965.EPI-10-0940.
109. Kowall B, Stang A, Rathmann W, Kostev K. No reduced risk of overall, colorectal, lung, breast, and prostate cancer with metformin therapy in diabetic patients: database analyses from Germany and the UK. Pharmacoepidemiol Drug Saf. 2015;24(8):865–74. doi:10.1002/pds.3823.
110. Franciosi M, Lucisano G, Lapice E, Strippoli GF, Pellegrini F, Nicolucci A. Metformin therapy and risk of cancer in patients with type 2 diabetes: systematic review. PLoS One. 2013;8(8):e71583. doi:10.1371/journal.pone.0071583.
111. Zhang P, Li H, Tan X, Chen L, Wang S. Association of metformin use with cancer incidence and mortality: a meta-analysis. Cancer Epidemiol. 2013;37(3):207–18. doi:10.1016/j.canep.2012.12.009.
112. Yu H, Yin L, Jiang X, Sun X, Wu J, Tian H, Gao X, He X. Effect of metformin on cancer risk and treatment outcome of prostate cancer: a meta-analysis of epidemiological observational studies. PLoS One. 2014;9(12):e116327. doi:10.1371/journal.pone.0116327.
113. Stopsack KH, Ziehr DR, Rider JR, Giovannucci EL. Metformin and prostate cancer mortality: a meta-analysis. Cancer Causes Control. 2016;27(1):105–13. doi:10.1007/s10552-015-0687-0.
114. Raval AD, Thakker D, Vyas A, Salkini M, Madhavan S, Sambamoorthi U. Impact of metformin on clinical outcomes among men with prostate cancer: a systematic review and meta-analysis. Prostate Cancer Prostatic Dis. 2015;18(2):110–21. doi:10.1038/pcan.2014.52.
115. Coyle C, Cafferty FH, Vale C, Langley RE. Metformin as an adjuvant treatment for cancer: a systematic review and meta-analysis. Ann Oncol. 2016;27(12):2184–95. doi:10.1093/annonc/mdw410.
116. Deng D, Yang Y, Tang X, Skrip L, Qiu J, Wang Y, Zhang F. Association between metformin therapy and incidence, recurrence and mortality of prostate cancer: evidence from a meta-analysis. Diabetes Metab Res Rev. 2015;31(6):595–602. doi:10.1002/dmrr.2645.
117. Nobes JP, Langley SE, Klopper T, Russell-Jones D, Laing RW. A prospective, randomized pilot study evaluating the effects of metformin and lifestyle intervention on patients with prostate cancer receiving androgen deprivation therapy. BJU Int. 2012;109(10):1495–502. doi:10.1111/j.1464-410X.2011.10555.x.
118. Chen YB, Chen Q, Wang Z, Zhou J. Insulin therapy and risk of prostate cancer: a systematic review and meta-analysis of observational studies. PLoS One. 2013;8(11):e81594. doi:10.1371/journal.pone.0081594.
119. Hsieh MC, Lee TC, Cheng SM, Tu ST, Yen MH, Tseng CH. The influence of type 2 diabetes and glucose-lowering therapies on cancer risk in the Taiwanese. Exp Diabetes Res. 2012;2012:413782. doi:10.1155/2012/413782.
120. Qiu H, Rhoads GG, Berlin JA, Marcella SW, Demissie K. Initial metformin or sulphonylurea exposure and cancer occurrence among patients with type 2 diabetes mellitus. Diabetes Obes Metab. 2013;15(4):349–57. doi:10.1111/dom.12036.
121. Onitilo AA, Stankowski RV, Berg RL, Engel JM, Glurich I, Williams GM, Doi SA. Type 2 diabetes mellitus, glycemic control, and cancer risk. Eur J Cancer Prev. 2014;23(2):134–40. doi:10.1097/CEJ.0b013e3283656394.
122. Hitron A, Adams V, Talbert J, Steinke D. The influence of antidiabetic medications on the development and progression of prostate cancer. Cancer Epidemiol. 2012;36(4):e243–50. doi:10.1016/j.canep.2012.02.005.
123. Haring A, Murtola TJ, Talala K, Taari K, Tammela TL, Auvinen A. Antidiabetic drug use and prostate cancer risk in the Finnish Randomized Study of Screening for Prostate Cancer. Scand J Urol. 2017;51(1):5–12. doi:10.1080/21681805.2016.1271353.

124. Frohlich E, Wahl R. Chemotherapy and chemoprevention by thiazolidinediones. Biomed Res Int. 2015;2015:845340. doi:10.1155/2015/845340.
125. Matsuyama M, Yoshimura R. Peroxisome proliferator-activated receptor-gamma is a potent target for prevention and treatment in human prostate and testicular cancer. PPAR Res. 2008;2008:249849. doi:10.1155/2008/249849.
126. Erdmann E, Harding S, Lam H, Perez A. Ten-year observational follow-up of PROactive: a randomized cardiovascular outcomes trial evaluating pioglitazone in type 2 diabetes. Diabetes Obes Metab. 2016;18(3):266–73. doi:10.1111/dom.12608.
127. Lewis JD, Habel LA, Quesenberry CP, Strom BL, Peng T, Hedderson MM, Ehrlich SF, Mamtani R, Bilker W, Vaughn DJ, Nessel L, Van Den Eeden SK, Ferrara A. Pioglitazone use and risk of bladder cancer and other common cancers in persons with diabetes. JAMA. 2015;314(3):265–77. doi:10.1001/jama.2015.7996.
128. Boxall N, Bennett D, Hunger M, Dolin P, Thompson PL. Evaluation of exposure to pioglitazone and risk of prostate cancer: a nested case-control study. BMJ Open Diabetes Res Care. 2016;4(1):e000303. doi:10.1136/bmjdrc-2016-000303.
129. Kernan WN, Viscoli CM, Furie KL, Young LH, Inzucchi SE, Gorman M, Guarino PD, Lovejoy AM, Peduzzi PN, Conwit R, Brass LM, Schwartz GG, Adams HP Jr, Berger L, Carolei A, Clark W, Coull B, Ford GA, Kleindorfer D, O'Leary JR, Parsons MW, Ringleb P, Sen S, Spence JD, Tanne D, Wang D, Winder TR, Investigators IT. Pioglitazone after ischemic stroke or transient ischemic attack. N Engl J Med. 2016;374(14):1321–31. doi:10.1056/NEJMoa1506930.
130. Platz EA, Clinton SK, Giovannucci E. Association between plasma cholesterol and prostate cancer in the PSA era. Int J Cancer. 2008;123(7):1693–8. doi:10.1002/ijc.23715.
131. Platz EA, Till C, Goodman PJ, Parnes HL, Figg WD, Albanes D, Neuhouser ML, Klein EA, Thompson IM Jr, Kristal AR. Men with low serum cholesterol have a lower risk of high-grade prostate cancer in the placebo arm of the prostate cancer prevention trial. Cancer Epidemiol Biomark Prev. 2009;18(11):2807–13. doi:10.1158/1055-9965.EPI-09-0472.
132. Farwell WR, D'Avolio LW, Scranton RE, Lawler EV, Gaziano JM. Statins and prostate cancer diagnosis and grade in a veterans population. J Natl Cancer Inst. 2011;103(11):885–92. doi:10.1093/jnci/djr108.
133. Shafique K, McLoone P, Qureshi K, Leung H, Hart C, Morrison DS. Cholesterol and the risk of grade-specific prostate cancer incidence: evidence from two large prospective cohort studies with up to 37 years' follow up. BMC Cancer. 2012;12:25. doi:10.1186/1471-2407-12-25.
134. Mondul AM, Clipp SL, Helzlsouer KJ, Platz EA. Association between plasma total cholesterol concentration and incident prostate cancer in the CLUE II cohort. Cancer Causes Control. 2010;21(1):61–8. doi:10.1007/s10552-009-9434-8.
135. Mondul AM, Weinstein SJ, Virtamo J, Albanes D. Serum total and HDL cholesterol and risk of prostate cancer. Cancer Causes Control. 2011;22(11):1545–52. doi:10.1007/s10552-011-9831-7.
136. Kok DE, van Roermund JG, Aben KK, den Heijer M, Swinkels DW, Kampman E, Kiemeney LA. Blood lipid levels and prostate cancer risk; a cohort study. Prostate Cancer Prostatic Dis. 2011;14(4):340–5. doi:10.1038/pcan.2011.30.
137. Iso H, Ikeda A, Inoue M, Sato S, Tsugane S, Group JS. Serum cholesterol levels in relation to the incidence of cancer: the JPHC study cohorts. Int J Cancer. 2009;125(11):2679–86. doi:10.1002/ijc.24668.
138. Eichholzer M, Stahelin HB, Gutzwiller F, Ludin E, Bernasconi F. Association of low plasma cholesterol with mortality for cancer at various sites in men: 17-y follow-up of the prospective Basel study. Am J Clin Nutr. 2000;71(2):569–74.
139. Wallace RB, Rost C, Burmeister LF, Pomrehn PR. Cancer incidence in humans: relationship to plasma lipids and relative weight. J Natl Cancer Inst. 1982;68(6):915–8.
140. Chyou PH, Nomura AM, Stemmermann GN, Kato I. Prospective study of serum cholesterol and site-specific cancers. J Clin Epidemiol. 1992;45(3):287–92.
141. Hiatt RA, Fireman BH. Serum cholesterol and the incidence of cancer in a large cohort. J Chronic Dis. 1986;39(11):861–70.

142. Steenland K, Nowlin S, Palu S. Cancer incidence in the National Health and Nutrition Survey I. Follow-up data: diabetes, cholesterol, pulse and physical activity. Cancer Epidemiol Biomark Prev. 1995;4(8):807–11.
143. Knekt P, Reunanen A, Aromaa A, Heliovaara M, Hakulinen T, Hakama M. Serum cholesterol and risk of cancer in a cohort of 39,000 men and women. J Clin Epidemiol. 1988;41(6):519–30.
144. Morris DL, Borhani NO, Fitzsimons E, Hardy RJ, Hawkins CM, Kraus JF, Labarthe DR, Mastbaum L, Payne GH. Serum cholesterol and cancer in the Hypertension Detection and Follow-up Program. Cancer. 1983;52(9):1754–9.
145. Ahn J, Lim U, Weinstein SJ, Schatzkin A, Hayes RB, Virtamo J, Albanes D. Prediagnostic total and high-density lipoprotein cholesterol and risk of cancer. Cancer Epidemiol Biomark Prev. 2009;18(11):2814–21. doi:10.1158/1055-9965.EPI-08-1248.
146. Kitahara CM, Berrington de Gonzalez A, Freedman ND, Huxley R, Mok Y, Jee SH, Samet JM. Total cholesterol and cancer risk in a large prospective study in Korea. J Clin Oncol. 2011;29(12):1592–8. doi:10.1200/JCO.2010.31.5200.
147. Van Hemelrijck M, Garmo H, Holmberg L, Walldius G, Jungner I, Hammar N, Lambe M. Prostate cancer risk in the Swedish AMORIS study: the interplay among triglycerides, total cholesterol, and glucose. Cancer. 2011;117(10):2086–95. doi:10.1002/cncr.25758.
148. Van Hemelrijck M, Walldius G, Jungner I, Hammar N, Garmo H, Binda E, Hayday A, Lambe M, Holmberg L. Low levels of apolipoprotein A-I and HDL are associated with risk of prostate cancer in the Swedish AMORIS study. Cancer Causes Control. 2011;22(7):1011–9. doi:10.1007/s10552-011-9774-z.
149. Gu Q, Paulose-Ram R, Burt VL, Kit BK. Prescription cholesterol-lowering medication use in adults aged 40 and over: United States, 2003–2012. NCHS Data Brief. 2014;177:1–8.
150. Moon H, Hill MM, Roberts MJ, Gardiner RA, Brown AJ. Statins: protectors or pretenders in prostate cancer? Trends Endocrinol Metab. 2014;25(4):188–96. doi:10.1016/j.tem.2013.12.007.
151. Alfaqih MA, Allott EH, Hamilton RJ, Freeman MR, Freedland SJ. The current evidence on statin use and prostate cancer prevention: are we there yet? Nat Rev Urol. 2017;14(2):107–19. doi:10.1038/nrurol.2016.199.
152. Bansal D, Undela K, D'Cruz S, Schifano F. Statin use and risk of prostate cancer: a meta-analysis of observational studies. PLoS One. 2012;7(10):e46691. doi:10.1371/journal.pone.0046691.
153. Lustman A, Nakar S, Cohen AD, Vinker S. Statin use and incident prostate cancer risk: does the statin brand matter? A population-based cohort study. Prostate Cancer Prostatic Dis. 2014;17(1):6–9. doi:10.1038/pcan.2013.34.
154. Jespersen CG, Norgaard M, Friis S, Skriver C, Borre M. Statin use and risk of prostate cancer: a Danish population-based case-control study, 1997–2010. Cancer Epidemiol. 2014;38(1):42–7. doi:10.1016/j.canep.2013.10.010.
155. Kantor ED, Lipworth L, Fowke JH, Giovannucci EL, Mucci LA, Signorello LB. Statin use and risk of prostate cancer: results from the Southern Community Cohort Study. Prostate. 2015;75(13):1384–93. doi:10.1002/pros.23019.
156. Freedland SJ, Hamilton RJ, Gerber L, Banez LL, Moreira DM, Andriole GL, Rittmaster RS. Statin use and risk of prostate cancer and high-grade prostate cancer: results from the REDUCE study. Prostate Cancer Prostatic Dis. 2013;16(3):254–9. doi:10.1038/pcan.2013.10.
157. Platz EA, Tangen CM, Goodman PJ, Till C, Parnes HL, Figg WD, Albanes D, Neuhouser ML, Klein EA, Lucia MS, Thompson IM Jr, Kristal AR. Statin drug use is not associated with prostate cancer risk in men who are regularly screened. J Urol. 2014;192(2):379–84. doi:10.1016/j.juro.2014.01.095.
158. Chan JM, Litwack-Harrison S, Bauer SR, Daniels NA, Wilt TJ, Shannon J, Bauer DC. Statin use and risk of prostate cancer in the prospective Osteoporotic Fractures in Men (MrOS) Study. Cancer Epidemiol Biomark Prev. 2012;21(10):1886–8. doi:10.1158/1055-9965.EPI-12-0816.
159. Tan P, Wei S, Yang L, Tang Z, Cao D, Liu L, Lei J, Fan Y, Gao L, Wei Q. The effect of statins on prostate cancer recurrence and mortality after definitive therapy: a systematic review and meta-analysis. Sci Rep. 2016;6:29106. doi:10.1038/srep29106.

160. Meng Y, Liao YB, Xu P, Wei WR, Wang J. Statin use and mortality of patients with prostate cancer: a meta-analysis. Onco Targets Ther. 2016;9:1689–96. doi:10.2147/OTT.S97993.
161. Wright JL, Kwon EM, Ostrander EA, Montgomery RB, Lin DW, Vessella R, Stanford JL, Mostaghel EA. Expression of SLCO transport genes in castration-resistant prostate cancer and impact of genetic variation in SLCO1B3 and SLCO2B1 on prostate cancer outcomes. Cancer Epidemiol Biomark Prev. 2011;20(4):619–27. doi:10.1158/1055-9965.EPI-10-1023.
162. Mostaghel E, Nelson PS, Nelson C, Montgomery RB. Intraprostatic steroidogenic enzymes—letter. Cancer Res. 2010;70(20):8247–8249.; author reply 9–50. doi:10.1158/0008-5472.CAN-10-1458.
163. Harshman LC. Mind the gap: what is driving the survival disparity between the sexes in bladder cancer? Cancer. 2016;122(13):1966–70. doi:10.1002/cncr.30027.
164. Harshman LC, Wang X, Nakabayashi M, Xie W, Valenca L, Werner L, Yu Y, Kantoff AM, Sweeney CJ, Mucci LA, Pomerantz M, Lee GS, Kantoff PW. Statin use at the time of initiation of androgen deprivation therapy and time to progression in patients with hormone-sensitive prostate cancer. JAMA Oncol. 2015;1(4):495–504. doi:10.1001/jamaoncol.2015.0829.
165. Boegemann M, Schlack K, Fischer AK, Gerss J, Steinestel J, Semjonow A, Schrader AJ, Krabbe LM. Influence of statins on survival outcome in patients with metastatic castration resistant prostate cancer treated with abiraterone acetate. PLoS One. 2016;11(9):e0161959. doi:10.1371/journal.pone.0161959.
166. Fitzpatrick AL, Daling JR, Furberg CD, Kronmal RA, Weissfeld JL. Hypertension, heart rate, use of antihypertensives, and incident prostate cancer. Ann Epidemiol. 2001;11(8):534–42.
167. Rosenberg L, Rao RS, Palmer JR, Strom BL, Stolley PD, Zauber AG, Warshauer ME, Shapiro S. Calcium channel blockers and the risk of cancer. JAMA. 1998;279(13):1000–4.
168. Lindgren AM, Nissinen AM, Tuomilehto JO, Pukkala E. Cancer pattern among hypertensive patients in North Karelia. Finland J Hum Hypertens. 2005;19(5):373–9. doi:10.1038/sj.jhh.1001834.
169. Friedman GD. Blood pressure and heart rate: no evidence for a positive association with prostate cancer. Ann Epidemiol. 1997;7(7):486–9.
170. Hole DJ, Hawthorne VM, Isles CG, McGhee SM, Robertson JW, Gillis CR, Wapshaw JA,Lever AF. Incidence of and mortality from cancer in hypertensive patients. BMJ. 1993;306(6878):609–11.
171. Batty GD, Shipley MJ, Marmot MG, Davey Smith G, Whitehall S. Blood pressure and site-specific cancer mortality: evidence from the original Whitehall study. Br J Cancer. 2003;89(7):1243–7. doi:10.1038/sj.bjc.6601255.
172. Martin RM, Vatten L, Gunnell D, Romundstad P. Blood pressure and risk of prostate cancer: Cohort Norway (CONOR). Cancer Causes Control. 2010;21(3):463–72. doi:10.1007/s10552-009-9477-x.
173. Pai PY, Hsieh VC, Wang CB, Wu HC, Liang WM, Chang YJ, Wu TN. Long term antihypertensive drug use and prostate cancer risk: a 9-year population-based cohort analysis. Int J Cardiol. 2015;193:1–7. doi:10.1016/j.ijcard.2015.05.042.
174. Stocks T, Hergens MP, Englund A, Ye W, Stattin P. Blood pressure, body size and prostate cancer risk in the Swedish Construction Workers cohort. Int J Cancer. 2010;127(7):1660–8. doi:10.1002/ijc.25171.
175. Palm D, Lang K, Niggemann B, Drell TL, Masur K, Zaenker KS, Entschladen F. The norepinephrine-driven metastasis development of PC-3 human prostate cancer cells in BALB/c nude mice is inhibited by beta-blockers. Int J Cancer. 2006;118(11):2744–9. doi:10.1002/ijc.21723.
176. Ronquist G, Rodriguez LA, Ruigomez A, Johansson S, Wallander MA, Frithz G, Svardsudd K. Association between captopril, other antihypertensive drugs and risk of prostate cancer. Prostate. 2004;58(1):50–6. doi:10.1002/pros.10294.
177. Rodriguez C, Jacobs EJ, Deka A, Patel AV, Bain EB, Thun MJ, Calle EE. Use of blood-pressure-lowering medication and risk of prostate cancer in the Cancer Prevention Study II Nutrition Cohort. Cancer Causes Control. 2009;20(5):671–9. doi:10.1007/s10552-008-9280-0.

178. Friis S, Sorensen HT, Mellemkjaer L, McLaughlin JK, Nielsen GL, Blot WJ, Olsen JH. Angiotensin-converting enzyme inhibitors and the risk of cancer: a population-based cohort study in Denmark. Cancer. 2001;92(9):2462–70.
179. Lindholm LH, Anderson H, Ekbom T, Hansson L, Lanke J, Dahlof B, de Faire U, Forsen K, Hedner T, Linjer E, Schersten B, Wester P, Moller T. Relation between drug treatment and cancer in hypertensives in the Swedish Trial in Old Patients with Hypertension 2: a 5-year, prospective, randomised, controlled trial. Lancet. 2001;358(9281):539–44.
180. Perron L, Bairati I, Harel F, Meyer F. Antihypertensive drug use and the risk of prostate cancer (Canada). Cancer Causes Control. 2004;15(6):535–41. doi:10.1023/B:CACO.0000036152.58271.5e.
181. Lever AF, Hole DJ, Gillis CR, McCallum IR, McInnes GT, MacKinnon PL, Meredith PA, Murray LS, Reid JL, Robertson JW. Do inhibitors of angiotensin-I-converting enzyme protect against risk of cancer? Lancet. 1998;352(9123):179–84. doi:10.1016/S0140-6736(98)03228-0.
182. Morote J, Planas J. Antihypertensive drugs and the risk of prostate cancer. Eur Urol. 2011;60(6):1309–10. doi:10.1016/j.eururo.2011.09.009.
183. Vezina RM, Lesko SM, Rosenberg L, Shapiro S. Calcium channel blocker use and the risk of prostate cancer. Am J Hypertens. 1998;11(12):1420–5.
184. Kemppainen KJ, Tammela TL, Auvinen A, Murtola TJ. The association between antihypertensive drug use and incidence of prostate cancer in Finland: a population-based case-control study. Cancer Causes Control. 2011;22(10):1445–52. doi:10.1007/s10552-011-9819-3.
185. Yoon C, Yang HS, Jeon I, Chang Y, Park SM. Use of angiotensin-converting-enzyme inhibitors or angiotensin-receptor blockers and cancer risk: a meta-analysis of observational studies. CMAJ. 2011;183(14):E1073–84. doi:10.1503/cmaj.101497.
186. Sipahi I, Debanne SM, Rowland DY, Simon DI, Fang JC. Angiotensin-receptor blockade and risk of cancer: meta-analysis of randomised controlled trials. Lancet Oncol. 2010;11(7):627–36. doi:10.1016/S1470-2045(10)70106-6.
187. Collaboration ARBT. Effects of telmisartan, irbesartan, valsartan, candesartan, and losartan on cancers in 15 trials enrolling 138,769 individuals. J Hypertens. 2011;29(4):623–35. doi:10.1097/HJH.0b013e328344a7de.
188. Pahor M, Guralnik JM, Ferrucci L, Corti MC, Salive ME, Cerhan JR, Wallace RB, Havlik RJ. Calcium-channel blockade and incidence of cancer in aged populations. Lancet. 1996;348(9026):493–7. doi:10.1016/S0140-6736(96)04277-8.
189. Jick H, Jick S, Derby LE, Vasilakis C, Myers MW, Meier CR. Calcium-channel blockers and risk of cancer. Lancet. 1997;349(9051):525–8. doi:10.1016/S0140-6736(97)80084-0.
190. Sorensen HT, Olsen JH, Mellemkjaer L, Marie A, Steffensen FH, McLaughlin JK, Baron JA. Cancer risk and mortality in users of calcium channel blockers. A cohort study. Cancer. 2000;89(1):165–70.
191. Debes JD, Roberts RO, Jacobson DJ, Girman CJ, Lieber MM, Tindall DJ, Jacobsen SJ. Inverse association between prostate cancer and the use of calcium channel blockers. Cancer Epidemiol Biomark Prev. 2004;13(2):255–9.
192. Thomas JA 2nd, Gerber L, Banez LL, Moreira DM, Rittmaster RS, Andriole GL, Freedland SJ. Prostate cancer risk in men with baseline history of coronary artery disease: results from the REDUCE Study. Cancer Epidemiol Biomark Prev. 2012;21(4):576–81. doi:10.1158/1055-9965.EPI-11-1017.
193. Lin H, Juang JL, Wang PS. Involvement of Cdk5/p25 in digoxin-triggered prostate cancer cell apoptosis. J Biol Chem. 2004;279(28):29302–7. doi:10.1074/jbc.M403664200.
194. Stoffer SS, Hynes KM, Jiang NS, Ryan RJ. Digoxin and abnormal serum hormone levels. JAMA. 1973;225(13):1643–4.
195. Newman RA, Yang P, Pawlus AD, Block KI. Cardiac glycosides as novel cancer therapeutic agents. Mol Interv. 2008;8(1):36–49. doi:10.1124/mi.8.1.8.
196. McConkey DJ, Lin Y, Nutt LK, Ozel HZ, Newman RA. Cardiac glycosides stimulate Ca^{2+} increases and apoptosis in androgen-independent, metastatic human prostate adenocarcinoma cells. Cancer Res. 2000;60(14):3807–12.

197. Yeh JY, Huang WJ, Kan SF, Wang PS. Inhibitory effects of digitalis on the proliferation of androgen dependent and independent prostate cancer cells. J Urol. 2001;166(5):1937–42.
198. Zhang H, Qian DZ, Tan YS, Lee K, Gao P, Ren YR, Rey S, Hammers H, Chang D, Pili R, Dang CV, Liu JO, Semenza GL. Digoxin and other cardiac glycosides inhibit HIF-1alpha synthesis and block tumor growth. Proc Natl Acad Sci USA. 2008;105(50):19579–86. doi:10.1073/pnas.0809763105.
199. Platz EA, Yegnasubramanian S, Liu JO, Chong CR, Shim JS, Kenfield SA, Stampfer MJ, Willett WC, Giovannucci E, Nelson WG. A novel two-stage, transdisciplinary study identifies digoxin as a possible drug for prostate cancer treatment. Cancer Discov. 2011;1(1):68–77. doi:10.1158/2159-8274.CD-10-0020.
200. Wright JL, Hansten PD, Stanford JL. Is digoxin use for cardiovascular disease associated with risk of prostate cancer? Prostate. 2014;74(1):97–102. doi:10.1002/pros.22733.
201. Kaapu KJ, Murtola TJ, Maattanen L, Talala K, Taari K, Tammela TL,Auvinen A. Prostate cancer risk among users of digoxin and other antiarrhythmic drugs in the Finnish Prostate Cancer Screening Trial. Cancer Causes Control. 2016;27(2):157–64. doi:10.1007/s10552-015-0693-2.
202. Karasneh RA, Murray LJ, Hughes CM, Cardwell CR. Digoxin use after diagnosis of prostate cancer and survival: a population-based cohort study. Pharmacoepidemiol Drug Saf. 2016;25(9):1099–103. doi:10.1002/pds.4018.
203. Flahavan EM, Sharp L, Bennett K, Barron TI. A cohort study of digoxin exposure and mortality in men with prostate cancer. BJU Int. 2014;113(2):236–45. doi:10.1111/bju.12287.
204. Kaapu KJ, Ahti J, Tammela TL, Auvinen A, Murtola TJ. Sotalol, but not digoxin is associated with decreased prostate cancer risk: a population-based case-control study. Int J Cancer. 2015;137(5):1187–95. doi:10.1002/ijc.29470.
205. Hayden M, Pignone M, Phillips C, Mulrow C. Aspirin for the primary prevention of cardiovascular events: a summary of the evidence for the U.S. Preventive Services Task Force. Ann Intern Med. 2002;136(2):161–72.
206. Hsu AL, Ching TT, Wang DS, Song X, Rangnekar VM, Chen CS. The cyclooxygenase-2 inhibitor celecoxib induces apoptosis by blocking Akt activation in human prostate cancer cells independently of Bcl-2. J Biol Chem. 2000;275(15):11397–403.
207. Kirschenbaum A, Liu X, Yao S, Levine AC. The role of cyclooxygenase-2 in prostate cancer. Urology. 2001;58(2 Suppl 1):127–31.
208. Liu Y, Chen JQ, Xie L, Wang J, Li T, He Y, Gao Y, Qin X, Li S. Effect of aspirin and other non-steroidal anti-inflammatory drugs on prostate cancer incidence and mortality: a systematic review and meta-analysis. BMC Med. 2014;12:55. doi:10.1186/1741-7015-12-55.
209. Wright JL, Chery L, Holt S, Lin DW, Luedeke M, Rinckleb AE, Maier C, Stanford JL. Aspirin and NSAID use in association with molecular subtypes of prostate cancer defined by TMPRSS2:ERG fusion status. Prostate Cancer Prostatic Dis. 2016;19(1):53–6. doi:10.1038/pcan.2015.49.
210. Pierce BL, Plymate S, Ostrander EA, Stanford JL. Diabetes mellitus and prostate cancer risk. Prostate. 2008;68(10):1126–32. doi:10.1002/pros.20777.
211. Fukui M, Tanaka M, Kadono M, Imai S, Hasegawa G, Yoshikawa T, Nakamura N. Serum prostate-specific antigen levels in men with type 2 diabetes. Diabetes Care. 2008;31(5):930–1. doi:10.2337/dc07-1962.
212. Muller H, Raum E, Rothenbacher D, Stegmaier C, Brenner H. Association of diabetes and body mass index with levels of prostate-specific antigen: implications for correction of prostate-specific antigen cutoff values? Cancer Epidemiol Biomark Prev. 2009;18(5):1350–6. doi:10.1158/1055-9965.EPI-08-0794.
213. Werny DM, Saraiya M, Gregg EW. Prostate-specific antigen values in diabetic and nondiabetic US men, 2001–2002. Am J Epidemiol. 2006;164(10):978–83. doi:10.1093/aje/kwj311.
214. Fowke JH, Motley SS, Cookson MS, Concepcion R, Chang SS, Wills ML, Smith JA Jr. The association between body size, prostate volume and prostate-specific antigen. Prostate Cancer Prostatic Dis. 2007;10(2):137–42. doi:10.1038/sj.pcan.4500924.

215. Jayalath VH, Ireland C, Fleshner NE, Hamilton RJ, Jenkins DJ. The relationship between metformin and serum prostate-specific antigen levels. Prostate. 2016;76(15):1445–53. doi:10.1002/pros.23228.
216. Werny DM, Thompson T, Saraiya M, Freedman D, Kottiri BJ, German RR, Wener M. Obesity is negatively associated with prostate-specific antigen in U.S. men, 2001–2004. Cancer Epidemiol Biomark Prev. 2007;16(1):70–6. doi:10.1158/1055-9965.EPI-06-0588.
217. Banez LL, Hamilton RJ, Partin AW, Vollmer RT, Sun L, Rodriguez C, Wang Y, Terris MK, Aronson WJ, Presti JC Jr, Kane CJ, Amling CL, Moul JW, Freedland SJ. Obesity-related plasma hemodilution and PSA concentration among men with prostate cancer. JAMA. 2007;298(19):2275–80. doi:10.1001/jama.298.19.2275.
218. Culp S, Porter M. The effect of obesity and lower serum prostate-specific antigen levels on prostate-cancer screening results in American men. BJU Int. 2009;104(10):1457–61. doi:10.1111/j.1464-410X.2009.08646.x.
219. Hekal IA, Ibrahiem EI. Obesity-PSA relationship: a new formula. Prostate Cancer Prostatic Dis. 2010;13(2):186–90. doi:10.1038/pcan.2009.53.
220. Hamilton RJ, Goldberg KC, Platz EA, Freedland SJ. The influence of statin medications on prostate-specific antigen levels. J Natl Cancer Inst. 2008;100(21):1511–8. doi:10.1093/jnci/djn362.
221. Wright JL, Lin DW, Stanford JL. The effect of demographic and clinical factors on the relationship between BMI and PSA levels. Prostate. 2011;71(15):1631–7. doi:10.1002/pros.21380.
222. Andriole GL, Bostwick DG, Brawley OW, Gomella LG, Marberger M, Montorsi F, Pettaway CA, Tammela TL, Teloken C, Tindall DJ, Somerville MC, Wilson TH, Fowler IL, Rittmaster RS, Group RS. Effect of dutasteride on the risk of prostate cancer. N Engl J Med. 2010;362(13):1192–202. doi:10.1056/NEJMoa0908127.

Chapter 4
Adipokines and Prostate Cancer

Cheryl L. Thompson and MacKenzie Reece

Abstract Adipokines (adipocytokines) have been suggested to play a role in the well-established association of obesity and prostate cancer. Adipokines are secreted by adipose tissue and dysregulated in obese individuals. Given their association with multiple pathways, it has been hypothesized that adipokines mediate the association between obesity and prostate cancer risk and aggressiveness. Mechanistic studies have provided good evidence of the role of leptin in prostate cancer cellular proliferation. In clinical studies, circulating levels of many adipokines have been associated with risk of prostate cancer, however many of these have been met with mixed results or suffered from small sample sizes, so there remains significant opportunities for more research in the area. In contrast, there has been evidence that inherited genetic variation in adipokines and their receptors may increase prostate cancer risk, with strong evidence particularly for *LEP* and *TNFa*. However, more studies in this area are needed as well. Although there is room for more research to understand the role of adipokines in clinical prostate cancer management, it is reasonable to hypothesize that adipokines can help manage the association between obesity and prostate cancer. With growing rates of obesity, in turn the impact of adipokines on prostate cancer risk and progression will increase. Thus, understanding adipokines in relation to prostate cancer may provide therapeutic and preventative measures to reduce the risk and progression of prostate cancer.

Keywords Adipokines • Prostate cancer • Leptin • Adiponectin • IL-6 • VEGF • TNF-α

C.L. Thompson (✉)
Department of Nutrition, Case Western Reserve University,
10900 Euclid Avenue, Cleveland, OH 44106-4971, USA
e-mail: Cheryl.l.thompson@case.edu

M. Reece
Department of Anatomy, Case Western Reserve University,
10900 Euclid Avenue, Cleveland, OH 44106, USA
e-mail: mjr192@case.edu

© Springer International Publishing AG 2018

E.A. Platz, N.A. Berger (eds.), *Energy Balance and Prostate Cancer*, Energy Balance and Cancer 14, DOI 10.1007/978-3-319-64940-5_4

Introduction

As outlined in previous chapters, the association of obesity with prostate cancer has been an active area of research over the past few decades. More and more evidence suggests that obesity plays a role in not only risk of prostate cancer [1], but prostate cancer aggressiveness [2, 3], as well as outcomes among prostate cancer patients [4]. With growing rates of obesity both in the United States and worldwide, it is important to understand the underlying biology of this association to minimize the impact of obesity on prostate cancer outcomes.

Adipokines are one of the mechanisms suggested to play a role in the association of prostate cancer and obesity [5]. Adipokines, sometimes referred to as adipocytokines, are signaling proteins secreted by adipose tissue. As expected, higher levels of adipokines are found in overweight and obese individuals. The signaling of adipokines alters multiple biological processes, and thus their actions have led many to hypothesize their role as mediators of the association between obesity and prostate cancer.

The goal of this chapter is to review the literature surrounding the association of adipokines and prostate cancer, from risk of prostate cancer to prostate cancer recurrence and survival, from both basic science and epidemiological perspectives. Although there are many adipokines that are dysregulated in obesity and insulin resistance [6, 7], and at least 15 associated with cancer [8], for the purposes of this chapter, we will study the ones more well researched with respect to cancer, particularly IL-6, TNF-α, VEGF, leptin and adiponectin (Fig. 4.1).

Adipokines and Obesity

Although previously thought to simply store excess energy, adipose tissue is now widely recognized to be an endocrine organ that secretes a number of signaling cytokines. These are collectively referred to as adipokines. Emerging research suggests that these signaling molecules play an important role in a number of biological

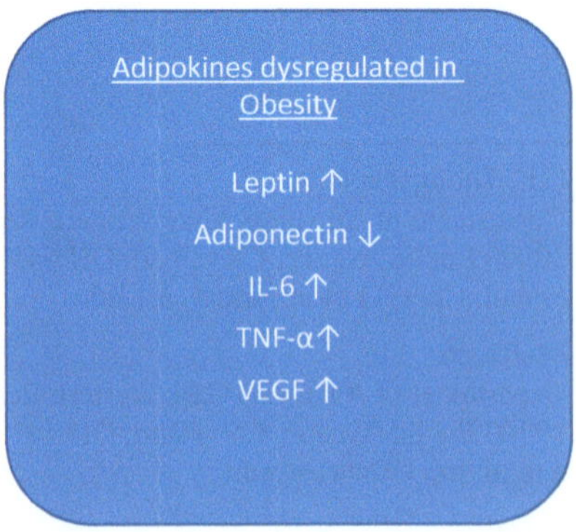

Fig. 4.1 Select adipokines in obesity

processes, and thus their function is hypothesized to mediate a number of the processes associated with energy dysregulation. Further, adipokines circulate throughout the body. Consequently their role is not limited to adipose tissue. Interestingly, particularly with respect to prostate cancer, adipokines are also important in hormonal regulation [8].

Adipokines also have a known role in inflammation, one of the key biological processes underlying the six hallmarks of cancer [9], through both paracrine and endocrine action. Many adipokines have been shown to be involved in inflammation [10], and emerging evidence suggests that obese individuals are in a constant low-grade inflammatory state, and the adipokines released by the adipose tissue have both pro-inflammatory and anti-inflammatory properties [11]. In obesity, the pro-inflammatory properties take over, resulting in this inflammatory state. In fact, obese individuals have higher levels of C-reactive protein (CRP) and IL-6 [12]. It is interesting to note the strong interaction between adipocytes and adipokines with immune-inflammatory cells. For example, it is now known that macrophages are present in adipose tissue, with increased numbers in obesity [12].

The role of individual adipokines in inflammation and immune response have also been studied. Leptin has been shown to regulate T-cell activation, as well as to protect T cells from apoptosis [13]. In mouse studies, leptin deficiency is associated with lower levels of inflammation and reduced immune responses [13]. Adiponectin inhibits IL-6 production in macrophages [14], and promotes the activation of I-L10 and IL-1RA [15]. Thus, there is a clear connection between adipokines and inflammation.

The association of insulin resistance and adipokines is also well established. Adiponectin regulates insulin sensitivity and is lower in individuals with type 2 diabetes [16], which is also related to inflammation. Indeed, the close interaction between obesity and insulin resistance with inflammation and immune response appears to be strongly driven by adipokines [17–20]. Indeed, this relationship may be key to the underlying relationship between adipokine and prostate cancer.

Adipokines and Risk of Prostate Cancer

Leptin

Although secreted by other tissues as well, leptin is secreted primarily by adipose tissue and controls signaling to the brain associated with hunger. The classic example of the role of leptin is the *ob/ob* mouse, with mutations in the leptin gene resulting in lack of leptin production. These mice are always hungry and suffer from extreme obesity. Low levels of leptin are meant to trigger hunger to save depleting fat store. With higher circulating levels of leptin, you feel more satiated. Leptin has been shown to be correlated with body fat and is thus higher in obese individuals [21]. However, in obesity, there is a decreased sensitivity to leptin, and thus obese individuals need more leptin to feel full, often referred to as "leptin resistance" [22].

Studies have shown increases in proliferation in androgen-dependent prostate cancer cell lines when treated with leptin [23]. Somasundar et al. showed data from two prostate cancer cells lines that illustrated the increase in proliferation upon exposure to leptin, via suppression of apoptosis. In additional studies, the same group provides further data suggesting that this association is due to activation of *PI3K* and/or *MAPK* pathways [24].

In addition to these mechanistic studies, epidemiological studies have suggested that higher circulating leptin levels are associated with increased prostate cancer risk [25, 26], with higher leptin levels being associated with up to 2.6 times the risk. However, the results have been inconsistent [27, 28], and quintile analyses do not show a convincing trend [26]. It will be important for further work to be done in this area, particularly in larger samples, to clarify this association and help understand the role of leptin in prostate cancer carcinogenesis.

In addition to circulating levels of leptin, individual variations in the Leptin (*LEP*) and Leptin receptor (*LEPR*) genes have been associated with prostate cancer risk. A recent meta-analysis of the G2548A polymorphism in *LEP* found that this variant was statistically significantly associated with both risk of prostate cancer (OR 1.26, 95% CI 1.05–1.51 under a recessive model) as well as overall cancer risk (1.19, 95% CI 1.00–1.41 under a recessive model) [29]. Other variations in both the *LEP* and *LEPR* genes have been suggested to be associated with prostate cancer risk, but recent meta-analyses have suggested an overall lack of sufficient evidence at this time [29, 30].

Adiponectin

Adiponectin is a major adipokine that, in contrast to other adipokines, is down-regulated in obese individuals [31]. It is also down-regulated in type 2 diabetes [31], and mice with a knockout of the adiponectin gene have significant insulin resistance [32]. Adiponectin acts with respect to metabolic conditions through a couple of mechanisms. High levels of adiponectin both increase fatty acid oxidation and inhibit glucose production in the liver [33].

A variety of molecular studies have shown the effect of adiponectin on prostate cancer. Bub et al. demonstrated that certain forms of adiponectin can inhibit growth of prostate cancer cells [34]. Interestingly, they also showed that adiponectin suppresses leptin and insulin-like growth factor-1 (IGF1), both of which increase growth of prostate cancer cells [34]. Other groups have noted the increase in motility of prostate cancer cell lines when treated with adiponectin [35], which was mediated through the upregulation of the *NF-κB, p38* and *AMPK* pathways. Still others have implicated the *AKT/mTOR* pathway in the relationship between adiponectin and prostate cancer [36].

In a small epidemiological study, circulating levels of adiponectin were inversely associated with prostate cancer risk [37]. Although circulating adiponectin levels were similarly correlated in a number of other cancers [38], others have found no association [28], and, given the limited data, much more work will need to be done to understand the association of circulating adiponectin with risk of prostate cancer, particularly in studies with larger sample sizes.

Genetic epidemiological studies have suggested that genetic variation in the adiponectin gene (*ADIPOQ*) and the two receptors of adiponectin (*ADIPOR1* and *ADIPOR2*) are associated with risk of prostate cancer. In a nested case-control study from the Physicians' Health Study, four of the twelve single nucleotide polymorphisms (SNPs) in *ADIPOQ* were associated with risk of prostate cancer, of which two (rs266729 and rs182052) and were also associated with circulating levels of adiponectin [39]. In another study, Kaklamani et al. found that haplotypes in *ADIPOQ* and *ADIPOR1* were associated with prostate cancer risk [40]. A third study noted the association with some of these same SNPs with prostate cancer in Chinese Han men [41]. However, in a study of African Americans, no SNPs in these three genes were associated with risk of prostate cancer [42], although it is important to note that this study included only 131 prostate cancer cases and 344 controls and did not include most of the previously associated SNPs. Further studies will need to be done to assess population differences in these associations and help explain these findings.

Although there is clearly evidence of the association of adiponectin with prostate cancer, it's important to note that, as studies have demonstrated, it is not a one-to-one association. Adiponectin has a complex relationship with other reproductive hormones and adipokines [43], many of which may interact to influence risk of prostate cancer. For example, it has been shown that leptin and adiponectin interact to regulate prostate cancer cell growth [44], which evidence further suggests that this cell growth is through targeting of *p53* and *BCL-2* [44].

TNF-α

Tumor Necrosis Factor-alpha (TNF-α) is an inflammatory adipokine secreted from activated monocytes, macrophages, neutrophils, T cells, and NK cells. It also has a well-established association with obesity and insulin resistance, and obese individuals have about 2.5 times the expression of TNF-α in their adipose tissue compared to non-obese individuals [45]. TNF- α is generally accepted to contribute the low grade inflammation observed in obesity due to the infiltration of macrophages [46].

TNF-α mechanistically has been shown to factor in increasing prostate cancer tumorigenesis by promoting inflammation and angiogenesis, while at the same time it has been shown to inhibit growth and induce apoptosis [47], a well-established paradoxical role observed in a number of cancers [48]. This dual role of TNF-α in prostate cancer may be due to the context in which TNF-α is studied [47, 49], and studies have even found different effects in different cell lines. For example, one study found that PC3 prostate cancer cells were resistant to TNF-α-induced apoptosis whereas LNCaP cells were not [50]. They further found that the resistance of the pro-apoptotic pathway in PC3 cells was mediated by NF-kB survival pathway, while the cells that were sensitive (LNCap) to TNF-α did not induce phosphorylation and resulting in apoptosis [50].

In a very small, early clinical study, serum TNF-α was not found to differ between metastatic prostate cancer patients and healthy controls [51]. However, due to the very small sample size, it would be important to investigate this association further.

The *TNFa* gene has been mapped to the major histocompatibility complex III (MHC III) region on chromosome 6p21.3 [52]. Previous studies have shown polymorphisms at the promoter region lead to an increased constitutive and inducible expression of TNF-α in comparison of polymorphic mutants at the TNF-α promoter region to the wild type [53]. Recently, there have been several studies suggesting that multiple SNPs within the gene itself or the promoter region of *TNFa*, including *TNFa* -308G/A and *TNFa* -238C/T [52] are associated with prostate cancer risk. A recent meta-analysis of 14 studies of the *TNFa* 308 G/A polymorphism (5757 patients and 6137 control subjects) and the *TNFa* -238 G/A polymorphism (1967 patients and 2004 control subjects) was conducted [54]. Results suggested that the *TNFa* -238G/A is not associated with risk of prostate cancer , but the *TNFa* -308G/A polymorphism had a significant association with prostate cancer risk [54]. They noted that individuals with one or more A variants in this SNP were about 50% more likely to develop prostate cancer [54].

VEGF

Vascular endothelial growth factor (VEGF), which was previously known as vascular permeability factor (VPF), is a signaling protein that is secreted to stimulate angiogenesis, increase microvascular permeability and endothelial cell growth, proliferation, migration, and differentiation in order to create new blood vessels during embryonic development, injury or repair of tissues, and hypoxic conditions with an increase in transcription factor hypoxia-inducible factor-1 and mRNA stability factors for VEGF [55]. In cancer, VEGF plays an important role in tumor neovascularization as well as tumor proliferation [55].

Many studies have looked at VEGF in serum as a biomarker for prostate cancer. In one study of 44 patients with prostate cancer, 57 with benign disease and 57 controls, they found that VEGF levels were substantially higher among prostate cancer patients, and correlated with PSA levels [56]. However, a more recent review suggested that overall there does not seem to be a good level of evidence suggesting circulating VEGF can distinguish between prostate cancer patients and controls [57].

A number of studies have also investigated the association between inherited variations in *VEGF* with risk of prostate cancer. One study looked at five polymorphisms in *VEGF* (rs833061, rs3025039, rs2010963, 1154G/A, and 2578C/A) in 702 men with prostate cancer and 702 controls, and found none were associated with prostate cancer risk [58]. In another study evaluating single gene and joint effects of genetic variants on prostate cancer risk in a case-control study that comprised of 193 African-American men with prostate cancer and 666 African-American controls, they found although no single variant was associated with overall prostate cancer risk, *VEGF* 2482T combined with *VEGFR* (the *VEGF* receptor) IVS6 + 54 loci were associated with risk of prostate cancer [59].

IL-6

Interleukin-6 (IL-6) is an inflammatory cytokine that is secreted by adipocytes, as well as visceral tissue such as prostate cancer and prostate stromal cells. IL-6 is responsible for acute inflammation, regulation of B and T-cells, as well as cell growth and viability [60]. The release of IL-6 can be stimulated by multiple factors including infectious agents, epithelial cell injury, urine reflux, systemic diseases, and diet [60]. The most common signaling of IL-6 involves the release of STAT-3 proteins. This release in turn induces transcription of growth factors and cytokines that have been associated with inflammation-related cancer [60]. Since it is known that IL-6 is secreted from adipocytes, and the concentration of IL-6 is directly proportional to obesity and insulin resistance, it is hypothesized that IL-6 is the mediator between obesity and an increased risk of prostate cancer [5]. Some research has shown that IL-6 secretion in high concentrations may lead to increased risk of prostate cancer, with a possible link between obesity, but the major signaling pathways involved in IL-6 and prostate cancer must be studied further. However, it is important to note that it is unlikely that there is a single mechanism for the IL-6 pathway in regards to prostate cancer, as other studies have shown that other proteins are likely involved as well [5].

IL-6 is of particular interest to prostate cancer because it has been noted that patients with untreated metastatic or castration-resistant prostate cancer have higher levels in comparison to healthy patients [61]. In a previous in-vitro study using the prostate cancer cell line LNCaP, long-term treatment with IL-6 at high concentrations (5 ng/ml) resulted in a higher basal cell proliferation rate than LNCaP cells without IL-6 added [62]. The cellular response in the LNCaP prostate cancer cells with IL-6 added lead to a reduction of an inhibitory growth response [62]. Thus, this could represent a mechanism for the carcinogenesis of prostate cells through the transition of IL-6 as a growth inhibitor to a growth stimulator.

Clinical studies of IL-6 in prostate cancer have shown elevation of circulating IL-6 among prostate cancer patients when compared to healthy men, or men with benign prostatic disease [63]. Another study of 80 prostate cancer patients found an association between extent of disease, including tumor burden and circulating IL-6 [64]. However, not all studies have come to the same conclusion [28, 65], and more research should be done to understand this association.

A recent analysis of multiple polymorphisms in *IL6* found that the less common allele of rs10499563 was associated with an increased prostate cancer risk in a Chinese population [66]. In another very recent study, which also utilized a Chinese population, the rs1800796 SNP (-572G/C) was found to confer a 30% increased risk of prostate cancer, with stronger effect among non-smoking individuals [67]. However, other studies have not found associations [65]. Overall, the genetic epidemiology of the *IL6* gene and prostate cancer risk has not been fully studied.

Adipokines in Prostate Cancer Aggressiveness

Prostate cancer is often a very indolent, slow-growing disease, and active surveillance (regular surveillance for disease progression without active treatment) is a common treatment plan for many patients. However, some patients develop aggressive forms of prostate cancer which ultimately leads to metastasis and mortality. Because of this, understanding the biology of prostate cancer aggressiveness is very important. Obesity is not only associated with overall risk of prostate cancer, but it seems to be associated more strongly with aggressive disease [68]. Thus adipokines as they relate to prostate cancer aggressiveness are of interest to many investigators.

Leptin

A number of studies have suggested leptin could pay a role in the link between obesity and aggressiveness of prostate cancer. In a study utilizing the DU145 and PC-3 androgen-resistant cell lines, Hoda et al. observed a dose-dependent effect of leptin on proliferation [69]. This same group followed this up and suggested that leptin may act through *PI3K/Akt* signaling to phosphorylate FOXO1 resulting in inactivation [70]. Another group provided evidence that suggests that there is a complex interaction of insulin and leptin, whereas although leptin generally inhibits prostate cancer growth, insulin prevents leptin from this action in RM1 cells [71]. In an interesting study investigating the adipocyte "secretome", Moreira et al. investigate the association of leptin and insulin on proliferation of androgen independent prostate cancer cells. However, they observed no effect of leptin on cell proliferation rates [72].

In a clinical study of prostate cancer patients, higher levels of circulating leptin was observed among patients with higher Gleason scores as well as more advanced disease [25]. However, others have not observed similar associations [73].

Adiponectin

In a recent study of 311 men with advanced prostate cancer and 413 men with localized prostate cancer in the United Kingdom, Burton et al. showed that circulating adiponectin was inversely associated with prostate cancer stage, but only among overweight and obese men [73]. This confirmed earlier reports [37, 74] and provides increasing evidence of the association between plasma adiponectin and prostate cancer stage, although the evidence for an association with Gleason score is still somewhat debated [37, 73–75]. Another recent study sought to investigate the association of plasma adiponectin in risk of aggressive prostate cancer and found no association [76].

Although the evidence for the association between inherited genetic variants in adiponectin and its receptors with prostate cancer risk is strong, there is less evidence of their association with Gleason score or tumor stage [39]. However, this area has not had much research done and more studies will need to be completed before we can draw definitive conclusions.

VEGF and IL-6

In a study of hypoxia-induced aggressiveness of prostate cancer cells, Bao et al. found that the aggressiveness is associated with increased expression of both VEGF and IL-6, and that this pathway could also contribute to the epithelial-to-mesenchymal transition in these cells [77].

Very few clinical or epidemiological studies have investigated the role of VEGF or IL-6 with prostate cancer aggressiveness. One exception was a study of African-American prostate cancer patients and controls, where they found that carriers of the *VEGF* -2482T allele had a threefold increase in the risk of developing a more aggressive of prostate cancer [59]. More will need to be done to investigate the clinical utility of both circulating VEGF and IL-6 as well as polymorphisms within these genes or their receptors with respect to prostate cancer aggressiveness.

Adipokines and Prostate Cancer Outcomes

Leptin

Although no study to date has investigated the association of circulating leptin with prostate cancer recurrence or survival, genetic studies have provided data suggesting a role of leptin in prostate cancer outcomes. A recent study identified a SNP in *LEPR*, along with four other SNPs in other genes, which were associated with prostate cancer-specific mortality [78]. Much more work needs to be done in the area of genetic association of *LEP* and *LEPR* with prostate cancer progression and/or mortality, as well as in the area of the association of circulating or tumor levels of leptin with outcomes.

Adiponectin

Circulating levels of adiponectin have been associated with prostate cancer mortality. In reviewing data from the Physician's Health Study, pre-diagnostic plasma adiponectin was associated with both less aggressive cancer and lower prostate cancer mortality [79], and this result was limited to obese men, similar to the Burton et al study, which found the association of adiponectin with prostate cancer aggressiveness to be only in obese men [73].

Although the research on genetic variation in *ADIPOQ*, *ADIPOR1* and *ADIPOR2* with outcomes in prostate cancer has been largely unexplored, there has been one exception. In a study of three variants in *ADIPOQ* and biochemical recurrence among prostate cancer patients receiving a radical prostatectomy, Gu et al. noted that variants of the rs182052 SNP were statistically significantly associated with recurrence [80]. Future studies will be needed to confirm as well as to identify other SNPs in these genes that might not have been captured in this single study.

TNF-α

Clinical studies of prostate cancer patients have shown that TNF-α levels were associated with tumor burden in a study of 80 prostate cancer patients, and elevated in patients with metastatic disease [64]. This same study showed that individual rises in serum TNF-α were associated with progression [64], however other studies have not shown an association [51]. To our knowledge, however, no study has looked at either circulating levels of TNF-α or genetic variations in TNF-α as predictors of prostate cancer survival, recurrence or progression.

VEGF

Many prognostic clinical features have been associated with VEGF. Plasma VEGF concentrations have been shown to be highest among patients with metastatic disease, which is not surprising given the well-established role of VEGF in neovascularization [81]. Others have studied the expression of VEGF in the prostate tumor and found it to be associated with Gleason score and/or biochemical failure [82, 83]. VEGF also seems to play a critical role in metastasis, particularly to the bone [84].

The predictive relationship between circulating VEGF and prostate cancer outcomes have been examined in a number of clinical studies. A recent meta-analysis that included 12 studies and over 1700 patients showed that circulating VEGF expression was a good predictor for cancer-specific survival and biomedical failure in prostate cancer patients [85]. However, although showing a trend, levels of VEGF were not statistically significant predictor of overall survival, progression-free survival and disease free survival [85], and others have found no association overall [86]. Further studies will have to see if VEGF could be used in combination with other biomarkers or clinical features to predict outcomes among prostate cancer patients.

Interestingly, polymorphisms in *VEGF*, specifically the -634C/G SNP, have been associated with progression free survival among prostate cancer patients treated with metronomic cyclophosphamide [87].

IL-6

There is growing evidence that circulating levels of IL-6 are correlated with prostate cancer prognosis. An earlier epidemiological study showed that high serum IL-6 (>7 pg/ml) levels are associated with prognostic factors as well as overall survival among prostate cancer patients [88]. In this study, their data suggest that serum IL-6 was an independent factor for prostate cancer prognosis, as well as a surrogate for extent of disease. Other studies have also correlated IL-6 levels with tumor burden [51], or with having metastases to the bone [89].

Importantly, there is also a good amount of evidence supporting the involvement of IL-6 in the transition from hormone-dependent to castrate-resistant [60]. IL-6 has been shown to increase activity of the androgen receptor (AR), and, conversely, bicalutamide, an androgen blocker, inhibits IL-6 [62]. Other studies using prostate cancer models have showed similar interplay between AR and IL6 as well [90, 91].

Summary

In summary, many adipokines have been suggested to exert a mediating effect between obesity and prostate cancer. Although the relationship between obesity and prostate cancer is undoubtedly complex, adipokines are likely to play a significant role. Indeed, many of the associations found in studies of adipokines and risk and outcomes from prostate cancer are in addition to obesity, suggesting that there are likely to be other mediators as well.

It is important to note that for a vast majority of adipokines, current clinical studies of tumor adipokine expression or circulating adipokine levels have generally been small, often retrospective, utilize different types of patients, and thus it is not surprising that they have come to differing conclusions. Additional large-scale clinical and epidemiological research should be done to help us understand the utility of these biomarkers in diagnosing and caring for prostate cancer patients.

Similarly, a number of genetic epidemiological studies have investigated the association between inherited variation in adipokine genes or genes encoding their receptors. We have summarized these in Table 4.1. There is good evidence in the literature for the association of variants in *LEP* and *TGFa* with prostate cancer risk. However, for many of the other genes, there either appears to be no association or the studies to date have had mixed findings. Regardless, from these studies we can conclude that there are at least some inherited variations in adipokines that may help explain some of their relationships with prostate cancer.

With growing rates of obesity, the effect of obesity on prostate cancer should be expected to increase as well. While the last couple decades of research has greatly expanded our knowledge of how adipokines influence prostate cancer development and progression, there is still quite a bit left unanswered, particularly on the clinical side. Understanding the role of adipokines in prostate cancer can help us develop

Table 4.1 Summary of association of adipokine genes with prostate cancer risk

	Reference(s)
Genes with meta-analysis level evidence	
LEP (Leptin)	[29]
TNFα (Tumor necrosis factor alpha)	[54]
Genes with some evidence	
ADIPOQ (Adiponectin)	[39, 40]
IL6 (Interleukin 6)	[65–67]
Genes with limited evidence to date	
LEPR (Leptin Receptor)	[29, 30]
ADIPOR1 (Adiponectin receptor 1)	[39, 42]
ADIPOR2 (Adiponectin receptor 2)	[39, 42]
VEGF (Vascular endothelial growth factor)	[58, 59]

Genes of the five adipokines in this chapter and their level of evidence for association of inherited variation in them with prostate cancer risk

novel therapeutics and/or preventive measures to reduce the impact of obesity on prostate cancer incidence and mortality.

References

1. Snowdon DA, Phillips RL, Choi W. Diet, obesity, and risk of fatal prostate cancer. Am J Epidemiol. 1984;120:244–50.
2. Gong Z, Neuhouser ML, Goodman PJ, et al. Obesity, diabetes, and risk of prostate cancer: results from the prostate cancer prevention trial. Cancer Epidemiol Biomarkers Prev. 2006;15:1977–83.
3. Rodriguez C, Freedland SJ, Deka A, et al. Body mass index, weight change, and risk of prostate cancer in the Cancer Prevention Study II Nutrition Cohort. Cancer Epidemiol Biomarkers Prev. 2007;16:63–9.
4. Cao Y, Ma J. Body mass index, prostate cancer-specific mortality, and biochemical recurrence: a systematic review and meta-analysis. Cancer Prev Res (Phila). 2011;4:486–501.
5. Mistry T, Digby JE, Desai KM, Randeva HS. Obesity and prostate cancer: a role for adipokines. Eur Urol. 2007;52:46–53.
6. Leal Vde O, Mafra D. Adipokines in obesity. Clin Chim Acta. 2013;419:87–94.
7. Fain JN, Madan AK, Hiler ML, et al. Comparison of the release of adipokines by adipose tissue, adipose tissue matrix, and adipocytes from visceral and subcutaneous abdominal adipose tissues of obese humans. Endocrinology. 2004;145:2273–82.
8. Lee CH, Woo YC, Wang Y, et al. Obesity, adipokines and cancer: an update. Clin Endocrinol (Oxf). 2015;83:147–56.
9. Hanahan D, Weinberg RA. Hallmarks of cancer: the next generation. Cell. 2011;144:646–74.
10. Trayhurn P, Wood IS. Adipokines: inflammation and the pleiotropic role of white adipose tissue. Br J Nutr. 2004;92:347–55.
11. Mancuso P. The role of adipokines in chronic inflammation. Immunotargets Ther. 2016;5:47–56.
12. Fantuzzi G. Adipose tissue, adipokines, and inflammation. J Allergy Clin Immunol. 2005;115:911–9. quiz 920
13. Fantuzzi G, Faggioni R. Leptin in the regulation of immunity, inflammation, and hematopoiesis. J Leukoc Biol. 2000;68:437–46.

14. Kumada M, Kihara S, Ouchi N, et al. Adiponectin specifically increased tissue inhibitor of metalloproteinase-1 through interleukin-10 expression in human macrophages. Circulation. 2004;109:2046–9.
15. Wolf AM, Wolf D, Rumpold H, et al. Adiponectin induces the anti-inflammatory cytokines IL-10 and IL-1RA in human leukocytes. Biochem Biophys Res Commun. 2004;323:630–5.
16. Beltowski J. Adiponectin and resistin—new hormones of white adipose tissue. Med Sci Monit. 2003;9:RA55–61.
17. Antuna-Puente B, Feve B, Fellahi S, Bastard JP. Adipokines: the missing link between insulin resistance and obesity. Diabetes Metab. 2008;34:2–11.
18. Bastard JP, Maachi M, Lagathu C, et al. Recent advances in the relationship between obesity, inflammation, and insulin resistance. Eur Cytokine Netw. 2006;17:4–12.
19. Kwon H, Pessin JE. Adipokines mediate inflammation and insulin resistance. Front Endocrinol (Lausanne). 2013;4:71.
20. Rabe K, Lehrke M, Parhofer KG, Broedl UC. Adipokines and insulin resistance. Mol Med. 2008;14:741–51.
21. Considine RV, Sinha MK, Heiman ML, et al. Serum immunoreactive-leptin concentrations in normal-weight and obese humans. N Engl J Med. 1996;334:292–5.
22. Pan H, Guo J, Su Z. Advances in understanding the interrelations between leptin resistance and obesity. Physiol Behav. 2014;130:157–69.
23. Onuma M, Bub JD, Rummel TL, Iwamoto Y. Prostate cancer cell-adipocyte interaction: leptin mediates androgen-independent prostate cancer cell proliferation through c-Jun NH2-terminal kinase. J Biol Chem. 2003;278:42660–7.
24. Somasundar P, Frankenberry KA, Skinner H, et al. Prostate cancer cell proliferation is influenced by leptin. J Surg Res. 2004;118:71–82.
25. Saglam K, Aydur E, Yilmaz M, Goktas S. Leptin influences cellular differentiation and progression in prostate cancer. J Urol. 2003;169:1308–11.
26. Stattin P, Soderberg S, Hallmans G, et al. Leptin is associated with increased prostate cancer risk: a nested case-referent study. J Clin Endocrinol Metab. 2001;86:1341–5.
27. Stattin P, Kaaks R, Johansson R, et al. Plasma leptin is not associated with prostate cancer risk. Cancer Epidemiol Biomarkers Prev. 2003;12:474–5.
28. Baillargeon J, Platz EA, Rose DP, et al. Obesity, adipokines, and prostate cancer in a prospective population-based study. Cancer Epidemiol Biomarkers Prev. 2006;15:1331–5.
29. He J, Xi B, Ruiter R, et al. Association of LEP G2548A and LEPR Q223R polymorphisms with cancer susceptibility: evidence from a meta-analysis. PLoS One. 2013;8:e75135.
30. Shi H, Shu H, Huang C, et al. Association of LEPR K109R polymorphisms with cancer risk: a systematic review and pooled analysis. J BUON. 2014;19:847–54.
31. Arita Y, Kihara S, Ouchi N, et al. Paradoxical decrease of an adipose-specific protein, adiponectin, in obesity. Biochem Biophys Res Commun. 1999;257:79–83.
32. Matsuzawa Y, Shimomura I, Kihara S, Funahashi T. Importance of adipocytokines in obesity-related diseases. Horm Res. 2003;60(Suppl 3):56–9.
33. Lihn AS, Pedersen SB, Richelsen B. Adiponectin: action, regulation and association to insulin sensitivity. Obes Rev. 2005;6:13–21.
34. Bub JD, Miyazaki T, Iwamoto Y. Adiponectin as a growth inhibitor in prostate cancer cells. Biochem Biophys Res Commun. 2006;340:1158–66.
35. Tang CH, Lu ME. Adiponectin increases motility of human prostate cancer cells via adipoR, p38, AMPK, and NF-kappaB pathways. Prostate. 2009;69:1781–9.
36. Barb D, Neuwirth A, Mantzoros CS, Balk SP. Adiponectin signals in prostate cancer cells through Akt to activate the mammalian target of rapamycin pathway. Endocr Relat Cancer. 2007;14:995–1005.
37. Goktas S, Yilmaz MI, Caglar K, et al. Prostate cancer and adiponectin. Urology. 2005;65:1168–72.
38. Kelesidis I, Kelesidis T, Mantzoros CS. Adiponectin and cancer: a systematic review. Br J Cancer. 2006;94:1221–5.

39. Dhillon PK, Penney KL, Schumacher F, et al. Common polymorphisms in the adiponectin and its receptor genes, adiponectin levels and the risk of prostate cancer. Cancer Epidemiol Biomarkers Prev. 2011;20:2618–27.
40. Kaklamani V, Yi N, Zhang K, et al. Polymorphisms of ADIPOQ and ADIPOR1 and prostate cancer risk. Metabolism. 2011;60:1234–43.
41. Gu CY, Li QX, Zhu Y, et al. Genetic variations of the ADIPOQgene and risk of prostate cancer in Chinese Han men. Asian J Androl. 2014;16:878–83.
42. Beebe-Dimmer JL, Zuhlke KA, Ray AM, et al. Genetic variation in adiponectin (ADIPOQ) and the type 1 receptor (ADIPOR1), obesity and prostate cancer in African Americans. Prostate Cancer Prostatic Dis. 2010;13:362–8.
43. Mistry T, Digby JE, Chen J, et al. The regulation of adiponectin receptors in human prostate cancer cell lines. Biochem Biophys Res Commun. 2006;348:832–8.
44. Mistry T, Digby JE, Desai KM, Randeva HS. Leptin and adiponectin interact in the regulation of prostate cancer cell growth via modulation of p53 and bcl-2 expression. BJU Int. 2008;101:1317–22.
45. Hotamisligil GS, Arner P, Caro JF, et al. Increased adipose tissue expression of tumor necrosis factor-alpha in human obesity and insulin resistance. J Clin Invest. 1995;95:2409–15.
46. Tzanavari T, Giannogonas P, Karalis KP. TNF-alpha and obesity. Curr Dir Autoimmun. 2010;11:145–56.
47. Tse BW, Scott KF, Russell PJ. Paradoxical roles of tumour necrosis factor-alpha in prostate cancer biology. Prostate Cancer. 2012;2012:128965.
48. Balkwill F. Tumour necrosis factor and cancer. Nat Rev Cancer. 2009;9:361–71.
49. Wang X, Lin Y. Tumor necrosis factor and cancer, buddies or foes? Acta Pharmacol Sin. 2008;29:1275–88.
50. Chopra DP, Menard RE, Januszewski J, Mattingly RR. TNF-alpha-mediated apoptosis in normal human prostate epithelial cells and tumor cell lines. Cancer Lett. 2004;203:145–54.
51. Adler HL, McCurdy MA, Kattan MW, et al. Elevated levels of circulating interleukin-6 and transforming growth factor-beta1 in patients with metastatic prostatic carcinoma. J Urol. 1999;161:182–7.
52. Fargion S, Valenti L, Dongiovanni P, et al. Tumor necrosis factor alpha promoter polymorphisms influence the phenotypic expression of hereditary hemochromatosis. Blood. 2001;97:3707–12.
53. El-Tahan RR, Ghoneim AM, El-Mashad N. TNF-alpha gene polymorphisms and expression. Springerplus. 2016;5:1508.
54. Ma L, Zhao J, Li T, et al. Association between tumor necrosis factor-alpha gene polymorphisms and prostate cancer risk: a meta-analysis. Diagn Pathol. 2014;9:74.
55. McMahon G. VEGF receptor signaling in tumor angiogenesis. Oncologist. 2000;5(Suppl 1):3–10.
56. Sharif MR, Shaabani A, Mahmoudi H, et al. Association of the serum vascular endothelial growth factor levels with benign prostate hyperplasia and prostate malignancies. Nephrourol Mon. 2014;6:e14778.
57. Botelho F, Pina F, Lunet N. VEGF and prostatic cancer: a systematic review. Eur J Cancer Prev. 2010;19:385–92.
58. Langsenlehner T, Langsenlehner U, Renner W, et al. Single nucleotide polymorphisms and haplotypes in the gene for vascular endothelial growth factor and risk of prostate cancer. Eur J Cancer. 2008;44:1572–6.
59. VanCleave TT, Moore JH, Benford ML, et al. Interaction among variant vascular endothelial growth factor (VEGF) and its receptor in relation to prostate cancer risk. Prostate. 2010;70:341–52.
60. Nguyen DP, Li J, Tewari AK. Inflammation and prostate cancer: the role of interleukin 6 (IL-6). BJU Int. 2014;113:986–92.
61. Wise GJ, Marella VK, Talluri G, Shirazian D. Cytokine variations in patients with hormone treated prostate cancer. J Urol. 2000;164:722–5.

62. Hobisch A, Ramoner R, Fuchs D, et al. Prostate cancer cells (LNCaP) generated after long-term interleukin 6 (IL-6) treatment express IL-6 and acquire an IL-6 partially resistant phenotype. Clin Cancer Res. 2001;7:2941–8.
63. Drachenberg DE, Elgamal AA, Rowbotham R, et al. Circulating levels of interleukin-6 in patients with hormone refractory prostate cancer. Prostate. 1999;41:127–33.
64. Michalaki V, Syrigos K, Charles P, Waxman J. Serum levels of IL-6 and TNF-alpha correlate with clinicopathological features and patient survival in patients with prostate cancer. Br J Cancer. 2004;90:2312–6.
65. Pierce BL, Biggs ML, DeCambre M, et al. C-reactive protein, interleukin-6, and prostate cancer risk in men aged 65 years and older. Cancer Causes Control. 2009;20:1193–203.
66. Chen J, Ying XM, Huang XM, et al. Association between polymorphisms in selected inflammatory response genes and the risk of prostate cancer. Onco Targets Ther. 2016;9:223–9.
67. Huang WJ, Wu LJ, Min ZC, et al. Interleukin-6-572G/C polymorphism and prostate cancer susceptibility. Genet Mol Res. 2016;15:447–53.
68. Freedland SJ, Platz EA. Obesity and prostate cancer: making sense out of apparently conflicting data. Epidemiol Rev. 2007;29:88–97.
69. Hoda MR, Theil G, Mohammed N, et al. The adipocyte-derived hormone leptin has proliferative actions on androgen-resistant prostate cancer cells linking obesity to advanced stages of prostate cancer. J Oncol. 2012;2012:280386.
70. Noda T, Kikugawa T, Tanji N, et al. Longterm exposure to leptin enhances the growth of prostate cancer cells. Int J Oncol. 2015;46:1535–42.
71. Ribeiro AM, Pereira S, Andrade S, et al. Insulin prevents leptin inhibition of RM1 prostate cancer cell growth. Pathol Oncol Res. 2012;18:499–507.
72. Moreira A, Pereira SS, Costa M, et al. Adipocyte secreted factors enhance aggressiveness of prostate carcinoma cells. PLoS One. 2015;10:e0123217.
73. Burton A, Martin RM, Holly J, et al. Associations of adiponectin and leptin with stage and grade of PSA-detected prostate cancer: the ProtecT study. Cancer Causes Control. 2013;24:323–34.
74. Sher DJ, Oh WK, Jacobus S, et al. Relationship between serum adiponectin and prostate cancer grade. Prostate. 2008;68:1592–8.
75. Freedland SJ, Sokoll LJ, Platz EA, et al. Association between serum adiponectin, and pathological stage and grade in men undergoing radical prostatectomy. J Urol. 2005;174:1266–70.
76. Stevens VL, Jacobs EJ, Sun J, Gapstur SM. No association of plasma levels of adiponectin and c-peptide with risk of aggressive prostate cancer in the Cancer Prevention Study II Nutrition Cohort. Cancer Epidemiol Biomarkers Prev. 2014;23:890–2.
77. Bao B, Ahmad A, Kong D, et al. Hypoxia induced aggressiveness of prostate cancer cells is linked with deregulated expression of VEGF, IL-6 and miRNAs that are attenuated by CDF. PLoS One. 2012;7:e43726.
78. Lin DW, FitzGerald LM, Fu R, et al. Genetic variants in the LEPR, CRY1, RNASEL, IL4, and ARVCF genes are prognostic markers of prostate cancer-specific mortality. Cancer Epidemiol Biomarkers Prev. 2011;20:1928–36.
79. Li H, Stampfer MJ, Mucci L, et al. A 25-year prospective study of plasma adiponectin and leptin concentrations and prostate cancer risk and survival. Clin Chem. 2010;56:34–43.
80. Gu C, Qu Y, Zhang G, et al. A single nucleotide polymorphism in ADIPOQ predicts biochemical recurrence after radical prostatectomy in localized prostate cancer. Oncotarget. 2015;6:32205–11.
81. Duque JL, Loughlin KR, Adam RM, et al. Plasma levels of vascular endothelial growth factor are increased in patients with metastatic prostate cancer. Urology. 1999;54:523–7.
82. Erkal EY, Bora H, Tepeoglu M, Akmansu M. Role of vascular endothelial growth factor in clinically localized prostate cancer treated with radiation therapy. Balkan Med J. 2014;31:43–9.
83. Wu TT, Wang JS, Jiann BP, et al. Expression of vascular endothelial growth factor in Taiwanese benign and malignant prostate tissues. J Chin Med Assoc. 2007;70:380–4.
84. Roberts E, Cossigny DA, Quan GM. The role of vascular endothelial growth factor in metastatic prostate cancer to the skeleton. Prostate Cancer. 2013;2013:418340.

85. Liu ZQ, Fang JM, Xiao YY, et al. Prognostic role of vascular endothelial growth factor in prostate cancer: a systematic review and meta-analysis. Int J Clin Exp Med. 2015;8:2289–98.
86. Pan L, Baek S, Edmonds PR, et al. Vascular endothelial growth factor (VEGF) expression in locally advanced prostate cancer: secondary analysis of radiation therapy oncology group (RTOG) 8610. Radiat Oncol. 2013;8:100.
87. Orlandi P, Fontana A, Fioravanti A, et al. VEGF-A polymorphisms predict progression-free survival among advanced castration-resistant prostate cancer patients treated with metronomic cyclophosphamide. Br J Cancer. 2013;109:957–64.
88. Nakashima J, Tachibana M, Horiguchi Y, et al. Serum interleukin 6 as a prognostic factor in patients with prostate cancer. Clin Cancer Res. 2000;6:2702–6.
89. Shariat SF, Andrews B, Kattan MW, et al. Plasma levels of interleukin-6 and its soluble receptor are associated with prostate cancer progression and metastasis. Urology. 2001;58:1008–15.
90. Zhang J, Pugh TD, Stebler B, et al. Orchiectomy increases bone marrow interleukin-6 levels in mice. Calcif Tissue Int. 1998;62:219–26.
91. Tsui KH, Lin YF, Chen YH, et al. Mechanisms by which interleukin-6 regulates prostate-specific antigen gene expression in prostate LNCaP carcinoma cells. J Androl. 2011;32:383–93.

Chapter 5
Cross-Sectional Epidemiology and Intervention Studies of Mediators of the Energy Imbalance-Prostate Cancer Association

Mieke Van Hemelrijck and Sabine Rohrmann

Abstract This chapter discusses both cross-sectional and intervention studies investigating how indicators of energy imbalance—energy intake, physical activity, and obesity—and their interventions—dietary restriction or exercise—are associated with potential mediators of the association between energy imbalance and prostate cancer risk and progression. We focus on biomarkers of pathways involved in energy metabolism—insulin growth factor-1, lipogenic pathway, prostaglandins, vasoactive intestinal peptide (VIP), sex steroid hormones, leptin and adipokines, irisin, epigenetics, telomere length, inflammation, and vitamin D—as the potential mediators. Despite a wide variety of both cross-sectional and intervention studies available, current findings are rather inconsistent for most of these potential mediators. Physical activity and dietary restriction have been inversely associated with insulin and lipid metabolism as well as inflammation in both observational and intervention studies. Prostaglandins and VIP have been investigated less frequently, whereas the numerous studies on sex steroid hormones are unclear about the effects of physical activity. Similarly, leptin and adiponectin have been studied frequently with inconsistent findings. Irisin is predominantly inversely linked with indicators the energy imbalance. Epigenetics and telomere length are two emerging areas of research in the context of energy imbalance with promising results from intervention studies. Finally, despite the potentially beneficial health effects of vitamin D, few studies have investigated how reducing energy imbalance may affect its circulating levels. We expect that the ongoing "Mechanisms research project" of the

M. Van Hemelrijck, PhD
Division of Cancer Studies, King's College London, Guy's Hospital,
3rd Floor Bermondsey Wing, London, UK
e-mail: mieke.vanhemelrijck@kcl.ac.uk

S. Rohrmann, PhD (✉)
Division of Chronic Disease Epidemiology, Epidemiology, Biostatistics and Prevention Institute, University of Zurich, Zurich, Switzerland
e-mail: sabine.rohrmann@uzh.ch

© Springer International Publishing AG 2018
E.A. Platz, N.A. Berger (eds.), *Energy Balance and Prostate Cancer*, Energy Balance and Cancer 14, DOI 10.1007/978-3-319-64940-5_5

World Cancer Research Fund, through a standardized review of research on the biological mechanisms underlying the effects of lifestyle factors influencing energy imbalance on prostate cancer risk and progression, will point to information gaps for more research and may identify targets for intervention.

Keywords Diet • Exercise • Cross-sectional studies • Intervention studies • Obesity

Introduction

This chapter discusses both cross-sectional and intervention studies investigating how indicators of energy imbalance—energy intake, physical activity, and obesity—and their interventions—dietary restriction or exercise—are associated with potential mediators of the association between energy balance and prostate cancer risk and progression. We focus on biomarkers of pathways involved in energy metabolism—insulin growth factor-1 (IGF-1), lipogenic pathway, prostaglandins, vasoactive intestinal peptide (VIP), sex steroid hormones, leptin and adipokines, irisin, epigenetics, telomere length, inflammation, and vitamin D—as the potential mediators. The first section of this chapter describes these potential mediators. The second section reviews cross-sectional studies investigating the mediators in relation to indicators of energy imbalance. The last section summarizes studies evaluating the effects of diet and exercise interventions on these mediators.

Potential Mediators of the Energy Imbalance-Prostate Cancer Associations

Energy metabolism could play a role in prostate cancer proliferation and progression through many different biological mechanisms. Before discussing cross-sectional and intervention studies evaluating these biological mechanisms in relation to indicators or interventions of energy imbalance, we provide a very brief overview of those potential mediators most commonly thought to link energy imbalance and prostate cancer risk and progression.

Insulin and the Insulin-Like Growth Factor (IGF) Family

Insulin, a polypeptide produced by beta cells in the pancreas, is involved in regulation of energy metabolism. It regulates glucose concentration by triggering glucose absorption by muscle, fat, and liver cells from the blood. Additionally, it is involved in regulating lipogenesis [1]. It has mitogenic and growth-stimulatory properties, such that hyperinsulinemia is thought be a risk factor for cancer.

IGF-1, a peptide hormone, that is thought to have a role in cell differentiation, proliferation, and apoptosis [2]. IGF-1 is mainly carried in the blood bound to

IGF-binding protein 3 (IGFBP3), such that the clearance of IGF-1 is reduced and its supply to target cells is prolonged [3]. With respect to prostate cancer, however, results are ambiguous ranging from inverse associations [4] and null findings [5, 6] to positive associations [7]. Nevertheless, a meta-analysis of 17 prospective and 2 cross-sectional studies confirmed a positive association between circulating levels of IGF-1 and the risk of prostate cancer [8].

Lipogenic Pathway

De novo synthesis of fatty acids has been observed in several types of cancer cells, including prostate cancer. Fatty acid synthase (FASN) is the major enzyme of lipogenesis and catalyzes the nicotinamide adenine dinucleotide phosphate (NADPH)-dependent condensation of acetyl-CoA and malonyl-CoA to produce predominantly 16-carbon palmitic acid [9]. Many cancers overexpress FASN, and some studies have shown that its overexpression is also associated with poor survival of cancer patients [10], including prostate cancer [11, 12].

In contrast to normal prostate epithelial cells, prostate cancer cells do not show increased aerobic glycolysis. Increased de novo synthesis of lipids is hence thought to be an early event of the disease, as shown by upregulation and increased activity of lipogenic enzymes (i.e., FASN) [13, 14], which are also regulated by some of the major cancer-driving signaling pathways: PTEN, PI3K, and AKT. Several studies have therefore also investigated the role of serum lipids (e.g. triglycerides, total cholesterol, high-density lipoprotein (HDL) and low-density lipoprotein (LDL) cholesterol) and risk and progression of prostate cancer [15].

Peroxisome proliferator-activated receptor gamma (PPARγ) is a nuclear receptor that is selectively expressed in adipose tissue. It has an important role in adipocyte differentiation, energy storage, insulin sensitization, and fatty acid metabolism [16].

Prostaglandins

Prostaglandin is one of the many stimulators thought to drive adipogenesis. It is of interest to prostate carcinogenesis, as it can also lower cell proliferation and therefore have tumor promoting effects [17].

Vasoactive Intestinal Peptide (VIP)

VIP is a neuropeptide that is widely distributed in the central nervous system and in the gastrointestinal tract neurons. Physiologically, it is important with respect to a variety of gastrointestinal functions such as mucosal ion transport, vasodilatation, and mucosal inflammatory immune responses. In animal models, VIP has been shown to play a role in the control of appetite, feeding behavior, and the age-dependent change of body phenotype, e.g., body fat mass gain and lean mass loss [18]. In addition to its role in glucose metabolism and modulation of the immune system, VIP has been suggested to play a role in the development of cancer through regulation of proliferation and cell differentiation [19]. VIP receptors are expressed on a number of human tumor cell types, including prostate cancer [20]. In prostate cancer cell lines, VIP stimulates cell proliferation and invasiveness [21].

Sex Steroid Hormones

Even though testosterone is considered to play a role in prostate cancer risk and progression, it is still unclear how circulating levels of sex steroid hormones affect this. A meta-analysis of 18 prospective studies did not show any impact of circulating hormones on prostate cancer risk [22]. However, in the context of energy balance and prostate cancer, testosterone and other sex steroid hormones may be potential mediators as there is cross-talk with energy homeostasis, e.g., excess adipose tissue results in increased conversion of testosterone to estradiol [23].

Leptin and Adipokines

Leptin, a hormone secreted by adipose tissue, helps to regulate energy homeostasis. Exogenous levels of circulating leptin have been shown to stimulate the growth of prostate cancer cells [24]. Leptin is one of many adipokines, i.e. cytokines secreted by adipose tissue, thought to be involved in the link between energy regulation and prostate carcinogenesis [25]. However, results are rather heterogeneous with respect to an association with prostate cancer in epidemiological studies [5].

Irisin

Another hormone recently suggested to link energy imbalance and cancer is irisin, also called the "exercise hormone", as it has been shown to be involved in thermogenesis and energy expenditure [26].

Epigenetic Modifications

Epigenetic modifications, including hyper- and hypomethylation of select genes or genomewide, has recently been shown to be one of the potential mechanistic linking lifestyle-related factors and prostate cancer [27]. For example, several components of the epigenetic machinery require intermediates of cellular metabolism for enzymatic function. Moreover, specific epigenetic influences of dietary glucose and lipid consumption have been observed across several organs and pathways associated with metabolism [28].

Telomeres

Telomeres are repetitive DNA sequences that protect the ends of chromosomes from degradation and recombination. Over the lifetime, they become shorter and finally dysfunctional, but cancer cells typically have the ability to maintain telomeres, which enhances viability. Because telomeres shorten with each round of replication, factors that increase the rate of proliferation, including possibly energy imbalance, would produce accelerating telomere shortening. Several studies have examined the association of telomere length, usually measured in peripheral blood lymphocytes, and cancer risk. For prostate cancer, whether an association between telomere length and prostate cancer risk exists is uncertain. The Health Professionals Follow-up Study [29] and the Prostate, Lung, Colorectal and Ovarian (PLCO) Cancer Screening trial [30] both possibly found that men with shorter telomere length had a lower, rather than higher, risk of prostate cancer, whereas no association between telomere length and prostate cancer risk or mortality was observed in a Danish study [31]. Note that it is unclear what telomere length in circulating leukocytes reflects relative to tissue telomere length.

Inflammation

Inflammatory cytokines are circulating factors implicated as key mediators for the effects of energy imbalance on carcinogenesis [32]. Shivappa and colleagues examined the ability of a newly developed dietary inflammatory index (DII) to predict prostate cancer risk and found that men in the fourth quartile of the DDI, as compared to men in the lowest quartile, have a 33% higher risk of developing prostate cancer [33]. These findings thus suggested that a pro-inflammatory diet may be a risk factor for prostate cancer.

Vitamin D

Preclinical evidence links vitamin D and cancer, suggesting that vitamin D has antiproliferative effects via mechanisms such the induction of G0/G1 cell cycle arrest, differentiation, and apoptosis [34]. Vitamin D has also been implicated in energy metabolism [35].

Observational Studies of Mediators of Energy Imbalance: Prostate Cancer Associations

This section reviews observational studies focused on the associations of indicators of energy imbalance (i.e., energy intake, physical activity, and obesity) with the above-listed mediators of the energy imbalance-prostate cancer association. In contrast to physical activity and obesity, only a few studies have reported on the associations for energy intake—either total energy intake or more specifically macronutrient intake, in particular fat intake, with the mediators.

Energy Intake

The association between energy intake and circulating **IGF-1** has been examined cross-sectionally in some studies. For example, in the Health Professionals Follow-up Study, energy intake was positively related to plasma IGF-1 level in normal weight men, but no association was observed in overweight or obese men [36]. No such association was observed in the Multiethnic Cohort [37] or the European Prospective Investigation into Cancer and Nutrition (EPIC) cohort [38], although these and other studies observed associations of other dietary components, in particular dairy consumption with IGF-1 concentrations (e.g. [38, 39, 88]).

A small study among 112 healthy Greek men examined the association between diet and **sex steroid hormones** cross-sectionally [40]; total energy intake was not associated with either testosterone or estradiol concentration. Similarly, no associations were seen in a British study of 696 middle-aged men [41].

Studies that cross-sectionally examined energy intake and blood concentrations of **leptin** generally observed no associations. In the Health Professionals Follow-up Study, men in the highest quintile of leptin concentration had higher intakes of total and saturated fat than men in the lowest quintile, but there was no difference in energy intake [42]. There were also no associations between energy intake and leptin concentration in the Multiethnic Cohort [43] or the EPIC cohort [38]. In the cross-sectional INTERLIPID study, total dietary energy intake was not significantly related with leptin concentration among normal weight and overweight participants, but in those with body mass index (BMI) ≥ 30 kg/m^2, total energy intake was significantly inversely related with leptin concentrations independent of body weight and physical activity [44]. No associations of total energy intake with circulating concentrations of **adiponectin** were observed in a study among Greek university students [45] or among 532 middle-aged men of the Health Professionals Follow-up Study [46].

Only one study cross-sectionally examined circulating **irisin** concentration and energy intake; no association was observed [47].

In a longitudinal study that included 405 young adult men and 204 women, baseline energy intake was inversely associated with follow-up **leukocyte telomere**

length in men, but not in women [48]. In another longitudinal study among 101 women and 47 men aged 20–59 years, no difference in telomere length over a 10-year follow-up period was observed between those participants who gained weight and those who kept their body weight constant [49]. **Epigenetic modifications** have, to our knowledge, not been examined in connection with total energy intake. However, in an analysis of 149 participants of the North Texas Healthy Heart Study a prudent dietary pattern rich in vegetables and fruits was associated with a lower prevalence of DNA hypomethylation [50].

The number of studies that examined the association between energy intake and **inflammation markers** in the general population is rather small. In a study with 151 middle-aged Greek participants, no association between energy intake and serum concentrations of C-reactive protein (CRP), a non-specific marker of inflammation, was observed, but better diet quality was inversely associated with lower CRP levels [47]. In an analysis of the National Health and Nutrition Examination Survey (NHANES), diet composition, including energy intake, had only little or no association with CRP concentration [51].

Physical Activity

In several cross-sectional studies, physical activity was related to lower concentrations of **insulin or C-peptide** [52–55], although not all studies showed statistically significant associations after adjustment for confounders [56]. NHANES analyses showed inverse associations of different types and levels of physical activity, even light activity, with fasting insulin concentrations [57, 58]. Physical activity increases muscle glucose uptake and muscle insulin sensitivity in the post-exercise period, which is thought to be due to increased sarcolemmal content of the glucose transporter GLUT4 [59].

Associations of physical activity with the **IGF system** components are inconsistent. In the Coronary Artery Risk Development in Young Adults Study (CARDIA) cohort, increased physical activity was associated with a decrease in IGFBP-3, but was not associated with IGF-1 [60]. In a German cross-sectional study, peak exercise capacity was not associated with IGF-1 concentration in men [61], whereas a study among Asian men observed an inverse association between physical activity and IGF-1 concentrations [39]. It has been speculated that differences by race/ethnicity, age or different categorization of the exposure variables, in particular obesity and physical activity, might explain the heterogeneity in results.

Several studies provided evidence that physical activity and fitness levels are generally associated with **blood lipids** [62]. In a study of 183 nonsmoking white men (35–53 years old), waist circumference was inversely associated with HDL cholesterol, where physical fitness was positively associated with HDL. Stratified by obesity status and fitness level, those men who were fat and fit had higher HDL levels than those who were fat and unfit [63]. A study of 12 lean and 26 obese sedentary men and 18 master athletes (mean age 65 years) observed that total and LDL cholesterol levels were comparable between these three groups, but HDL cholesterol levels were higher in master athletes than in obese sedentary men and lean sedentary men, and in lean sedentary men than in obese sedentary men. Triglyceride concentrations were similar in master athletes and lean sedentary men, but higher in obese sedentary men [64]. However, the question of an interaction between obesity and physical fitness/activity is still understudied and, hence, a matter of debate.

In a cross-sectional analysis of NHANES III data, physical activity was positively associated with **total and free testosterone**, but not with **estradiol** or sex hormone-binding globulin **(SHBG)** concentrations [65]. In an analysis of continuous NHANES data, non-obese men with more physical activity had a reduced odds of low or low normal testosterone concentrations, but this was not seen in obese men [66]. A Danish cross-sectional study reported lower testosterone in men watching many hours of television, but no associations were observed for time spent in front of the computer or time spent on physical activity [67]. These examples illustrate that the associations of physical activity and sedentary behavior with circulating sex steroid concentration are still unclear.

In a cross-sectional study including 3640 non-diabetic British men aged 60–79 years, **leptin** concentrations decreased significantly with increasing physical activity [68]. Similar inverse associations were observed in the Health Professionals Follow-up Study [42] and the CARDIA study [69]. In the Miami Community Health Study, the inverse association between leptin and physical activity among men was independent of percent body fat and insulin, suggesting that activity may act directly on leptin or leptin resistance [70]. Associations of physical activity and **adiponectin** concentrations are less frequently studied than leptin. One Japanese study observed that circulating levels of adiponectin were positively correlated with physical fitness after taking BMI into account, but there was no association with physical activity per se [71], whereas an older Japanese study did see a positive association between physical activity and adiponectin concentrations [72].

In a Spanish cross-sectional study including 428 men and women, circulating **irisin** concentrations were higher in active than in sedentary individuals [73].

Quite a number of studies have examined associations between physical activity and **telomere length**. However, a review that included 37 studies concluded that the association remains unclear [74]. Although the authors noted a tendency toward an effect of exercise on telomere length, many of these results were not statistically significant. In the Copenhagen City Heart Study short telomere length was cross-sectionally associated with physical inactivity, but a change in leukocyte telomere length during 10 years was not associated [75].

In two US cohort studies, physical activity was inversely associated with plasma levels of the following **inflammatory markers**: sTNF-R1, sTNF-R2, interleukin-6 (IL-6), and CRP. However, adjustment for BMI and leptin attenuated most of these associations [55], suggesting that the association between physical activity and systemic inflammation is at least partly explained by a lower degree of obesity in physically active subjects.

Physical activity is positively associated with circulating **vitamin D** concentration, as observed in several epidemiological studies. For example, in an analysis of

NHANES data, an increase of 10 min of moderate-to-vigorous activity per day, irrespective of being self-reported or measured by accelerometer, was associated with an increase in circulating vitamin D levels [76]. The odds ratio (OR) for being vitamin D deficient (<20 ng/mL) comparing being insufficiently active with being sufficiently active was 1.32 (95% CI 1.11–1.57). Interestingly, these associations were not stronger for self-reported outdoor activities compared with indoor activities. Similarly, a French study showed an association between physical activity and vitamin D, even after adjusting for sun exposure and practice of outdoor hobbies or sports [77]. In contrast, in another US study, physical inactivity was a major modifiable predictor of low vitamin D status [78]. Effects of physical activity on serum phosphate concentrations and/or parathyroid hormone production are thought to increase vitamin D concentrations independent of sun exposure [79].

Obesity

Positive associations between overall obesity, expressed by BMI or abdominal obesity, with circulating levels of **insulin and C-peptide** have been reported in several cross-sectional studies [56, 80–82]. Several studies also examined cross-sectionally how **IGF-1** is associated with obesity. However, the findings observed are quite heterogeneous. In an analysis of NHANES III data, IGF-1 decreased with increasing BMI and waist circumference [83]. They did, however, not examine the association with IGFBP-3 or the ratio as an indicator of free IGF-1 concentration. In the CARDIA study, higher BMI, but not larger waist circumference, was associated with lower IGF-1; neither BMI nor waist circumference was related to IGFBP-3 concentrations [60]. Among 1142 male participants in the EPIC cohort, IGF-1 concentrations were associated with BMI in an "inverse" U-shaped manner: men with BMI of 26–27 kg/m^2 had the highest IGF-1 serum levels, but IGFBP-3 concentrations were not associated with BMI [84]. This pattern has also been reported in a Swedish study [85]. In a recent Danish study including 1493 men, circulating IGF-1 levels were inversely associated with all anthropometric markers adjusting for age, alcohol consumption, smoking and physical activity [86]; IGFBP-3 concentrations were not evaluated. In a German cohort, inverse linear and quadratic associations between anthropometric parameters and serum IGF-1 were found. Additionally, men with high waist circumference more often had low serum IGF-1 and less often had high serum IGF-1 levels compared to men with low waist circumference [87]. In a study among Chinese men, IGF-1 was positively associated with BMI, as was IGFBP-3 [39]. Other studies observed no associations of IGF-1 and/or IGFBP-3 concentration with obesity (for example, [88]).

Numerous studies have shown a cross-sectional association between obesity and **blood lipids** [89, 90]. Both overall obesity and abdominal obesity tend to be positively associated with total and LDL cholesterol as well as triglyceride concentrations, but inversely with HDL cholesterol.

Variations in the **fatty acid synthase** (*FASN*) gene in relation to differences in BMI have been examined in several studies. In non-diabetic Pima Indians, a Val1483Ile polymorphism (GTC to ATC) was associated with percentage of body fat. Compared with homozygotes for the Val variant, subjects with Ile/x had a lower mean percentage of body fat (30 ± 1% vs. 33 ± 1%, P = 0.002; adjusted for age, sex, and family membership), resulting in a lower mean carbohydrate oxidation rate [91]. In a German study, Caucasians boys with Ile/Val genotype compared to Val/Val had a lower BMI standard deviation score (SDS; −0.36 ± 0.29 vs 0.09 ± 0.05, P < 0.05), whereas the opposite was observed in girls (0.48 ± 0.19 vs 0.09 ± 0.05, P < 0.05) [92]. A third study, conducted among mostly Caucasian women, found that two SNPs in *FASN* were associated with obesity [93]. Lastly, a US study showed that men with the homozygous AA (vs. GG) variant of rs1127678 in *FASN* had an approximately 2% higher BMI [94]. A German study including 196 lean or obese participants observed that increased FASN gene expression in adipose tissue was linked to visceral fat accumulation, but also impaired insulin sensitivity and increased circulating fasting insulin, as well as an increase in IL-6, leptin and retinol binding-protein 4 [95].

A common missense polymorphism in ***PPARG*** is the Pro12Ala polymorphism. In a meta-analysis that included 25 studies, the combined results showed that the *PPARG* Pro12Ala polymorphism was positively associated with obesity (Ala vs. Pro: OR = 1.55, 95% CI 1.34–1.80; Pro/Ala vs. Pro/Pro: OR = 1.54, 95% CI 1.31–1.82; Ala/Ala & Pro/Ala vs. Pro/Pro: OR = 1.61, 95% CI 1.36–1.90) [16].

In a small Japanese study, plasma concentrations of **8-epi-prostaglandin F2alpha (PGF2α)** were significantly positively correlated with BMI, body fat weight, visceral and total fat area in obese and non-obese men [96]. A positive association of urinary PGF2a with visceral fat accumulation was also observed in another Japanese study [97]. In a small US study, higher BMI was positively associated with higher prostaglandin E2 (**PGE2**) concentration in rectal mucosa, whereas having more leisure-time physical activity was inversely associated with PGE2 concentration [98]. **Urinary 8-isoprostane** levels were positively associated with body weight and waist circumference in a small European study [99].

Hardly any epidemiological data exists on the association of **VIP** and energy imbalance in humans. A US study that included 1000 white participants used genome-wide analysis to examine factors that were associated with BMI and body fat mass [100]. Of the almost 1000 pathways analyzed, the VIP pathway was most strongly associated with fat mass and the third most strongly associated pathway with BMI.

Sex steroid hormones have been examined in much detail with respect to their association with obesity. In a review from 2010, 18 of the 20 studies observed inverse associations between testosterone concentration and BMI; 15 of 16 studies found SHBG also to be inversely related with BMI, and 10 of 12 reported an inverse relationship between free testosterone and BMI [101]. Four of the ten studies measuring estradiol observed a positive relationship with BMI, while the remaining studies did not observe any statistically significant association. Studies conducted in NHANES III and published after this review observed that increased body fat was associated with lower circulating levels of testosterone (total and free) and SHBG and higher circulating levels of free estradiol in men. This was true for body fat as measured by dual-energy X-ray absorptiometry [102], as well as anthropometric measures such as BMI and waist circumference [103]. In the BACH study, the authors observed the same associations cross-sectionally in men [104]. In addition, their longitudinal analyses support the hypothesis that body composition affects hormone levels and not the reverse.

Body weight and obesity have extensively been studied in relation to **leptin** concentrations with mostly positive associations (e.g., [56]). In one of the earliest studies, percent body fat was positively associated with leptin concentrations in a US population, but interestingly abdominal fat was not independently associated with leptin [105], which was confirmed in a later study among Japanese adults [106]. In 30 abdominally obese men with insulin resistance, most of the individual variation in serum leptin concentration was explained by the amount of subcutaneous abdominal adipose tissue, insulin sensitivity, and BMI [107]. The opposite is true for the association of body fat and obesity with blood concentrations of **adiponectin**: generally, inverse associations between indicators of obesity and adiponectin are observed in cross-sectional studies [108–110]. In a prospective study conducted among 247 healthy men from the Health Professionals Follow-up Study, men in the highest quintile of plasma leptin (mean = 12.1 ng/mL) weighed more, were less physically active, and had higher circulating insulin levels than men in the lowest quintile (mean = 2.7 ng/mL). After adjustments for baseline age, weight, height, smoking status, alcohol intake, and physical activity, each 10 ng/mL increase in plasma leptin concentration was associated with a 1.68 kg (95% CI 0.14–3.18 kg) weight gain over the 4-year follow-up period. The observed association between leptin level and weight gain was limited to men with a baseline BMI $\geq$ 25 kg/m^2 [111]. In the CARDIA study, leptin concentrations were positively associated with BMI [69]. However, 8-year weight change was not related to initial leptin concentration, but leptin change correlated highly with weight change. In a prospective Japanese study among 1003 middle-aged participants, a change in body weight over a 5-year period was inversely associated with the change in adiponectin concentration, such that men who reduced their body weight by 2 kg or more were 2.56 (95% CI 1.21–5.42) times more likely to be in the upper tertile of adiponectin change than those who gained $\geq$2 kg, independent of their baseline body weight [112]. The Rancho Bernardo Study also observed a positive association for changes in body weight with baseline leptin concentrations and an inverse association with baseline adiponectin [113]. However, the authors concluded that their results suggest that the levels of leptin and adiponectin may simply follow rather than influence an individual's weight changes.

In sedentary participants of a Spanish cross-sectional study, **irisin** levels were positively associated with BMI, but this association was not seen in physically active individuals [73]. Interestingly, neither percent fat mass nor waist-to-hip ratio was statistically significantly associated with irisin concentration in either group of participants. In a German study with 40 participants, obese individuals had higher plasma irisin concentrations compared to normal weight and anorexic patients.

Plasma irisin was also positively correlated with fat mass and fat-free mass [114]. In a study with 117 healthy women, circulating irisin concentrations were non-significantly positively correlated with BMI and more strongly positively associated with fat-free mass [115].

In a GWAS analysis, increased BMI in adults of European origin was associated with increased DNA **methylation** in white blood cells and in adipose tissue at the *HIF3A* locus, a component of the hypoxia inducible transcription factor (HIF) [116]. Associations between the methylation of genes with biologically plausible relationships to adiposity were detected in an epigenome-wide study conducted among US cohorts. Top differences in DNA methylation by obesity status were found for *CPT1A*, which encodes carnitine palmitoyltransferase 1A, the rate-limiting enzyme for mitochondrial fatty acid oxidation, *PHGDH*, which encodes the phosphoglycerate dehydrogenase enzyme that catalyzes the first step in the phosphorylation pathway of serine biosynthesis, *CD38*, an immunologically relevant gene expressed in CD41 T-cells, and long intergenic non-coding RNA 00263 [117]. This study, however, did not observe statistically significant associations between *HIF3A* methylation and obesity. In a small study with 73 obese patients, level of methylation of the adiponectin gene locus in subcutaneous adipose tissue was positively associated with BMI and waist circumference, whereas level of methylation of the leptin gene in white blood cells was inversely associated with BMI [118]. In a Spanish study that included 60 women, differences between normal-weight and overweight/obese individuals were observed in the methylation status of CpG sites of *CLOCK* (CpGs 1, 5–6, 8 and 11–14) and of *BMAL1* (CpGs 6–7, 8, 15 and 16–17) [119].

A meta-analysis on the association between obesity and **telomere length,** which included 12 studies, concluded that telomere length was statistically significantly shorter in obese than normal weight individuals, but the study also noted strong heterogeneity among the studies [120]. In a German cohort, weight gain during adulthood was inversely associated with leukocyte telomere length cross-sectionally, but there was no association between weight gain and change in telomere length over time. Looking at different compartments of adipose tissue, a German study that included 47 lean and 50 obese participants observed shorter telomere length in subcutaneous compared to visceral adipose tissue. Shorter telomere length in subcutaneous adipose tissue was entirely due to shorter telomere length in the stromal vascular fraction, compared to visceral adipose tissue [121]. A recent study in the Health Professionals Follow-up Study measured telomere length in cancer and benign cells of 596 prostate cancer patients. Overweight/obese men had 7.4% shorter telomeres in stromal cells than normal weight men. The least active men had shorter telomeres in stromal cells than more active men. Men who were overweight/obese and the least active had the shortest telomeres in stromal cells (20.7% shorter), compared with normal weight men who were the most active. Cancer cell telomere length and telomere length variability did not differ by measures of adiposity or activity [122]. The Copenhagen City Heart Study, which evaluated both cross-sectional and prospective associations, observed that short telomere leukocyte length was cross-sectionally associated with increased BMI, but change in telomere length over 10 years was not associated with BMI [75].

A wide range of **inflammatory markers** has been evaluated in the context of obesity. One of the most exhaustive studies so far was conducted within the Prostate, Lung, Ovarian and Colorectal Cancer Screening Trial [56]. Of 78 inflammation-related biomarkers, 12 were positively associated with BMI, including C-reactive protein (CRP) and soluble TNF receptor-II (sTNFR-II). However, no statistically significant associations were seen for IL-6 and IL-1Ra. In an analysis of the Framingham Heart Study, CRP and TNFRII were also associated with baseline BMI, whereas IL-6 was associated with waist circumference [123].

Vitamin D is widely discussed as a potential mediator of the association between obesity and cancer. In a meta-analysis of 12 observational studies, the random effects analyses showed a pooled RR of 1.52 (95% CI 1.33–1.73) for the association between low vitamin D status (<50 nmol/L) and obesity (BMI > 30 kg/m^2; OR = 1.52, 95% CI 1.33–1.73); however, the I^2 statistic suggested heterogeneity among the studies [124]. Different mechanisms might explain the inverse association between circulating vitamin D concentration and obesity. First, adipose tissue is considered a storage site for vitamin D, which is fat-soluble, leading to a lower blood concentration of vitamin D in individuals with higher fat mass [125]. Second, obese individuals less frequently engage in outdoor activities and/or may dress differently leading to lower endogenous vitamin D production [126].

Intervention Studies of Mediators of Energy Imbalance: Prostate Cancer Associations

The following section describes intervention studies for energy metabolism indicators aimed at altering any of the above-mentioned mediators of energy imbalance–prostate cancer associations. Interventions are categorized as diet or exercise interventions.

Diet Interventions

As we are interested in mediators of the energy imbalance–prostate cancer association, this section only focuses on calorie restriction diets. An overview of intervention studies published in the last 5 years is provided in Table 5.1, which summarizes the type of diet and the mediators investigated. The section below describes some of these studies in more detail.

Several of the mediators listed above have been studied together in a single intervention setting. For example, a study based on a 3-year long clinical intervention involving daily 100-kcal energy deficits for 122 overweight/obese participants observed that successful weight loss participants (reduction of at least 2 kg) exhibited significantly reduced **insulin**, **triglycerides, total and LDL cholesterol**, **free fatty acids**, and **leukocyte** count (P = 0.030) [127]. A small study based on 42 obese men and women who underwent eight weeks of (partial) formula diet (so that one meal per day was reduced to 300 kcal), showed significant decreases in levels of high-sensitive **CRP, IL-6, or TNF-α** [128]. Furthermore, serum IL-1β, IL-6, and urinary **PGF2α** were significantly reduced (45%, 30%, and 14%, respectively). In contrast, the unsuccessful weight loss group exhibited significant increases in percentage of body fat, waist circumference, oxidized LDL, and TNF-α, as well as a significant decrease in HDL. An 8-week intervention trial randomized 324 subjects to one of four energy-restricted diets (−30% relative to estimated requirements): salmon (3 × 150 g/week); cod (3 × 150 g/week); fish oil capsules (1.3 g/day); and control (sunflower oil capsules, no seafood). Overall, salmon consumption was most effective with a decrease in the following inflammation parameters: **high-sensitivity CRP**—32.0%; **IL-6**—18.4%; **prostaglandin F2 alpha**—18.5%; all P < 0.05. Cod consumption decreased high-sensitivity CRP and IL-6 (−21.5 and −10.8%, respectively, both P < 0.05). Changes in the other two groups were not significant [129].

Caloric restrictions have also been investigated with a focus on changes in **sex steroid hormones**. A dietary intervention with a very low calorie diet (800 kcal/day) for 12 weeks in 13 obese men was found to increase total testosterone (6.97 nmol/L to 13.21 nmol/L; P = 0.001) and SHBG (22.11–42.12 nmol/L; P = 0.001) concentrations in serum [130].

Additionally, **adiponectin** has been shown to be affected by dietary restriction. A 6 month behavioral intervention study comparing standard calorie- and fat-restricted diet and a calorie- and fat-restricted lacto-ovo-vegetarian diet including 143 overweight/obese adults showed that weight loss, irrespective of diet type, increased adiponectin levels [131]. Another study based on 82 health subjects showed that **leptin** levels decreased following a very low energy diet for 8 weeks [132].

Effects on **irisin** have been studied less. An intervention study based on 93 Caucasian adults diagnosed with metabolic syndrome showed depletion of irisin as well as serum lipid markers following an 8-week-long energy-restricted program [133].

To date no intervention study specifically focused on diet and **epigenetics** from a calorie restriction point of view. However, this is an area of interest as some studies in other fields have found promising results. For instance, Scoccianti et al. studied a group of 88 smokers randomly assigned to three diets: a normal isocaloric diet, a diet enriched in flavonoids and isothiocyanates, and a regimen consisting of a normal isocaloric diet supplemented with flavonoids (green tea and soy products) [134]. Three distinct patterns of methylation were observed, suggesting that the isocaloric diet may stabilize global epigenetic (LINE1 DNA methylation) patterns in peripheral white blood cells, but the study did not provide evidence for methylation changes in specific genes associated with this short-term dietary intervention [134].

Table 5.1 Overview of dietary intervention studies investigating effects on mediators of the energy imbalance-prostate cancer association

Study	Dietary intervention	Mediator studied
Acharya (2013) [131]	Standard calorie- and fat-restricted diet (STD-D) and a calorie- and fat-restricted lacto-ovo-vegetarian diet (LOV-D)	Adiponectin
Calbet (2014) [139]	Combining caloric restriction (CR: 3.2 kcal/kg body weight per day) with exercise (8-h walking + 45-min arm cranking per day) to induce an energy deficit of ~5000 kcal/day	IGF-1 Lipogenic pathway Sex steroid hormones Leptin
Camps (2015) [132]	Very low energy diet for 8 weeks	Leptin
Chae (2013) [127]	Daily 100-kcal calorie deficits	Lipogenic pathway Prostaglandin Inflammation
de la Iglesia (2014) [133]	8-week-long energy-restricted program (−30% of the energy requirements)	Lipogenic pathway Irisin
Hussain (2012) [140]	Low-carbohydrate ketogenic diet compared with the low-calorie diet	IGF-1 Lipogenic pathway
Goto (2014) [137]	Standard low-protein diet	Vitamin D
Ibero-Baraibar (2015) [136]	15% energy restricted diet for 4 weeks	Inflammation Vitamin D
Lecoultre (2011) [141]	Three forms of calorie restriction: 25% calorie restriction from baseline, same with exercise, or low calorie diet	Leptin
Moller (2015) [128]	(Partial) formula diet	Inflammation
Ornish (2013) [135]	Comprehensive lifestyle intervention	Telomere length
Ramel (2010) [129]	Four different energy restriction diets	Inflammation
Rock (2012) [138]	2-Year clinical trial of a weight-loss program	Vitamin D
Schulte (2014) [130]	Very low calorie diet (800 kcal/d) for 12 weeks	Sex steroid hormones
Tang (2013)	Prescribed weight-loss diet with 0.8 versus 1.4 g protein kg/day	IGF-1 Lipogenic pathway
Tapsell (2014) [142]	Two energy deficit healthy diet advice groups differing only by doubling the serving (portion) sizes of vegetables in the comparator group	IGF-1 Lipogenic pathway
Rezaeipour (2014) [143]	Negative calorie and low calorie diet with exercise	Lipogenic pathway
Ruth (2013) [144]	High fat, low carbohydrate diet compared to low fat high carbohydrate diet	IGF-1 Lipogenic pathway Adiponectin Inflammation

To our knowledge, only one pilot intervention study investigated how energy restriction affects **telomere length** [135]. Based on ten men in the intervention group (comprehensive lifestyle changes related to diet, activity, stress management, and social support) and 25 men in the control group, the intervention was associated with an increase in relative telomere length after 5 years of follow-up. These results point towards the need for larger randomized controlled trials.

Vitamin D has been investigated substantially in the context of obesity [124], however most intervention studies to date focus on the effects of vitamin D supplementation as an intervention rather than vitamin D levels as an outcome. A randomized study by Ibero-Baraibar et al. found that serum levels of vitamin D increased following a 15% energy-restricted diet for 4 weeks [136], whereas levels of markers of inflammation such as CRP, TNF-α, and IL-6 decreased. Another study evaluating the effects of a standard low-protein diet on 1,25-dihydroxyvitamin D levels in patients with early (n = 15) and advanced (n = 20) chronic kidney disease observed that the intervention increased levels in the early group, but decreased levels the advanced group [137]. Rock and colleagues assessed data from 383 overweight or obese women who participated in a 2-year clinical trial of a weight-loss program, in which 51% lost at least 5% of baseline weight by 24 months, 18% lost 5–10%, and 33% lost >10% [138]. By study end, 64% of overweight or obese women had recommended serum vitamin D concentrations of 20 ng/mL as well as 83% of those whose weight loss achieved a normal BMI. These findings suggest that weight loss is associated with increased serum vitamin D concentration in overweight or obese women.

Exercise Interventions

An overview of exercise intervention studies published in the last 5 years is provided in Table 5.2, summarizing the type of exercise and the mediators investigated. The section below describes some of these studies in more detail.

With respect to insulin, a meta-analysis synthesized the **insulin sensitivity** outcomes of supervised exercise interventions [145] using 78 reports and reported that the exercise intervention lead to a higher mean insulin sensitivity. Numerous studies have also reported that aerobic exercise reduces **serum lipid levels** such total and LDL cholesterol and increases HDL cholesterol [146–150].

Even though **prostaglandins** are suggested to be a mediator for the link between energy and prostate cancer, no exercise intervention studies have yet investigated effects on prostate tissue. For colon mucosa, no difference in mean prostaglandin concentrations in tissue between exercisers and controls was found in a 12-month randomized controlled trial (RCT) [151]. In contrast, an RCT based on 41 men and 22 women investigating concentrations of prostaglandin E2 in rectal mucosa found that higher BMI was associated with higher prostaglandin E2 levels and higher levels of leisure-time physical activity were inversely associated with prostaglandin E2 levels [98].

Table 5.2 Overview of exercise intervention studies investigating effects on mediators of the energy imbalance–prostate cancer association

Study	Exercise intervention	Mediator studied
Ackel-D'Elia (2014) [156]	Leisure physical activity, aerobic training and aerobic training plus resistance training	Leptin
Beavers (2013) [157, 164]	Control group, physical activity group, and physical activity and diet group	Inflammation
Cameron (2016) [158]	Acute 3-d isocaloric 25% energy depletion by dieting alone or by aerobic exercise alone	Leptin
Chan (2012) [163]	Exercise and nutrition, problem solving, and control arm	Vitamin D
Chow (2015) [150]	Tobacco, Exercise and Diet Messages (TEXT ME) trial	Lipogenic pathway
Conn (2014) [145]	Meta-analysis of supervised exercise interventions	Insulin
Gordon (2014) [146]	Aerobic exercise	Lipogenic pathway
Jakicic (2015) [148]	Six-month behavioural weight loss intervention that included weekly group sessions, a prescribed energy-restricted diet, and moderate to vigorous physical activity	Lipogenic pathway
Khoo (2013) [154]	Low volume and high volume moderate-intensity exercise	Sex steroid hormones
Kim (2015) [161]	Elastic band exercise program consisted of 12 weeks of 1-h session 2 days per week	Irisin
Lima (2015) [159]	Aerobic training and aerobic plus resistance training on the plasma levels of interleukin-6 (IL-6) and tumor necrosis factor alpha (TNF-α) of elderly hypertensive subjects	Inflammation
Maclaren (1995) [152]	90 min of treadmill running	Vasoactive Intestinal Peptide
Mendham (2014) [165]	Cycling, small-sided games, or sedentary control for 8 weeks	Inflammation
Monteiro (2015) [147]	Two randomized training groups, concurrent or aerobic, for 20 weeks	Lipogenic pathway
Sjogren (2014) [162]	The intervention group received individualized physical activity on prescription	Telomere length
Stoke (2013) [155]	Resistance, spring and endurance exercise	Sex steroid hormones
Tapsell (2015) [149]	12 month randomised controlled trial testing effects of a novel interdisciplinary lifestyle intervention versus usual care	Lipogenic pathway
Qiu (2015) [160]	Meta-analysis of chronic exercise training	Irisin

VIP has also been studied as a marker in exercise RCTs. A small study based on six male endurance runners and six male hockey players evaluated plasma VIP levels before and after 90 min of treadmill running and observed significant increases [152]. However, no other studies have investigated in detail the effects of physical activity on VIP levels.

With respect to **sex steroid hormones**, a recent RCT found no effect of lifelong training history on serum testosterone, cortisol, and SHBG when comparing 20 lifelong exercising males with 28 age-matched lifelong sedentary individuals [153]. However, another RCT comparing the effects of low volume and high volume moderate-intensity exercise among 90 men abdominally obese, sedentary Asian men only found an increase in testosterone for those in the high volume group (2.06 ± 0.46 nmol/L) [154]. These differences may be potentially due to the differences in type of exercise, as already suggested following another study investigating hormone responses to resistance, spring and endurance exercise in eight young men using a repeated measures design in which each subject served as his own control. The nature and magnitude of the hormone response were influenced by exercise type. For instance, only endurance and sprint exercise increased growth hormone, cortisol, prolactin and testosterone. Resistance exercise only increased testosterone and glucose [155].

Seventy two German obese adolescents randomized to leisure physical activity, aerobic training and aerobic training plus resistance training found a reduction in leptin levels for both aerobic training arms [156]. The already stated effect of a combination of physical activity and weight loss was also observed in a study from North Carolina measuring adiponectin, leptin, high-sensitivity interleukin (hsIL)-6, IL-6sR, IL-8, and soluble TNFR between a control group, physical activity group, and physical activity and diet group [157]. The combination of diet and physical activity reduced leptin and hsIL-6 levels more than physical activity alone. Another recent study based on ten male participants in a randomized crossover study of acute 3-day isocaloric 25% energy depletion by dieting alone or by aerobic exercise alone showed no changes in plasma concentrations of leptin over time [158]. Finally, an RCT based on 44 volunteers aged 60–75 studied changes in inflammatory blood markers over 10 weeks in an aerobic group, resistance plus aerobic group and control group. After the intervention, IL-6 was reduced in the aerobic group compared to the control group ($p = 0.04$), and TNF-α levels were lower only in the resistance plus aerobic group compared to the control group ($P = 0.01$) [159].

Exercise has also been found to reduce levels of **irisin**. A recent meta-analysis evaluated the effects of chronic exercise training on circulating irisin in adults. Three randomized controlled trials (RCTs) showed that chronic exercise training moderately and statistically significantly decreased circulating irisin level ($d = -0.46$; 95% CI −0.76 to −0.15) [160]. A more recent RCT based on female 50 participants over 65 years old found that resistance training might be an efficient intervention to increase irisin levels [161].

To our knowledge no intervention study has investigated the effects of exercise on **epigenetics**. Its effects on **telomere length** have been studied in one study that measured blood cells 6 months apart in 49 68-year-old, sedentary, overweight individuals taking part in a randomized controlled physical activity intervention trial [162]. Reduced sitting time was associated with telomere lengthening in blood cells in this sedentary population.

Finally, many studies have investigated the effects of **vitamin D** supplements on wellbeing, but few studies have focused on the effects of exercise on circulating vitamin D levels. A Taiwanese study based on 117 adults aged 65–79 years compared an exercise and nutrition arm and a problem-solving therapy arm to controls [163]. Those in the exercise and nutrition arm had larger increase in serum 25(OH) vitamin D levels than the other two groups (P = 0.006).

Conclusion

Despite a wide variety of both cross-sectional and intervention studies available, findings are rather inconsistent for most of the proposed mediators of the energy imbalance-prostate cancer association. General patterns from observational and/or intervention studies include potentially beneficial associations/effects of energy balance on insulin levels and lipid metabolism, inflammation, and irisin. Study results are inconsistent for energy balance and sex steroid hormones, leptin, and adiponectin. Few studies have been conducted on the link between energy balance and prostaglandins and VIP. Epigenetics and telomere length are emerging areas of research potentially influenced by energy balance with promising results from intervention studies. Despite the potentially beneficial health effects of vitamin D, few studies have investigated how reducing energy imbalance may affect its circulating levels.

Hence, there is a need for a standardized way of reviewing the vast amount of research on the biological processes (or mechanisms) underlying the effects of lifestyle factors on prostate cancer risk. The ongoing "Mechanisms research project" of the World Cancer Research Fund and the University of Bristol will in the future help us collate and review such research [166]. The teams are pioneering a new groundbreaking method of identifying mechanisms by which lifestyle factors cancer cause cancer in a comprehensive and systematic way. It involves a new online tool to automate the process and enable hundreds of thousands of studies to be identified and sifted. It will allow researchers to identify mechanistic studies on a specific exposure and outcome. The methods are currently being tested by researchers in the Netherlands and Germany, with a full validation study expected to take place next year [166].

References

1. Dimitriadis G, Mitrou P, Lambadiari V, Maratou E, Raptis SA. Insulin effects in muscle and adipose tissue. Diabetes Res Clin Pract. 2011;93(Suppl 1):S52–9.
2. Khandwala HM, McCutcheon IE, Flyvbjerg A, Friend KE. The effects of insulin-like growth factors on tumorigenesis and neoplastic growth. Endocr Rev. 2000;21(3):215–44.
3. Jones JI, Clemmons DR. Insulin-like growth factors and their binding proteins: biological actions. Endocr Rev. 1995;16(1):3–34.
4. Lai GY, Helzlsouer KJ, Clipp SL, Rifai N, Platz EA. Association between C-peptide concentration and prostate cancer incidence in the CLUE II Cohort Study. Cancer Prev Res. 2010;3(10):1334–41.

5. Lai GY, Giovannucci EL, Pollak MN, Peskoe SB, Stampfer MJ, Willett WC, et al. Association of C-peptide and leptin with prostate cancer incidence in the Health Professionals Follow-up Study. Cancer Causes Control. 2014;25(5):625–32.
6. Stevens VL, Jacobs EJ, Sun J, Gapstur SM. No association of plasma levels of adiponectin and c-peptide with risk of aggressive prostate cancer in the Cancer Prevention Study II Nutrition Cohort. Cancer Epidemiol Biomarkers Prev. 2014;23(5):890–2.
7. Neuhouser ML, Till C, Kristal A, Goodman P, Hoque A, Platz EA, et al. Finasteride modifies the relation between serum C-peptide and prostate cancer risk: results from the Prostate Cancer Prevention Trial. Cancer Prev Res (Phila). 2010;3(3):279–89.
8. Travis RC, Appleby PN, Martin RM, Holly JM, Albanes D, Black A, et al. A meta-analysis of individual participant data reveals an association between circulating levels of IGF-I and prostate cancer risk. Cancer Res. 2016;76(8):2288–300.
9. Liu H, Liu JY, Wu X, Zhang JT. Biochemistry, molecular biology, and pharmacology of fatty acid synthase, an emerging therapeutic target and diagnosis/prognosis marker. Int J Biochem Mol Biol. 2010;1(1):69–89.
10. Swinnen JV, Vanderhoydonc F, Elgamal AA, Eelen M, Vercaeren I, Joniau S, et al. Selective activation of the fatty acid synthesis pathway in human prostate cancer. Int J Cancer. 2000;88(2):176–9.
11. Shurbaji MS, Kalbfleisch JH, Thurmond TS. Immunohistochemical detection of a fatty acid synthase (OA-519) as a predictor of progression of prostate cancer. Hum Pathol. 1996;27(9):917–21.
12. Takahiro T, Shinichi K, Toshimitsu S. Expression of fatty acid synthase as a prognostic indicator in soft tissue sarcomas. Clin Cancer Res. 2003;9(6):2204–12.
13. Zadra G, Photopoulos C, Loda M. The fat side of prostate cancer. Biochim Biophys Acta. 2013;1831(10):1518–32.
14. Suburu J, Chen YQ. Lipids and prostate cancer. Prostaglandins Other Lipid Mediat. 2012;98(1-2):1–10.
15. Arthur R, Rodriguez-Vida A, Zadra G, Moller H, Van Hemelrijck M. Serum lipids as markers of prostate cancer occurrence and prognosis? Clin Lipidol. 2015;10(2):145–65.
16. Yao YS, Li J, Jin YL, Chen Y, He LP. Association between PPAR-gamma2 Pro12Ala polymorphism and obesity: a meta-analysis. Mol Biol Rep. 2015;42(6):1029–38.
17. Ali AT, Hochfeld WE, Myburgh R, Pepper MS. Adipocyte and adipogenesis. Eur J Cell Biol. 2013;92(6-7):229–36.
18. Vu JP, Larauche M, Flores M, Luong L, Norris J, Oh S, et al. Regulation of appetite, body composition, and metabolic hormones by vasoactive intestinal polypeptide (VIP). J Mol Neurosci. 2015;56(2):377–87.
19. Veljkovic M, Dopsaj V, Dopsaj M, Branch DR, Veljkovic N, Sakarellos-Daitsiotis MM, et al. Physical activity and natural anti-VIP antibodies: potential role in breast and prostate cancer therapy. PLoS One. 2011;6(11):e28304.
20. Reubi JC, Laderach U, Waser B, Gebbers JO, Robberecht P, Laissue JA. Vasoactive intestinal peptide/pituitary adenylate cyclase-activating peptide receptor subtypes in human tumors and their tissues of origin. Cancer Res. 2000;60(11):3105–12.
21. Moody TW, Nuche-Berenguer B, Jensen RT. Vasoactive intestinal peptide/pituitary adenylate cyclase activating polypeptide, and their receptors and cancer. Curr Opin Endocrinol Diabetes Obes. 2016;23(1):38–47.
22. Endogenous Hormones and Prostate Cancer Collaborative Group, Roddam AW, Allen NE, Appleby P, Key TJ. Endogenous sex hormones and prostate cancer: a collaborative analysis of 18 prospective studies. J Natl Cancer Inst. 2008;100(3):170–83.
23. Michalakis K, Mintziori G, Kaprara A, Tarlatzis BC, Goulis DG. The complex interaction between obesity, metabolic syndrome and reproductive axis: a narrative review. Metabolism. 2013;62(4):457–78.
24. Baillargeon J, Rose DP. Obesity, adipokines, and prostate cancer (review). Int J Oncol. 2006;28(3):737–45.

25. Paz-Filho G, Lim EL, Wong ML, Licinio J. Associations between adipokines and obesity-related cancer. Front Biosci (Landmark Ed). 2011;16:1634–50.
26. Provatopoulou X, Georgiou GP, Kalogera E, Kalles V, Matiatou MA, Papapanagiotou I, et al. Serum irisin levels are lower in patients with breast cancer: association with disease diagnosis and tumor characteristics. BMC Cancer. 2015;15(1):898.
27. Labbe DP, Zadra G, Ebot EM, Mucci LA, Kantoff PW, Loda M, et al. Role of diet in prostate cancer: the epigenetic link. Oncogene. 2015;34(36):4683–91.
28. Keating ST, El-Osta A. Epigenetics and metabolism. Circ Res. 2015;116(4):715–36.
29. Julin B, Shui I, Heaphy CM, Joshu CE, Meeker AK, Giovannucci E, et al. Circulating leukocyte telomere length and risk of overall and aggressive prostate cancer. Br J Cancer. 2015;112(4):769–76.
30. Mirabello L, Huang W-Y, Wong JYY, Chatterjee N, Reding D, David Crawford E, et al. The association between leukocyte telomere length and cigarette smoking, dietary and physical variables, and risk of prostate cancer. Aging Cell. 2009;8(4):405–13.
31. Weischer M, Nordestgaard BG, Cawthon RM, Freiberg JJ, Tybjaerg-Hansen A, Bojesen SE. Short telomere length, cancer survival, and cancer risk in 47102 individuals. J Natl Cancer Inst. 2013;105(7):459–68.
32. Anderson AS, Key TJ, Norat T, Scoccianti C, Cecchini M, Berrino F, et al. European code against cancer 4th Edition: obesity, body fatness and cancer. Cancer Epidemiol. 2015;39(Suppl 1):S34–45.
33. Shivappa N, Bosetti C, Zucchetto A, Montella M, Serraino D, La Vecchia C, et al. Association between dietary inflammatory index and prostate cancer among Italian men. Br J Nutr. 2014;17:1–6.
34. Deeb KK, Trump DL, Johnson CS. Vitamin D signalling pathways in cancer: potential for anticancer therapeutics. Nat Rev Cancer. 2007;7(9):684–700.
35. Fraser DR. Vitamin D deficiency and energy metabolism. Endocrinology. 2015;156(6):1933–5.
36. Giovannucci E, Pollak M, Liu Y, Platz EA, Majeed N, Rimm EB, et al. Nutritional predictors of insulin-like growth factor I and their relationships to cancer in men. Cancer Epidemiol Biomarkers Prev. 2003;12(2):84–9.
37. DeLellis K, Rinaldi S, Kaaks RJ, Kolonel LN, Henderson B, Le Marchand L. Dietary and lifestyle correlates of plasma insulin-like growth factor-I (IGF-I) and IGF binding protein-3 (IGFBP-3): the multiethnic cohort. Cancer Epidemiol Biomarkers Prev. 2004;13(9):1444–51.
38. Crowe FL, Key TJ, Allen NE, Appleby PN, Roddam A, Overvad K, et al. The association between diet and serum concentrations of IGF-I, IGFBP-1, IGFBP-2, and IGFBP-3 in the European Prospective Investigation into Cancer and Nutrition. Cancer Epidemiol Biomarkers Prev. 2009;18(5):1333–40.
39. Probst-Hensch NM, Wang H, Goh VH, Seow A, Lee HP, Yu MC. Determinants of circulating insulin-like growth factor I and insulin-like growth factor binding protein 3 concentrations in a cohort of Singapore men and women. Cancer Epidemiol Biomarkers Prev. 2003;12(8):739–46.
40. Tamimi R, Mucci LA, Spanos E, Lagiou A, Benetou V, Trichopoulos D. Testosterone and oestradiol in relation to tobacco smoking, body mass index, energy consumption and nutrient intake among adult men. Eur J Cancer Prev. 2001;10(3):275–80.
41. Allen NE, Appleby PN, Davey GK, Key TJ. Lifestyle and nutritional determinants of bioavailable androgens and related hormones in British men. Cancer Causes Control. 2002;13(4):353–63.
42. Chu NF, Stampfer MJ, Spiegelman D, Rifai N, Hotamisligil GS, Rimm EB. Dietary and lifestyle factors in relation to plasma leptin concentrations among normal weight and overweight men. Int J Obes Relat Metab Disord. 2001;25(1):106–14.
43. DeLellis HK, Rinaldi S, Kaaks R, Kolonel L, Henderson B, Le Marchand L. Lifestyle and dietary correlates of plasma insulin-like growth factor binding protein-1 (IGFBP-1), leptin, and C-peptide: the Multiethnic Cohort. Nutr Cancer. 2007;58(2):136–45.

44. Nakamura Y, Ueshima H, Okuda N, Murakami Y, Miura K, Kita Y, et al. Serum leptin and total dietary energy intake: the INTERLIPID Study. Eur J Nutr. 2013;52(6):1641–8.
45. Yannakoulia M, Yiannakouris N, Bluher S, Matalas AL, Klimis-Zacas D, Mantzoros CS. Body fat mass and macronutrient intake in relation to circulating soluble leptin receptor, free leptin index, adiponectin, and resistin concentrations in healthy humans. J Clin Endocrinol Metab. 2003;88(4):1730–6.
46. Pischon T, Girman CJ, Rifai N, Hotamisligil GS, Rimm EB. Association between dietary factors and plasma adiponectin concentrations in men. Am J Clin Nutr. 2005;81(4):780–6.
47. Park KH, Zaichenko L, Peter P, Davis CR, Crowell JA, Mantzoros CS. Diet quality is associated with circulating C-reactive protein but not irisin levels in humans. Metabolism. 2014;63(2):233–41.
48. Kark JD, Goldberger N, Kimura M, Sinnreich R, Aviv A. Energy intake and leukocyte telomere length in young adults. Am J Clin Nutr. 2012;95(2):479–87.
49. Bunout D, Barrera G, de la Maza MP, Leiva L, Hirsch S. Effect of weight maintenance or gain in a 10 years period over telomere length, sirtuin 1 and 6 expression and carotid intima media thickness. J Hum Nutr Diet. 2015;28(2):155–64.
50. Zhang FF, Morabia A, Carroll J, Gonzalez K, Fulda K, Kaur M, et al. Dietary patterns are associated with levels of global genomic DNA methylation in a cancer-free population. J Nutr. 2011;141(6):1165–71.
51. Austin GL, Krueger PM. Increasing the percentage of energy from dietary sugar, fats, and alcohol in adults is associated with increased energy intake but has minimal association with biomarkers of cardiovascular risk. J Nutr. 2013;143(10):1651–8.
52. Li Y, Meng L, Miao Q, Sato Y. Association between physical activity and serum C-peptide levels among the elderly. Geriatr Gerontol Int. 2014;14(3):647–53.
53. Feskens EJ, Loeber JG, Kromhout D. Diet and physical activity as determinants of hyperinsulinemia: the Zutphen Elderly Study. Am J Epidemiol. 1994;140(4):350–60.
54. Fung TT, Hu FB, Yu J, Chu NF, Spiegelman D, Tofler GH, et al. Leisure-time physical activity, television watching, and plasma biomarkers of obesity and cardiovascular disease risk. Am J Epidemiol. 2000;152(12):1171–8.
55. Pischon T, Hankinson SE, Hotamisligil GS, Rifai N, Rimm EB. Leisure-time physical activity and reduced plasma levels of obesity-related inflammatory markers. Obes Res. 2003;11(9):1055–64.
56. Kitahara CM, Trabert B, Katki HA, Chaturvedi AK, Kemp TJ, Pinto LA, et al. Body mass index, physical activity, and serum markers of inflammation, immunity, and insulin resistance. Cancer Epidemiol Biomarkers Prev. 2014;23(12):2840–9.
57. Wolff-Hughes DL, Fitzhugh EC, Bassett DR, Churilla JR. Total activity counts and bouted minutes of moderate-to-vigorous physical activity: relationships with cardiometabolic biomarkers using 2003–2006 NHANES. J Phys Act Health. 2015;12(5):694–700.
58. Howard B, Winkler EA, Sethi P, Carson V, Ridgers ND, Salmon JO, et al. Associations of low- and high-intensity light activity with cardiometabolic biomarkers. Med Sci Sports Exerc. 2015;47(10):2093–101.
59. Maarbjerg SJ, Sylow L, Richter EA. Current understanding of increased insulin sensitivity after exercise—emerging candidates. Acta Physiol (Oxf). 2011;202(3):323–35.
60. Gapstur SM, Kopp P, Chiu BC, Gann PH, Colangelo LA, Liu K. Longitudinal associations of age, anthropometric and lifestyle factors with serum total insulin-like growth factor-I and IGF binding protein-3 levels in Black and White men: the CARDIA Male Hormone Study. Cancer Epidemiol Biomarkers Prev. 2004;13(12):2208–16.
61. Glaser S, Friedrich N, Ewert R, Schaper C, Krebs A, Dorr M, et al. Association of circulating IGF-I and IGFBP-3 concentrations and exercise capacity in healthy volunteers: results of the Study of Health in Pomerania. Growth Horm IGF Res. 2010;20(6):404–10.
62. Berg A, Halle M, Franz I, Keul J. Physical activity and lipoprotein metabolism: epidemiological evidence and clinical trials. Eur J Med Res. 1997;2(6):259–64.
63. O'Donovan G, Kearney E, Sherwood R, Hillsdon M. Fatness, fitness, and cardiometabolic risk factors in middle-aged white men. Metabolism. 2012;61(2):213–20.

64. Goldberg AP, Busby-Whitehead MJ, Katzel LI, Krauss RM, Lumpkin M, Hagberg JM. Cardiovascular fitness, body composition, and lipoprotein lipid metabolism in older men. J Gerontol A Biol Sci Med Sci. 2000;55(6):M342–9.
65. Shiels MS, Rohrmann S, Menke A, Selvin E, Crespo CJ, Rifai N, et al. Association of cigarette smoking, alcohol consumption, and physical activity with sex steroid hormone levels in US men. Cancer Causes Control. 2009;20(6):877–86.
66. Steeves JA, Fitzhugh EC, Bradwin G, McGlynn KA, Platz EA, Joshu CE. Cross-sectional association between physical activity and serum testosterone levels in US men: results from NHANES 1999–2004. Andrology 2016;4(3):465-472.
67. Priskorn L, Jensen TK, Bang AK, Nordkap L, Joensen UN, Lassen TH, et al. Is sedentary lifestyle associated with testicular function? A cross-sectional study of 1,210 men. Am J Epidemiol. 2016;184(4):284–94.
68. Wannamethee SG, Tchernova J, Whincup P, Lowe GD, Kelly A, Rumley A, et al. Plasma leptin: associations with metabolic, inflammatory and haemostatic risk factors for cardiovascular disease. Atherosclerosis. 2007;191(2):418–26.
69. Folsom AR, Jensen MD, Jacobs DR Jr, Hilner JE, Tsai AW, Schreiner PJ. Serum leptin and weight gain over 8 years in African American and Caucasian young adults. Obes Res. 1999;7(1):1–8.
70. Donahue RP, Zimmet P, Bean JA, Decourten M, DeCarlo Donahue RA, Collier G, et al. Cigarette smoking, alcohol use, and physical activity in relation to serum leptin levels in a multiethnic population: The Miami Community Health Study. Ann Epidemiol. 1999;9(2):108–13.
71. Miyatake N, Numata T, Murakami H, Kawakami R, Sanada K, Tabata I, et al. Circulating adiponectin levels are associated with peak oxygen uptake in Japanese. Environ Health Prev Med. 2014;19(4):279–85.
72. Tsukinoki R, Morimoto K, Nakayama K. Association between lifestyle factors and plasma adiponectin levels in Japanese men. Lipids Health Dis. 2005;4:27.
73. Moreno M, Moreno-Navarrete JM, Serrano M, Ortega F, Delgado E, Sanchez-Ragnarsson C, et al. Circulating irisin levels are positively associated with metabolic risk factors in sedentary subjects. PLoS One. 2015;10(4):e0124100.
74. Mundstock E, Zatti H, Louzada FM, Oliveira SG, Guma FT, Paris MM, et al. Effects of physical activity in telomere length: systematic review and meta-analysis. Ageing Res Rev. 2015;22:72–80.
75. Weischer M, Bojesen SE, Nordestgaard BG. Telomere shortening unrelated to smoking, body weight, physical activity, and alcohol intake: 4,576 general population individuals with repeat measurements 10 years apart. PLoS Genet. 2014;10(3):e1004191.
76. Wanner M, Richard A, Martin B, Linseisen J, Rohrmann S. Associations between objective and self-reported physical activity and vitamin D serum levels in the US population. Cancer Causes Control. 2015;26(6):881–91.
77. Touvier M, Deschasaux M, Montourcy M, Sutton A, Charnaux N, Kesse-Guyot E, et al. Determinants of vitamin D status in Caucasian adults: influence of sun exposure, dietary intake, sociodemographic, lifestyle, anthropometric, and genetic factors. J Invest Dermatol. 2015;135(2):378–88.
78. Brock K, Huang WY, Fraser DR, Ke L, Tseng M, Stolzenberg-Solomon R, et al. Low vitamin D status is associated with physical inactivity, obesity and low vitamin D intake in a large US sample of healthy middle-aged men and women. J Steroid Biochem Mol Biol. 2010;121(1-2):462–6.
79. Maimoun L, Sultan C. Effect of physical activity on calcium homeostasis and calciotropic hormones: a review. Calcif Tissue Int. 2009;85(4):277–86.
80. Haffner SM, Mykkanen L, Stern MP, Valdez RA, Heisserman JA, Bowsher RR. Relationship of proinsulin and insulin to cardiovascular risk factors in nondiabetic subjects. Diabetes. 1993;42(9):1297–302.
81. Seidell JC, Perusse L, Despres JP, Bouchard C. Waist and hip circumferences have independent and opposite effects on cardiovascular disease risk factors: the Quebec Family Study. Am J Clin Nutr. 2001;74(3):315–21.

82. Hanley AJ, McKeown-Eyssen G, Harris SB, Hegele RA, Wolever TM, Kwan J, et al. Cross-sectional and prospective associations between abdominal adiposity and proinsulin concentration. J Clin Endocrinol Metab. 2002;87(1):77–83.
83. Parekh N, Roberts CB, Vadiveloo M, Puvananayagam T, Albu JB, Lu-Yao GL. Lifestyle, anthropometric, and obesity-related physiologic determinants of insulin-like growth factor-1 in the Third National Health and Nutrition Examination Survey (1988–1994). Ann Epidemiol. 2010;20(3):182–93.
84. Crowe FL, Key TJ, Allen NE, Appleby PN, Overvad K, Gronbaek H, et al. A cross-sectional analysis of the associations between adult height, BMI and serum concentrations of IGF-I and IGFBP-1 -2 and -3 in the European Prospective Investigation into Cancer and Nutrition (EPIC). Ann Hum Biol. 2010 Aug 23.
85. Lukanova A, Soderberg S, Stattin P, Palmqvist R, Lundin E, Biessy C, et al. Nonlinear relationship of insulin-like growth factor (IGF)-I and IGF-I/IGF-binding protein-3 ratio with indices of adiposity and plasma insulin concentrations (Sweden). Cancer Causes Control. 2002;13(6):509–16.
86. Friedrich N, Thuesen B, Jorgensen T, Juul A, Spielhagen C, Wallaschofksi H, et al. The association between IGF-I and insulin resistance: a general population study in Danish adults. Diabetes Care. 2012;35(4):768–73.
87. Friedrich N, Rosskopf D, Brabant G, Volzke H, Nauck M, Wallaschofski H. Associations of anthropometric parameters with serum TSH, prolactin, IGF-I, and testosterone levels: results of the Study of Health in POMERANIA (SHIP). Exp Clin Endocrinol Diabetes. 2010;118(4):266–73.
88. Schoen RE, Schragin J, Weissfeld JL, Thaete FL, Evans RW, Rosen CJ, et al. Lack of association between adipose tissue distribution and IGF-1 and IGFBP-3 in men and women. Cancer Epidemiol Biomarkers Prev. 2002;11(6):581–6.
89. Howard BV, Ruotolo G, Robbins DC. Obesity and dyslipidemia. Endocrinol Metab Clin North Am. 2003;32(4):855–67.
90. Franssen R, Monajemi H, Stroes ES, Kastelein JJ. Obesity and dyslipidemia. Endocrinol Metab Clin North Am. 2008;37(3):623–33. viii
91. Kovacs P, Harper I, Hanson RL, Infante AM, Bogardus C, Tataranni PA, et al. A novel missense substitution (Val1483Ile) in the fatty acid synthase gene (FAS) is associated with percentage of body fat and substrate oxidation rates in nondiabetic Pima Indians. Diabetes. 2004;53(7):1915–9.
92. Korner A, Ma L, Franks PW, Kiess W, Baier LJ, Stumvoll M, et al. Sex-specific effect of the Val1483Ile polymorphism in the fatty acid synthase gene (FAS) on body mass index and lipid profile in Caucasian children. Int J Obes (Lond). 2007;31(2):353–8.
93. Campa D, Husing A, Chang-Claude J, Dostal L, Boeing H, Kroger J, et al. Genetic variability of the fatty acid synthase pathway is not associated with prostate cancer risk in the European Prospective Investigation on Cancer (EPIC). Eur J Cancer. 2011;47(3):420–7.
94. Nguyen PL, Ma J, Chavarro JE, Freedman ML, Lis R, Fedele G, et al. Fatty acid synthase polymorphisms, tumor expression, body mass index, prostate cancer risk, and survival. J Clin Oncol. 2010;28(25):3958–64.
95. Berndt J, Kovacs P, Ruschke K, Kloting N, Fasshauer M, Schon MR, et al. Fatty acid synthase gene expression in human adipose tissue: association with obesity and type 2 diabetes. Diabetologia. 2007;50(7):1472–80.
96. Urakawa H, Katsuki A, Sumida Y, Gabazza EC, Murashima S, Morioka K, et al. Oxidative stress is associated with adiposity and insulin resistance in men. J Clin Endocrinol Metab. 2003;88(10):4673–6.
97. Fujita K, Nishizawa H, Funahashi T, Shimomura I, Shimabukuro M. Systemic oxidative stress is associated with visceral fat accumulation and the metabolic syndrome. Circ J. 2006;70(11):1437–42.
98. Martinez ME, Heddens D, Earnest DL, Bogert CL, Roe D, Einspahr J, et al. Physical activity, body mass index, and prostaglandin E2 levels in rectal mucosa. J Natl Cancer Inst. 1999;91(11):950–3.

99. Costabile G, Della Pepa G, Bozzetto L, Annuzzi G, Vetrani C, Giacco R, et al. Urine 8-isoprostane in relation to adiposity and insulin resistance in individuals at high cardiometabolic risk. Metab Syndr Relat Disord. 2015;13(4):187–91.
100. Liu YJ, Guo YF, Zhang LS, Pei YF, Yu N, Yu P, et al. Biological pathway-based genome-wide association analysis identified the vasoactive intestinal peptide (VIP) pathway important for obesity. Obesity (Silver Spring). 2010;18(12):2339–46.
101. MacDonald AA, Herbison GP, Showell M, Farquhar CM. The impact of body mass index on semen parameters and reproductive hormones in human males: a systematic review with meta-analysis. Hum Reprod Update. 2010;16(3):293–311.
102. Trabert B, Graubard BI, Nyante SJ, Rifai N, Bradwin G, Platz EA, et al. Relationship of sex steroid hormones with body size and with body composition measured by dual-energy X-ray absorptiometry in US men. Cancer Causes Control. 2012;23(12):1881–91.
103. Rohrmann S, Shiels MS, Lopez DS, Rifai N, Nelson WG, Kanarek N, et al. Body fatness and sex steroid hormone concentrations in US men: results from NHANES III. Cancer Causes Control. 2011;22(8):1141–51.
104. Gates MA, Mekary RA, Chiu GR, Ding EL, Wittert GA, Araujo AB. Sex steroid hormone levels and body composition in men. J Clin Endocrinol Metab. 2013;98(6):2442–50.
105. Ostlund RE Jr, Yang JW, Klein S, Gingerich R. Relation between plasma leptin concentration and body fat, gender, diet, age, and metabolic covariates. J Clin Endocrinol Metab. 1996;81(11):3909–13.
106. Shimizu H, Shimomura Y, Hayashi R, Ohtani K, Sato N, Futawatari T, et al. Serum leptin concentration is associated with total body fat mass, but not abdominal fat distribution. Int J Obes Relat Metab Disord. 1997;21(7):536–41.
107. Johannsson G, Karlsson C, Lonn L, Marin P, Bjorntorp P, Sjostrom L, et al. Serum leptin concentration and insulin sensitivity in men with abdominal obesity. Obes Res. 1998;6(6):416–21.
108. Kotani K, Sakane N, Saiga K, Kato M, Ishida K, Kato Y, et al. Serum adiponectin levels and lifestyle factors in Japanese men. Heart Vessels. 2007;22(5):291–6.
109. Vilarrasa N, Vendrell J, Maravall J, Broch M, Estepa A, Megia A, et al. Distribution and determinants of adiponectin, resistin and ghrelin in a randomly selected healthy population. Clin Endocrinol (Oxf). 2005;63(3):329–35.
110. Choi KM, Lee J, Lee KW, Seo JA, Oh JH, Kim SG, et al. The associations between plasma adiponectin, ghrelin levels and cardiovascular risk factors. Eur J Endocrinol. 2004;150(5):715–8.
111. Chu NF, Spiegelman D, Yu J, Rifai N, Hotamisligil GS, Rimm EB. Plasma leptin concentrations and four-year weight gain among US men. Int J Obes Relat Metab Disord. 2001;25(3):346–53.
112. Arawaka N, Daimon M, Oizumi T, Jimbu Y, Kameda W, Yamaguchi H, et al. Correlation between change in body weight rather than current body weight and change in serum adiponectin levels in a Japanese population—The Funagata Study. Metabolism. 2006;55(3):324–30.
113. Langenberg C, Bergstrom J, Laughlin GA, Barrett-Connor E. Ghrelin, adiponectin, and leptin do not predict long-term changes in weight and body mass index in older adults: longitudinal analysis of the Rancho Bernardo Cohort. Am J Epidemiol. 2005;162(12):1189–97.
114. Stengel A, Hofmann T, Goebel-Stengel M, Elbelt U, Kobelt P, Klapp BF. Circulating levels of irisin in patients with anorexia nervosa and different stages of obesity—correlation with body mass index. Peptides. 2013;39:125–30.
115. Huh JY, Panagiotou G, Mougios V, Brinkoetter M, Vamvini MT, Schneider BE, et al. FNDC5 and irisin in humans: I. Predictors of circulating concentrations in serum and plasma and II. mRNA expression and circulating concentrations in response to weight loss and exercise. Metabolism. 2012;61(12):1725–38.
116. Dick KJ, Nelson CP, Tsaprouni L, Sandling JK, Aissi D, Wahl S, et al. DNA methylation and body-mass index: a genome-wide analysis. Lancet. 2014;383(9933):1990–8.
117. Aslibekyan S, Demerath EW, Mendelson M, Zhi D, Guan W, Liang L, et al. Epigenome-wide study identifies novel methylation loci associated with body mass index and waist circumference. Obesity (Silver Spring). 2015;23(7):1493–501.

118. Houde AA, Legare C, Biron S, Lescelleur O, Biertho L, Marceau S, et al. Leptin and adiponectin DNA methylation levels in adipose tissues and blood cells are associated with BMI, waist girth and LDL-cholesterol levels in severely obese men and women. BMC Med Genet. 2015;16:29.
119. Milagro FI, Gomez-Abellan P, Campion J, Martinez JA, Ordovas JM, Garaulet M. CLOCK, PER2 and BMAL1 DNA methylation: association with obesity and metabolic syndrome characteristics and monounsaturated fat intake. Chronobiol Int. 2012;29(9):1180–94.
120. Mundstock E, Sarria EE, Zatti H, Mattos Louzada F, Kich Grun L, Herbert Jones M, et al. Effect of obesity on telomere length: systematic review and meta-analysis. Obesity (Silver Spring). 2015;23(11):2165–74.
121. Muezzinler A, Mons U, Dieffenbach AK, Butterbach K, Saum KU, Schick M, et al. Body mass index and leukocyte telomere length dynamics among older adults: Results from the ESTHER cohort. Exp Gerontol. 2016;74:1–8.
122. Joshu CE, Peskoe SB, Heaphy CM, Kenfield SA, Van Blarigan EL, Mucci LA, et al. Prediagnostic obesity and physical inactivity are associated with shorter telomere length in prostate stromal cells. Cancer Prev Res (Phila). 2015;8(8):737–42.
123. Fontes JD, Yamamoto JF, Larson MG, Wang N, Dallmeier D, Rienstra M, et al. Clinical correlates of change in inflammatory biomarkers: The Framingham Heart Study. Atherosclerosis. 2013;228(1):217–23.
124. Shanmugalingam T, Crawley D, Bosco C, Melvin J, Rohrmann S, Chowdhury S, et al. Obesity and cancer: the role of vitamin D. BMC Cancer. 2014;14:712.
125. Blum M, Dolnikowski G, Seyoum E, Harris SS, Booth SL, Peterson J, et al. Vitamin D(3) in fat tissue. Endocrine. 2008;33(1):90–4.
126. Kull M, Kallikorm R, Lember M. Body mass index determines sunbathing habits: implications on vitamin D levels. Intern Med J. 2009;39(4):256–8.
127. Chae JS, Paik JK, Kang R, Kim M, Choi Y, Lee SH, et al. Mild weight loss reduces inflammatory cytokines, leukocyte count, and oxidative stress in overweight and moderately obese participants treated for 3 years with dietary modification. Nutr Res. 2013;33(3):195–203.
128. Moller K, Ostermann AI, Rund K, Thoms S, Blume C, Stahl F, et al. Influence of weight reduction on blood levels of C-reactive protein, tumor necrosis factor-alpha, interleukin-6, and oxylipins in obese subjects. Prostaglandins Leukot Essent Fatty Acids. 2016;106:39–49.
129. Ramel A, Martinez JA, Kiely M, Bandarra NM, Thorsdottir I. Effects of weight loss and seafood consumption on inflammation parameters in young, overweight and obese European men and women during 8 weeks of energy restriction. Eur J Clin Nutr. 2010;64(9):987–93.
130. Schulte DM, Hahn M, Oberhauser F, Malchau G, Schubert M, Heppner C, et al. Caloric restriction increases serum testosterone concentrations in obese male subjects by two distinct mechanisms. Horm Metab Res. 2014;46(4):283–6.
131. Acharya SD, Brooks MM, Evans RW, Linkov F, Burke LE. Weight loss is more important than the diet type in improving adiponectin levels among overweight/obese adults. J Am Coll Nutr. 2013;32(4):264–71.
132. Camps SG, Verhoef SP, Westerterp KR. Leptin and energy restriction induced adaptation in energy expenditure. Metabolism. 2015;64(10):1284–90.
133. de la Iglesia R, Lopez-Legarrea P, Crujeiras AB, Pardo M, Casanueva FF, Zulet MA, et al. Plasma irisin depletion under energy restriction is associated with improvements in lipid profile in metabolic syndrome patients. Clin Endocrinol (Oxf). 2014;81(2):306–11.
134. Scoccianti C, Ricceri F, Ferrari P, Cuenin C, Sacerdote C, Polidoro S, et al. Methylation patterns in sentinel genes in peripheral blood cells of heavy smokers: influence of cruciferous vegetables in an intervention study. Epigenetics. 2011;6(9):1114–9.
135. Ornish D, Lin J, Chan JM, Epel E, Kemp C, Weidner G, et al. Effect of comprehensive lifestyle changes on telomerase activity and telomere length in men with biopsy-proven low-risk prostate cancer: 5-year follow-up of a descriptive pilot study. Lancet Oncol. 2013;14(11):1112–20.
136. Ibero-Baraibar I, Navas-Carretero S, Abete I, Martinez JA, Zulet MA. Increases in plasma 25(OH)D levels are related to improvements in body composition and blood pressure

in middle-aged subjects after a weight loss intervention: longitudinal study. Clin Nutr. 2015;34(5):1010–7.

137. Goto S, Nakai K, Kono K, Yonekura Y, Ito J, Fujii H, et al. Dietary phosphorus restriction by a standard low-protein diet decreased serum fibroblast growth factor 23 levels in patients with early and advanced stage chronic kidney disease. Clin Exp Nephrol. 2014;18(6):925–31.
138. Rock CL, Emond JA, Flatt SW, Heath DD, Karanja N, Pakiz B, et al. Weight loss is associated with increased serum 25-hydroxyvitamin D in overweight or obese women. Obesity (Silver Spring). 2012;20(11):2296–301.
139. Calbet JA, Ponce-Gonzalez JG, Perez-Suarez I, de la Calle HJ, Holmberg HC. A time-efficient reduction of fat mass in 4 days with exercise and caloric restriction. Scand J Med Sci Sports. 2015;25(2):223–33.
140. Hussain TA, Mathew TC, Dashti AA, Asfar S, Al-Zaid N, Dashti HM. Effect of low-calorie versus low-carbohydrate ketogenic diet in type 2 diabetes. Nutrition. 2012;28(10):1016–21.
141. Lecoultre V, Ravussin E, Redman LM. The fall in leptin concentration is a major determinant of the metabolic adaptation induced by caloric restriction independently of the changes in leptin circadian rhythms. J Clin Endocrinol Metab. 2011;96(9):E1512–6.
142. Tapsell LC, Batterham MJ, Thorne RL, O'Shea JE, Grafenauer SJ, Probst YC. Weight loss effects from vegetable intake: a 12-month randomised controlled trial. Eur J Clin Nutr. 2014;68(7):778–85.
143. Rezaeipour M, Apanasenko GL, Nychyporuk VI. Investigating the effects of negative-calorie diet compared with low-calorie diet under exercise conditions on weight loss and lipid profile in overweight/obese middle-aged and older men. Turk J Med Sci. 2014;44(5):792–8.
144. Ruth MR, Port AM, Shah M, Bourland AC, Istfan NW, Nelson KP, et al. Consuming a hypocaloric high fat low carbohydrate diet for 12 weeks lowers C-reactive protein, and raises serum adiponectin and high density lipoprotein-cholesterol in obese subjects. Metabolism. 2013;62(12):1779–87.
145. Conn VS, Koopman RJ, Ruppar TM, Phillips LJ, Mehr DR, Hafdahl AR. Insulin sensitivity following exercise interventions: systematic review and meta-analysis of outcomes among healthy adults. J Prim Care Community Health. 2014;5(3):211–22.
146. Gordon B, Chen S, Durstine JL. The effects of exercise training on the traditional lipid profile and beyond. Curr Sports Med Rep. 2014;13(4):253–9.
147. Monteiro PA, Chen KY, Lira FS, Saraiva BT, Antunes BM, Campos EZ, et al. Concurrent and aerobic exercise training promote similar benefits in body composition and metabolic profiles in obese adolescents. Lipids Health Dis. 2015;14:153.
148. Jakicic JM, King WC, Marcus MD, Davis KK, Helsel D, Rickman AD, et al. Short-term weight loss with diet and physical activity in young adults: The IDEA study. Obesity (Silver Spring). 2015;23(12):2385–97.
149. Tapsell LC, Lonergan M, Martin A, Batterham MJ, Neale EP, HealthTrack ST. Interdisciplinary lifestyle intervention for weight management in a community population (HealthTrack study): Study design and baseline sample characteristics. Contemp Clin Trials. 2015;45(Pt B):394–403.
150. Chow CK, Redfern J, Hillis GS, Thakkar J, Santo K, Hackett ML, et al. Effect of lifestyle-focused text messaging on risk factor modification in patients with coronary heart disease: a randomized clinical trial. JAMA. 2015;314(12):1255–63.
151. Abrahamson PE, King IB, Ulrich CM, Rudolph RE, Irwin ML, Yasui Y, et al. No effect of exercise on colon mucosal prostaglandin concentrations: a 12-month randomized controlled trial. Cancer Epidemiol Biomarkers Prev. 2007;16(11):2351–6.
152. MacLaren DP, Raine NM, O'Connor AM, Buchanan KD. Human gastrin and vasoactive intestinal polypeptide responses to endurance running in relation to training status and fluid ingested. Clin Sci (Lond). 1995;89(2):137–43.
153. Hayes LD, Sculthorpe N, Herbert P, Baker JS, Hullin DA, Kilduff LP, et al. Resting steroid hormone concentrations in lifetime exercisers and lifetime sedentary males. Aging Male. 2015;18(1):22–6.

154. Khoo J, Tian HH, Tan B, Chew K, Ng CS, Leong D, et al. Comparing effects of low- and high-volume moderate-intensity exercise on sexual function and testosterone in obese men. J Sex Med. 2013;10(7):1823–32.
155. Stokes KA, Gilbert KL, Hall GM, Andrews RC, Thompson D. Different responses of selected hormones to three types of exercise in young men. Eur J Appl Physiol. 2013;113(3):775–83.
156. Ackel-D'Elia C, Carnier J, Bueno CR Jr, Campos RM, Sanches PL, Clemente AP, et al. Effects of different physical exercises on leptin concentration in obese adolescents. Int J Sports Med. 2014;35(2):164–71.
157. Beavers KM, Ambrosius WT, Nicklas BJ, Rejeski WJ. Independent and combined effects of physical activity and weight loss on inflammatory biomarkers in overweight and obese older adults. J Am Geriatr Soc. 2013;61(7):1089–94.
158. Cameron JD, Goldfield GS, Riou ME, Finlayson GS, Blundell JE, Doucet E. Energy depletion by diet or aerobic exercise alone: impact of energy deficit modality on appetite parameters. Am J Clin Nutr. 2016;103(4):1008–16.
159. Lima LG, Bonardi JM, Campos GO, Bertani RF, Scher LM, Louzada-Junior P, et al. Effect of aerobic training and aerobic and resistance training on the inflammatory status of hypertensive older adults. Aging Clin Exp Res. 2015;27(4):483–9.
160. Qiu S, Cai X, Sun Z, Schumann U, Zugel M, Steinacker JM. Chronic exercise training and circulating irisin in adults: a meta-analysis. Sports Med. 2015;45(11):1577–88.
161. Kim HJ, So B, Choi M, Kang D, Song W. Resistance exercise training increases the expression of irisin concomitant with improvement of muscle function in aging mice and humans. Exp Gerontol. 2015;70:11–7.
162. Sjogren P, Fisher R, Kallings L, Svenson U, Roos G, Hellenius ML. Stand up for health—avoiding sedentary behaviour might lengthen your telomeres: secondary outcomes from a physical activity RCT in older people. Br J Sports Med. 2014;48(19):1407–9.
163. Chan DC, Tsou HH, Yang RS, Tsauo JY, Chen CY, Hsiung CA, et al. A pilot randomized controlled trial to improve geriatric frailty. BMC Geriatr. 2012;12:58.
164. Beavers KM, Beavers DP, Newman JJ, Anderson AM, Loeser RF Jr, Nicklas BJ, et al. Effects of total and regional fat loss on plasma CRP and IL-6 in overweight and obese, older adults with knee osteoarthritis. Osteoarthritis Cartilage. 2015;23(2):249–56.
165. Mendham AE, Duffield R, Marino F, Coutts AJ. Small-sided games training reduces CRP, IL-6 and leptin in sedentary, middle-aged men. Eur J Appl Physiol. 2014;114(11):2289–97.
166. World Cancer Research Fund. Mechanisms Research Project. 2016 [cited 2016 .22 September]; Available from: http://www.wcrf-uk.org/uk/our-research/mechanisms-research-project.

Chapter 6
Impact of Metabolic Factors on Screening, Early Detection, and Management of Prostate Cancer

Daniel S. Han and J. Kellogg Parsons

Abstract In this chapter, we review the influence of energy imbalance on prostate cancer screening, diagnosis, and management. The influence of obesity on prostate cancer screening, diagnosis, and management is substantial and complex. Obese men have lower serum PSA, a tool to used to screen for prostate cancer, and larger prostate volume, which may lead to a reduced likelihood that an extant, but occult tumor without lethal potential is ever detected, while that same delay may lead to more advanced stages of disease at diagnosis and corresponding increases in prostate cancer mortality. Obesity can adversely affect the efficacy and safety of the treatment of prostate cancer with surgery or radiation. Development of an optimal framework to guide decision-making for prostate cancer screening, risk stratification, and management in obese men is needed.

Keywords Prostate cancer screening • Prostate cancer management • Body mass index • Prostate specific antigen • Prostate volume

Introduction

Since the advent of widespread prostate cancer screening with prostate-specific antigen (PSA) and digital rectal examination (DRE) in the 1990s, the incidence of advanced disease at time of diagnosis has decreased by 80% [1] and age-adjusted prostate cancer mortality has decreased by approximately 40% [2]. Although potentially due in part to lead time bias after earlier detection, decreased prostate cancer mortality has largely been attributed to treatment of screen-detected tumors [3–5]. Two randomized trials involving over 180,000 European men observed robust

D.S. Han, MD • J. Kellogg Parsons, MD, MHS (✉)
Moores Cancer Center, University of California San Diego Health,
3855 Health Sciences Drive, La Jolla, CA 92093, USA
e-mail: dsh004@ucsd.edu; k0parsons@mail.ucsd.edu

© Springer International Publishing AG 2018

E.A. Platz, N.A. Berger (eds.), *Energy Balance and Prostate Cancer*, Energy Balance and Cancer 14, DOI 10.1007/978-3-319-64940-5_6

overall survival benefits in those who underwent PSA screening, thus confirming its efficacy to diminish prostate cancer mortality [6–8].

Screened men who are at-risk for prostate cancer—i.e., those with high serum concentrations of PSA and/or an abnormal DRE—are offered trans-rectal or trans-perineal prostate biopsy using ultrasound guidance with or without magnetic resonance imaging (MRI). Men diagnosed with prostate cancer from biopsy are then risk-stratified according to a series of clinical variables—Gleason grade, PSA, and clinical staging—to guide treatment decisions. Treatments for early-stage, screen-detected prostate cancer include surveillance, surgery, radiation, and ablation with cryosurgery or high-intensity focused ultrasound.

Metabolic disturbances and modifiable risk factors of disease that result from energy imbalances—including body mass index (BMI) and obesity—can potentially influence PSA concentrations and other components of prostate cancer screening. In this chapter, we discuss the effects of metabolic factors on prostate cancer screening and diagnosis.

Prostate Cancer Screening: Concepts and Controversies

Prostate cancer population screening consists of periodic PSA testing and DRE. Prior to the availability of the PSA test, the DRE was the sole method for prostate cancer screening [9]. DRE is noted to have high inter-observer variability, poor sensitivity, and limited specificity [10]. The addition of PSA testing improves the positive predictive value of DRE for prostate cancer to as much as 83%, depending on PSA level [11]. DRE may potentially help identify aggressive cancers in patients with lower (<2.5 ng/mL) PSA values [12].

PSA is a serine protease secreted from acinar epithelial cells of the prostate and is a member of the kallikrein family. It circulates in serum via bound and unbound forms and is used to estimate the risk of prostate cancer. However, PSA is not a prostate cancer-specific biomarker: up to 75% of men with an elevated serum PSA between 4 and 10 ng/mL who undergo prostate biopsy do not have cancer [13].

In fact, aggressive screening, diagnosis, and treatment of early-stage prostate cancer has generated debate regarding *over-detection*: the diagnosis of screen-detected indolent prostate cancer that, left untreated, would otherwise not provoke symptoms or diminish overall or prostate cancer-specific survival. *Over-treatment* of screen-detected indolent cancers may expose patients to substantial risks of morbidity without a corresponding survival benefit [14]. In 2012, the U.S. Preventive Services Task Force (USPSTF) concluded from the available evidence that the potential harms of PSA testing outweigh its potential benefits and recommended against population-based screening for prostate cancer [15].

However, Level I evidence supports the benefits of screening. The European Randomized Study of Screening for Prostate Cancer (ERSPC) [6, 16] was a multinational trial of 182,160 men aged 55–69 years randomized to a control or screening arm from 1991 to 2003. Men in the screening arm underwent PSA testing every

2–4 years, with biopsy performed for PSA > 3.0 ng/mL. After a median follow-up of 11 years, the screening group had a 21% relative risk reduction in prostate cancer death; the number needed to screen to prevent 1 prostate cancer death was 1055. The Göteborg trial [7] was a population-based PSA screening study of 20,000 men aged 50–64 years randomized to biennial PSA screening versus control. In the screening arm, there was a 44% relative risk reduction in prostate cancer-specific mortality at a median follow-up of 14 years.

While a third randomized trial, the prostate arm of the U.S. Prostate, Lung, Colorectal, and Ovarian (PLCO) Cancer Screening Trial [17, 18], showed no benefit to screening, the PLCO could not effectively assess the effect of PSA-based screening on prostate cancer mortality because of excessive contamination of the control arm with screened men. For example, 74% of men in the control arm were screened at least once, and 44% of the men had at least 1 PSA test prior to the study. Thus, the PLCO arm could not effectively test whether a screening intervention reduced prostate cancer mortality.

Still, maximizing the early detection of prostate cancer will indeed increase the detection of both indolent and aggressive cancers among informed men who have elected to participate in a prostate cancer screening program [14]. To decrease prostate cancer mortality, yet mitigate against the potential morbidities of over-detection and over-treatment, a judicious, tailored approach to population screening using evidence-based guidelines for periodic PSA testing and DRE in appropriately counseled men is indicated.

Evidence-Based Guidelines for Prostate Cancer Screening

Several professional societies have published evidence-based guidelines for prostate cancer screening. The American Urological Association (AUA) recommends shared decision-making between physicians and men aged 55–69 years that weighs the risks and benefits, and proceeds based on the patient's preferences; it recommends against routine screening for average-risk men at the ages of 40–54 (www.auanet.org). There is no specific threshold of PSA that is an absolute indication for a biopsy; rather, the AUA recommends consideration of factors that may increase the PSA, such as prostate enlargement, inflammation, and patient age.

The National Comprehensive Cancer Network (NCCN) Guidelines for Early Detection of Prostate Cancer recommend a risk/benefit discussion with men aged 45–75 years and a baseline PSA and DRE to determine the frequency of future testing (www.nccn.org). A PSA level > 3.0 ng/mL and/or an abnormal DRE should prompt further evaluation, discussion, and consideration of prostate biopsy. Although currently not indicated as first-line screening tests, for patients and physicians who wish to further define the probability of biopsy-detectable cancer, the NCCN recommends consideration of newer biomarker tests that increase the specificity of prostate cancer detection. These assays include % free PSA [19], the Prostate Health Index (*phi*) [20], PCA-3 [21], and the 4-kallikrein (4 K) panel [22].

These tests may inform the decision to perform biopsy through improved specificity compared to total PSA for the detection of clinically significant prostate cancer.

Both the AUA and NCCN guidelines recommend consideration of upper age limits and life expectancy. The AUA guidelines do not recommend routine screening in patients older than 70 years of age or with a life expectancy less than 10–15 years; for the NCCN, the parameters are men older than 75 years of age and less than 10-year life expectancy.

Metabolic Factors and Prostate Cancer Screening: Obesity and PSA

Factors that influence serum PSA concentrations include age, prostate volume, infection, inflammation, and instrumentation acting on the prostate. PSA is known to be directly correlated with age; thus, age-adjusted PSA reference ranges have been proposed to make PSA a more discriminating tumor marker to detect prostate cancer in men of various ages [23]. For every cubic centimeter increase in prostate volume, PSA increases by approximately 4% [23]. Instrumentation that acts directly on the prostate, such as prostate biopsy and transurethral resection of the prostate (TURP), significantly increase serum PSA levels [24]. Urinary tract infections and prostatitis also affect PSA values.

Another factor that influences serum PSA concentrations, and thus potentially prostate cancer detection, is obesity. Evidence-based guidelines for prostate cancer screening and detection are based on population screening with PSA. Studies have consistently observed inverse associations of body mass index (BMI) and serum PSA. In a population-based study of almost 2800 men without prostate cancer, Baillargeon and colleagues observed that mean PSA decreased as BMI category increased: from 1.01 ng/mL in normal (<24.9 kg/m^2) BMI men to 0.69 ng/mL in morbidly obese (>40 kg/m^2) men [25]. Similarly, Barqawi and colleagues noted in a population-based study of nearly 4500 men that obese men (BMI > 30 kg/m^2) had significantly lower PSA levels compared to non-obese men (BMI < 30 kg/m^2) across all age groups [26].

Investigators have offered two theories to explain these associations of higher BMI with lower PSA. One is the *anti-androgen theory*: obese men have lower circulating concentrations of serum androgens compared to non-obese men, possibly as a result of increased peripheral aromatization of androgens to estrogen by adipose tissue—decreased serum androgens leads to decreased stimulation of PSA production by the prostate gland [27, 28]. The second is the *hemodilution theory*. This theory posits that obese patients have a larger circulating plasma volume, which dilutes serum PSA and thus decreases observed serum PSA concentrations. In a study of approximately 14,000 men with prostate cancer who underwent radical prostatectomy, Bañez and colleagues observed that obese males with BMI >35 kg/m^2 had higher estimated plasma volumes and lower PSA concentrations [29]. Furthermore, obese patients had similar or even greater PSA mass (the calculated amount of PSA circulating in serum) compared to men of normal weight. These investigators suggested that this lends further credence to the hemodilution theory, since if the anti-androgen theory were true, obese males should theoretically have less PSA mass than that of normal-weight males. These findings have been validated in other populations [30], most notably 28,000 men in the prostate arm of the PLCO trial [31].

Regardless of etiology, inverse associations of obesity with PSA could potentially result in diminished screening detection of localized—but clinically significant—cancers in obese men and to corresponding increases in the incidence of advanced disease in this population. Indeed, higher BMI has been linked with increased risk of prostate cancer-specific mortality [32] and increased probability of aggressive prostate cancer at time of diagnosis [33]. These data suggest that clinicians should consider lowering PSA thresholds for performing prostate biopsy in obese patients. Rundle and Neugut proposed PSA biopsy thresholds of ≥4.0 ng/mL, ≥3.5 ng/mL, and ≥3.1 ng/mL for non-obese, obese, and morbidly obese men, respectively [30].

Still, the clinical implications of these findings remain unclear. The latest version of the PCPT prostate cancer risk calculator no longer takes BMI into account as a variable (http://deb.uthscsa.edu/URORiskCalc/Pages/calcs.jsp). However, a previously developed BMI-adjusted PCPT prostate cancer risk calculator was analyzed by Liang and colleagues in an external validation study using 3258 men from the SELECT Trial who underwent prostate biopsy [34]. They found that for men without a family history of prostate cancer, increased BMI was not associated with risk of prostate cancer incidence but was significantly associated with high-grade disease. For men with known family history of prostate cancer, increasing BMI was independently associated with increased risk of both prostate cancer incidence and high-grade disease. The authors concluded that practitioners should consider including BMI as a factor during clinical assessment of prostate cancer risk, especially for patients with known family history of prostate cancer. However, none of the three major evidence-based clinical guidelines for urologists—AUA, NCCN, and European Association of Urology (www.uroweb.org)—currently recommend specific PSA screening parameters for obese patients.

Metabolic Factors and Prostate Cancer Diagnosis: Prostate Volume and Biopsy

Screened men with elevated PSA and/or abnormal DRE may undergo prostate biopsy for cancer diagnosis. Unlike diagnostic biopsy for most other solid organ tumors, standard-of-care prostate biopsy is performed without image guidance or selective targeting of suspect lesions. This practice, known as *systematic* biopsy, renders prostate cancer diagnosis susceptible to variations in prostate volume: a prostate tumor, particularly a smaller one, is more likely to be detected in a smaller volume prostate than a comparably sized tumor in a larger volume prostate [35, 36].

Metabolic factors may influence prostate volume and thus bias cancer detection. Multiple studies have shown that higher BMI is associated with increased prostate volume [37–39]. In the Baltimore Longitudinal Study of Aging, each 1 kg/m^2 increase in BMI corresponded to a 0.41 cc increase in MRI-measured prostate volume [40]. Patients with elevated fasting glucose levels (>110 mg/dL) and also men diagnosed with diabetes had a higher likelihood of prostate enlargement. In a study of BMI, PSA, and prostate volume in 1414 men undergoing radical prostatectomy, Freedland and colleagues observed a direct association of BMI and prostate size in younger men [28]. Similarly, in 13,343 men undergoing radical prostatectomy, Kopp and colleagues noted that preoperative BMI was associated with increased prostate weight: for each 1 kg/m^2 increase in BMI, prostate weight increased by 0.45 g (95% CI 0.35–0.55, P-trend <0.001) [41]. In addition, compared with men with BMI < 25 kg/m^2, men with a BMI ≥ 35 kg/m^2 had a 40% increased probability of prostate weight of at least 40 g and a 70% increased probability of prostate weight of at least 50 g.

These data suggest that metabolic-induced variations in prostate volume may potentially bias prostate cancer detection in a manner similar to PSA in obese men. Because prostate cancer is harder to detect in larger volume prostates, metabolic disturbances associated with increased prostate volume—notably obesity—might delay detection of clinically significant disease and worsen clinical outcomes. There are, however, no data to directly support this concept.

Metabolic Factors and Prostate Cancer Incidence

While there is no direct evidence of prostate cancer detection bias associated with metabolically-induced alterations in PSA and prostate volume, there are indirect data: several studies have observed associations of obesity with increased risk of aggressive prostate cancer, which would support the concept that obesity delays prostate cancer diagnosis. In 2952 men from the CaPSURE registry, Kane and colleagues noted that overweight, obese, and very obese men had an increased risk of aggressive prostate cancer at time of diagnosis [42]. Amling and colleagues analyzed 860 patients with prostate cancer from multiple institutions treated with radical prostatectomy and found that obese patients presented at a younger age, had higher mean Gleason scores, had a higher chance of Gleason sum ≥ 7 (i.e., clinically significant) disease, and decreased chance of organ-confined disease [43]. Furthermore, on multivariable logistic regression, BMI was independently associated with Gleason sum. In 363 patients who underwent radical prostatectomy, Rohrmann and colleagues also found that the risk of high-grade cancer increased with BMI, especially among men less than 50 years of age [44].

Other studies have observed associations of obesity with prostate cancer mortality. In the Cancer Prevention Studies I (n = 381,638) and II (n = 434,630), prostate cancer mortality was significantly higher for obese (BMI > 30 kg/m^2) than non-obese (BMI < 25 kg/m^2) men in multivariable models [45]. Furthermore, prostate cancer mortality was over 30% higher in the heaviest (BMI 18.50–22.99 kg/m^2) compared to the leanest (BMI < 18.50 kg/m^2) men.

In contrast, BMI appears to be inversely associated with incident prostate cancer. In a meta-analysis of 12 prospective studies on localized prostate cancer (n = 1,033,009) and 13 prospective studies on advanced prostate cancer (n = 1,080,790) assessing the association of BMI and prostate cancer, Discacciati et al. reported that obesity conferred a decreased risk of localized disease, while it increased the risk for advanced prostate cancer [46]. One interpretation of these data would be that diminished PSA and increased prostate volume in obese relative to non-obese men reduces the likelihood that an extant, but occult tumor without lethal potential is ever detected, while that same delay leads to more advanced stages of disease at diagnosis and corresponding increases in prostate cancer mortality.

Of note, an alternative explanation of these data is that associations of obesity with prostate cancer may, all or in part, be causal. That is, both the biology of adiposity and detection bias may potentially contribute to the observed inverse associations of obesity with incident localized disease and positive associations for advanced disease and mortality (http://www.wcrf.org/int/research-we-fund/continuous-update-project-findings-reports/prostate-cancer).

Additional energy balance associated-factors—diet and physical activity—may also be associated with prostate cancer risk, although at this time the evidence is insufficient to be conclusive (http://www.wcrf.org/int/research-we-fund/continuous-update-project-findings-reports/prostate-cancer). Specifically, fat intake has been linked to increased risk. In a population-based case-control study from Utah that analyzed dietary intake in 358 patients with prostate cancer vs 679 controls, West et al. found an odds ratio of 2.9 for aggressive disease in older males 68–74 years of age with high dietary fat intake [47]. Le Marchand et al. studied a cohort of 20,316 men from Hawaii and found elevated relative risks of prostate cancer with consumption of beef (RR 1.6), milk (RR 1.4), and overall high-fat animal products (RR 1.6) [48]. Overall, the data regarding the association of physical activity and prostate cancer risk suggests an inverse association. In a meta-analysis of the literature studying physical activity and its association with cancer, Friedenreich found that the majority of the studies available in the literature suggest a beneficial effect of physical activity on prostate cancer [49]. The majority of the studies showed a 10–30% decreased risk of prostate cancer. Additionally, multiple large population-based studies report an inverse association between physical activity and prostate cancer risk [50–52].

With respect to prostate cancer outcomes after the diagnosis, a study by Friedenreich and colleagues analyzed 830 prostate cancer patients prospectively up to 17 years and examined prostate cancer survival in relation to post-diagnosis physical activity [53]. Post-diagnosis physical activity was significantly associated with lower all-cause mortality risk (HR 0.58) and lower prostate cancer-specific mortality risk (HR 0.56). No significant associations were found between physical activity and risk of first recurrence/progression, however.

As stated previously, the clinical significance of these findings remain unclear. There are no evidence-based guidelines that factor obesity, dietary intake, physical activity, and their association with higher-grade disease and increased mortality in clinical decision-making for prostate cancer screening.

Energy Balance and Management of Prostate Cancer

The main initial options for treating clinically localized prostate cancer with curative intent are surgery and radiation. Obesity has also been shown to potentially affect the efficacy and/or safety of these treatment modalities.

Obesity potentially places patients at risk of peri-operative surgical complications. Tjeertes and colleagues analyzed over 4000 patients who underwent surgery and found that obesity was associated with increased risks of surgical site infection, longer operative time, and increased surgical blood loss [54]. However, there was no difference in major post-operative complications, and obesity was actually associated with an overall improvement in 30-day complication rate and long-term survival. Xu and colleagues performed a meta-analysis of studies focused on outcomes of robotic-assisted laparoscopic radical prostatectomy in obese patients [55]. Obese men had significantly increased operative time and surgical blood loss, but the length of post-operative hospital stay and complication rates (overall, minor, major) did not differ significantly between obese and non-obese patients. Increased operative time is likely due to increased technical difficulty due to the patient's larger body habitus. Other studies have shown similar results by obesity status in both open (radical retropubic and radical perineal) [56] and laparoscopic prostatectomies [57].

While obesity has not been linked to an increase in major surgical complications, studies have shown that obesity is associated with an increased risk of positive surgical margins, increased risk of biochemical recurrence, and decreased progression-free survival. In a retrospective study of 1006 patients who either underwent radical retropubic prostatectomy (RRP) or radical perineal prostatectomy (RPP) at a single institution from 1988 to 2005, Fitzsimons and colleagues found that obese patients had an increased risk of positive surgical margins in both surgical approaches [56]. This was true even after controlling for pathologic disease severity. Ho and colleagues showed in a retrospective study of 1038 patients who underwent radical prostatectomy that obese patients had a higher PSA nadir after surgery and increased risk of biochemical recurrence compared to non-obese patients [58]. Freedland and colleagues corroborated the finding of an increased risk of biochemical recurrence in obese patients from a study of 1106 patients who underwent prostatectomy [59]. Possible reasons for suboptimal surgical disease control in obese men are both a higher risk of advanced disease and the increase in technical difficulty of the operation leading to a higher rate of positive surgical margins. There are currently no evidence-based guidelines for obesity and surgical management of prostate cancer.

Obesity has also been shown to adversely affect treatment outcomes after radiation treatment. Wang and colleagues analyzed 1442 patients with clinically located prostate cancer treated with intensity-modulated radiotherapy (IMRT) [60]. They found that increasing BMI was linked to increased risks of biochemical recurrence, distant metastases, prostate cancer-specific mortality, and overall mortality after IMRT. Stroup and colleagues analyzed outcomes of 1868 men who underwent primary external beam radiation therapy (EBRT) for clinically localized prostate cancer [61]. Utilizing the 2006 RTOG-ASTRO criteria, they observed that obesity was associated with greater odds of biochemical recurrence after EBRT. Keto and colleagues studied 287 men from the SEARCH database who underwent radical prostatectomy with neoadjuvant androgen deprivation therapy [62] and found that higher BMI (>25 kg/m^2) was associated with an increased risk of metastasis and trends towards increased risk of castrate-resistant disease and prostate cancer-specific mortality. These investigators postulated that one potential explanation for these observations was an increased plasma volume in obese men that dilutes the concentration of androgen deprivation drug distribution, thus decreasing its efficacy. Further studies need to be performed to further elucidate the effects of obesity on radiation treatment and neoadjuvant androgen deprivation. Similar to surgery, there are no evidence-based guidelines that include obesity as a factor when counseling patients towards radiation therapy.

Conclusions

In summary, the effect of energy balance, most notably obesity, on prostate cancer screening, diagnosis, and management is substantial and complex. Obesity has been clearly linked to decreased PSA and increased prostate volume, which may lead to decreased screen detection of clinically-significant, localized prostate cancer. Indeed, obese men have been shown to have a decreased risk of prostate cancer incidence but a higher risk of advanced disease at diagnosis, possibly, in part, due to detection bias causing a delay in diagnosis of localized disease until obese patients present with more advanced stages of disease. In addition, obese men have a higher risk of prostate cancer-specific mortality. Obesity has also been shown to adversely affect outcomes of prostate cancer treatment with surgery (increased risks of positive surgical margins and biochemical recurrence) and radiation (increased risks of biochemical recurrence, metastasis, prostate cancer-specific mortality, and overall mortality). Further studies are needed to delineate the mechanisms through which obesity confers these risks, and future prospective studies include development of an optimal framework to guide decision-making for prostate cancer screening, risk stratification, and management in obese men.

References

1. Catalona WJ. History of the discovery and clinical translation of prostate-specific antigen. Asian J Urol. 2014;1:12–4.
2. Cooperberg MR. Implications of the new AUA guidelines on prostate cancer detection in the U.S. Curr Urol Rep. 2014;15(7):420.
3. Jhaveri FM, Klein EA, Kupelian PA, et al. Declining rates of extracapsular extension after radical prostatectomy: evidence for continued stage migration. J Clin Oncol. 1999;17(10):3167–72.
4. Etzioni R, Gulati R, Tsodikov A, et al. The prostate cancer conundrum revisited: treatment changes and prostate cancer mortality declines. Cancer. 2012;118:5955–63.

5. Siegel R, Naishadham D, Jemal A. Cancer statistics, 2013. CA Cancer J Clin. 2013;63:11–30.
6. Schröder FH, Hugosson J, Roobol MJ, et al. Screening and prostate-cancer mortality in a randomized European study. N Engl J Med. 2009;360(13):1320–8.
7. Hugosson J, Carlsson S, Aus G, et al. Mortality results from the Göteberg randomised population-based prostate-cancer screening trial. Lancet Oncol. 2010;11:725–32.
8. Schröder FH, Hugosson J, Roobol MJ, et al. Screening and prostate cancer mortality: results of the European Randomized Study of Screening for Prostate Cancer (ERSPC) at 13 years of follow-up. Lancet. 2014;384:2027–35.
9. Catalona WJ, Richie JP, Ahmann FR, et al. Comparison of digital rectal examination and serum prostate specific antigen in the early detection of prostate cancer: results of a multicenter clinical trial of 6,630 men. J Urol. 1994;151:1283–90.
10. Schroder FH, van der Maas P, Beemsterboer P, et al. Evaluation of the digital rectal examination as a screening test for prostate cancer. Rotterdam section of the European Randomized Study of Screening for Prostate Cancer. J Natl Cancer Inst. 1998;90:1817–23.
11. Schröder FH, et al. Evaluation of the digital rectal examination as a screening test for prostate cancer. Rotterdam section of the European Randomized Study of Screening for Prostate Cancer. J Natl Cancer Inst. 1998 Dec 2;90(23):1817–23.
12. Hattangadi JA, Chen MH, D'Amico AV. Early detection of high-grade prostate cancer using digital rectal examination (DRE) in men with a prostate-specific antigen level of <2.5 ng/mL and the risk of death. BJU Int. 2012;110:1636–41.
13. Catalona WJ, Partin AW, Slawin KM, et al. Use of the percentage of free prostate-specific antigen to enhance differentiation of prostate cancer from benign prostatic disease: a prospective multicenter clinical trial. JAMA. 1998;279(19):1542–7.
14. McDonald ML, Parsons JK. The case for tailored prostate cancer screening: an NCCN perspective. J Natl Compr Cancer Netw. 2015 Dec;13(12):1576–158.
15. Moyer VA. US preventive services task force. Screening for prostate cancer: U.S. preventive services task force recommendation statement. Ann Intern Med. 2012;157:120–34.
16. Schröder FH, Hugosson J, Roobol MJ, et al. Prostate-cancer mortality at 11 years of follow-up. N Engl J Med. 2012;366(11):981–90.
17. Andriole GL, Crawford ED, Grubb RL, et al. Mortality results from a randomized prostate-cancer screening trial. N Engl J Med. 2009;360:1310–9.
18. Andriole GL, Crawford ED, Grubb RL, et al. Prostate cancer screening in the randomized prostate, lung, colorectal, and ovarian cancer screening trial: mortality results after 13 years of follow-up. J Natl Cancer Inst. 2012;104:1–8.
19. Partin AW, Brawer MK, Subong EN, et al. Prospective evaluation of percent free-PSA and complexed-PSA for early detection of prostate cancer. Prostate Cancer Prostatic Dis. 1998;1:197–203.
20. Filella X, Giménez N. Evaluation of [−2] proPSA and Prostate Health Index (phi) for the detection of prostate cancer: a systematic review and meta-analysis. Clin Chem Lab Med. 2013;51:729–39.
21. Gittelman MC, Hertzman B, Bailen J, et al. PCA3 molecular urine test as a predictor of repeat prostate biopsy outcome in men with previous negative biopsies: a prospective multicenter clinical study. J Urol. 2013 Jul;190(1):64–9.
22. Vickers AJ, Gupta A, Savage CJ, et al. A panel of kallikrein marker predicts prostate cancer in a large, population-based cohort followed for 15 years without screening. Cancer Epidemiol Biomark Prev. 2011;20:255–61.
23. Oesterling JE, Jacobsen SJ, Chute CG, et al. Serum prostate-specific antigen in a community-based population of healthy men. Establishment of age-specific reference ranges. JAMA. 1993;270(7):860–4.
24. Oesterling JE, Rice DC, Glenski WJ, et al. Effect of cystoscopy, prostate biopsy, and transurethral resection of prostate on serum prostate-specific antigen concentration. Urology. 1993;42(3):276–82.
25. Baillargeon J, Pollock BH, Kristal AR, et al. The association of body mass index and prostate-specific antigen in a population-based study. Cancer. 2005;103:1092–5.

26. Barqawi AB, Golden BK, O'Donnell C, et al. Observed effect of age and body mass index on total and complexed PSA: analysis from a national screening program. Urology. 2005;65(4):708–12.
27. Calle EE, Kaaks R. Overweight, obesity and cancer: epidemiological evidence and proposed mechanisms. Nat Rev. Cancer. 2004;4(8):579–91.
28. Freedland SJ, Platz EA, Presti JC Jr, et al. Obesity, serum prostate specific antigen and prostate size: implications for prostate cancer detection. J Urol. 2006;175:500–4.
29. Banez LL, Hamilton RJ, Partin AW, et al. Obesity-related plasma hemodilution and PSA concentration among men with prostate cancer. JAMA. 2007;298:2275–80.
30. Rundle A, Neugut AI. Obesity and screening PSA levels among men undergoing an annual physical exam. Prostate. 2008;68:373–80.
31. Grubb RL 3rd, Black A, Izmirlian G et al. Serum prostate-specific antigen hemodilution among obese men undergoing screening in the Prostate, Lung, Colorectal, and Ovarian Cancer Screening Trial. Cancer Epidemiol Biomark Prev 2009; 18: 748–751.
32. Calle EE, Rodriguez C, Walker-Thurmond K, Thun MJ. Overweight, obesity, and mortality from cancer in a prospectively studied cohort of U.S. adults. N Engl J Med. 2003;348(17):1625–38.
33. Kane CJ, Bassett WW, Sadetsky N, et al. Obesity and prostate cancer clinical risk factors at presentation: data from CaPSURE. J Urol. 2005 Mar;173(3):732–6.
34. Liang Y, Ketchum NS, Goodman PJ, et al. Is there a role for body mass index in assessment of prostate cancer risk on biopsy? J Urol. 2014 Oct;192(4):1094–9.
35. Cohen YC, Liu KS, Heyden NL, et al. Detection bias due to the effect of finasteride on prostate volume: a modeling approach for analysis of the Prostate Cancer Prevention Trial. J Natl Cancer Inst. 2007 Sep 19;99(18):1366–74.
36. Lucia MS, Epstein JI, Goodman PJ, et al. Finasteride and high-grade prostate cancer in the Prostate Cancer Prevention Trial. J Natl Cancer Inst. 2007;99(18):1375–83.
37. Park JH, Cho BL, Kwon HT, et al. Effect of body mass index and waist circumference on prostate specific antigen and prostate volume in a generally healthy Korean population. J Urol. 2009;182(1):106–10.
38. Xie LP, Bai Y, Zhang XZ, et al. Obesity and benign prostatic enlargement: a large observational study in China. Urology. 2007;69(4):680–4.
39. Fowke JH, Motley SS, Cookson MS, et al. The association between body size, prostate volume and prostate-specific antigen. Prostate Cancer Prostatic Dis. 2007;10(2):137–42.
40. Parsons JK, Carter HB, Partin AW, et al. Metabolic factors associated with benign prostatic hyperplasia. J Clin Endocrinol Metab. 2006;91(7):2562–8.
41. Kopp RP, Han M, Partin AW, et al. Obesity and prostate enlargement in men with localized prostate cancer. BJU Int. 2011;108(11):1750–5.
42. Kane CJ, Bassett WW, Sadetsky N, et al. Obesity and prostate cancer clinical risk factors at presentation: data from CaPSURE. J Urol. 2005;173(3):732–6.
43. Amling CL, Kane CJ, Riffenburgh RH, et al. Relationship between obesity and race in predicting adverse pathologic variables in patients undergoing radical prostatectomy. Urology. 2001;58(5):723–8.
44. Rohrmann S, Roberts WW, Walsh PC, et al. Family history of prostate cancer and obesity in relation to high-grade disease and extraprostatic extension in young men with prostate cancer. Prostate. 2003;55(2):140–6.
45. Rodriguez C, Patel AV, Calle EE, et al. Body mass index, height, and prostate cancer mortality in two large cohorts of adult men in the United States. Cancer Epidemiol Biomark Prev. 2001;10(4):345–53.
46. Discacciati A, Orsini N, Wolk A. Body mass index and incidence of localized and advanced prostate cancer—a dose-response meta-analysis of prospective studies. Ann Oncol. 2012;23(7):1665–71.
47. West DW, Slattery ML, Robison LM, et al. Adult dietary intake and prostate cancer risk in Utah: a case-control study with special emphasis on aggressive tumors. Cancer Causes Control. 1991;2:85–94.

48. Le Marchand L, Kolonel LN, Wilkens LR, et al. Animal fat consumption and prostate cancer: a prospective study in Hawaii. Epidemiology. 1994;5(3):276–82.
49. Friedenreich CM. Physical activity and cancer prevention: from observational to intervention research. Cancer Epidemiol Biomark Prev. 2001;10(4):287–301.
50. Patel AV, Rodriguez C, Jacobs EJ, et al. Recreational physical activity and risk of prostate cancer in a large cohort of US men. Cancer Epidemiol Biomark Prev. 2005 Jan;14(1):275–9.
51. Johnsen NF, Tjønneland A, Thomsen BL, et al. Physical activity and risk of prostate cancer in the European Prospective Investigation into Cancer and Nutrition (EPIC) cohort. Int J Cancer. 2009;125(4):902–8.
52. Nilsen TI, Romundstad PR, Vatten LJ. Recreational physical activity and risk of prostate cancer: a prospective population-based study in Norway (the HUNT study). Int J Cancer. 2006;119(12):2943–7.
53. Friedenreich CM, Wang Q, Neilson HK, et al. Physical activity and survival after prostate cancer. Eur Eurol. 2016;70(4):576–85.
54. Tjeertes EK, Hoeks SE, Beks SB, et al. Obesity—a risk factor for postoperative complications in general surgery? BMC Anesthesiol. 2015;15:112.
55. Xu T, Wang X, Xia L, et al. Robot-assisted prostatectomy in obese patients: how influential is obesity on operative outcomes? J Endourol. 2015;29(2):198–208.
56. Fitzsimons NJ, Sun LL, Philipp D, et al. A single-institution comparison between radical perineal and radical retropubic prostatectomy on perioperative and pathological outcomes for obese men: an analysis of the Duke Prostate Center Database. Urology. 2007;70(6):1146–51.
57. Eden CG, Chang CM, Gianduzzo T, et al. The impact of obesity on laparoscopic radical prostatectomy. BJU Int. 2006;98(6):1279–82.
58. Ho T, Gerber L, Aronson WJ, et al. Obesity, prostate-specific antigen nadir, and biochemical recurrence after radical prostatectomy: biology or technique? Results from the SEARCH database. Eur Urol. 2012;62(5):910–6.
59. Freedland SJ, Aronson WJ, Kane CJ, et al. Impact of obesity on biochemical control after radical prostatectomy for clinically localized prostate cancer: a report by the Shared Equal Access Regional Cancer Hospital Database Study Group. J Clin Oncol. February 2004;22(3):446–53.
60. Wang L, Murphy C, Ruth K, et al. Impact of obesity on outcomes after definitive dose escalated intensity modulated radiation therapy for localized prostate cancer. Cancer. 2015;121(17):3010–7.
61. Stroup SP, Cullen J, Auge BK, et al. Effect of obesity on prostate-specific antigen recurrence after radiation therapy for localized prostate cancer as measured by the 2006 Radiation Therapy Oncology Group-American Society for Therapeutic Radiation and Oncology (RTOG-ASTRO) Phoenix consensus definition. Cancer. 2007;110(5):1003–9.
62. Keto CJ, Aronson WJ, Terris MK, et al. Obesity is associated with castration-resistant disease and metastasis in men treated with androgen deprivation therapy after radical prostatectomy: results from the SEARCH database. BJU Int. 2012;110(4):492–8.

Chapter 7
Androgen Deprivation Therapy for Prostate Cancer: Effects on Body Composition and Metabolic Health

Grace Huang and Shehzad Basaria

Abstract Prostate cancer (PCa) is the most common malignancy diagnosed in American men. Androgen-deprivation therapy (ADT) has become the standard treatment for locally invasive, recurrent and metastatic PCa. Despite its effectiveness in lowering testosterone levels and improving survival in a subset of patients, ADT is associated with adverse effects including sexual dysfunction, vasomotor symptoms, anemia, osteoporosis and decreased quality of life. Altered body composition, resulting in reduced muscle mass and increased fat mass, is also frequently encountered in patients receiving ADT. As a result of these adverse changes in body composition, metabolic complications such as insulin resistance, diabetes, dyslipidemia and metabolic syndrome have also increased. These metabolic disturbances might be responsible for the increased cardiovascular morbidity and mortality seen in this patient population. Thus, screening, monitoring and treatment for cardiovascular risk factors (i.e. hyperglycemia, diabetes, hyperlipidemia, hypertension, obesity) in men receiving ADT might be prudent. Here we review the literature evaluating body composition changes as well as metabolic and cardiovascular complications of ADT.

Keywords Prostate cancer • Androgen deprivation therapy • Body composition • Insulin resistance • Hyperglycemia • Diabetes • Dyslipidemia • Metabolic syndrome • Cardiovascular disease

G. Huang, M.D. (✉)
Section on Men's Health, Aging and Metabolism, Brigham and Women's Hospital, Harvard Medical School, 221 Longwood Ave, BLI-541, Boston, MA 02115, USA
e-mail: ghuang7@partners.org

S. Basaria, M.D.
Brigham and Women's Hospital, Harvard Medical School, 221 Longwood Ave, BLI-541, Boston, MA 02115, USA
e-mail: sbasaria@partners.org

© Springer International Publishing AG 2018

E.A. Platz, N.A. Berger (eds.), *Energy Balance and Prostate Cancer*, Energy Balance and Cancer 14, DOI 10.1007/978-3-319-64940-5_7

Introduction

Prostate cancer (PCa) is the most common malignancy in American men and its incidence rose following the introduction of screening for prostate-specific antigen (PSA) levels, but the rate has declined recently following changed screening guidelines [1]. Since the description of its androgen-dependence, androgen-deprivation therapy (ADT) has been used in men with locally invasive, recurrent and metastatic PCa. Approximately 600,000 men in the United States alone are receiving ADT [2]. The aim of ADT is to suppress testosterone levels into the castrate range (<50 ng/dl; normal range 300–1000 ng/dl) [3]. The modalities of ADT include surgery (orchiectomy) or medical therapy (gonadotropin releasing hormone [GnRH] agonists or antagonists). Adjuvant use of ADT does improve survival in a subset of men with locally-invasive disease [4, 5], although recent trends suggest that ADT is now being used even in patients with early stage PCa and in those experiencing biochemical recurrence (rising PSA) despite no survival advantage having been shown in these patient populations. The use of ADT in the United States has increased in the past decade [6–9], hence, significant numbers of American men experience profound hypogonadism as a result of ADT.

Despite its effectiveness in improving mortality in a subset of patients, ADT is associated with numerous adverse effects including sexual dysfunction, vasomotor symptoms, poor quality of life, anemia, low bone density, increased fat mass, loss of muscle mass and strength as well as metabolic and cardiovascular complications [10, 11]. Here we summarize the adverse effects of androgen deprivation therapy with a focus on body composition changes and cardiometabolic complications (Fig. 7.1).

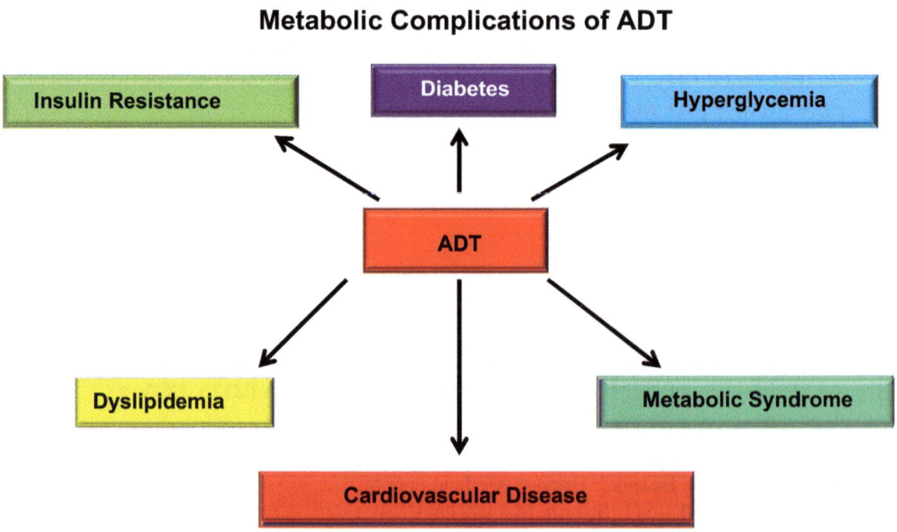

Fig. 7.1 Cardiometabolic complications of ADT

Hypogonadism, Body Composition and Cardiometabolic Health

Testosterone levels, after peaking in the second and third decade of life, decline gradually with advancing age [12]. In aging men, this decline in testosterone levels correlates with decreased lean body mass and increased fat mass which is reversed with testosterone replacement [13, 14]. Furthermore, low circulating testosterone levels in men have been associated with obesity [15], type 2 diabetes [16], metabolic syndrome [17], coronary artery disease [18] and cardiovascular events [19] in population studies. Intervention trials of testosterone administration in hypogonadal as well as eugonadal, young and older men have reported increases in lean body mass, decreases in whole body and visceral fat and improvement in cardiometabolic parameters. These observations are consistent with laboratory studies demonstrating that androgens stimulate mesenchymal pluripotent stem cells to commit to the myogenic lineage while inhibiting their differentiation into adipocytes [20] (Fig. 7.2). Data from preclinical models show that male mice with genetic disruption of the androgen receptor demonstrate insulin resistance, suggesting that androgens and/or androgen receptor signaling is important in the regulation of glucose metabolism [21]. Furthermore, low-density lipoprotein receptor-deficient mice undergoing orchiectomy develop atherosclerosis, which is attenuated by testosterone replacement [22]. These data support the mechanistic plausibility that androgen deficiency can result in adverse changes in body composition and metabolic dysregulation that could potentially lead to increased risk for cardiovascular disease (CVD).

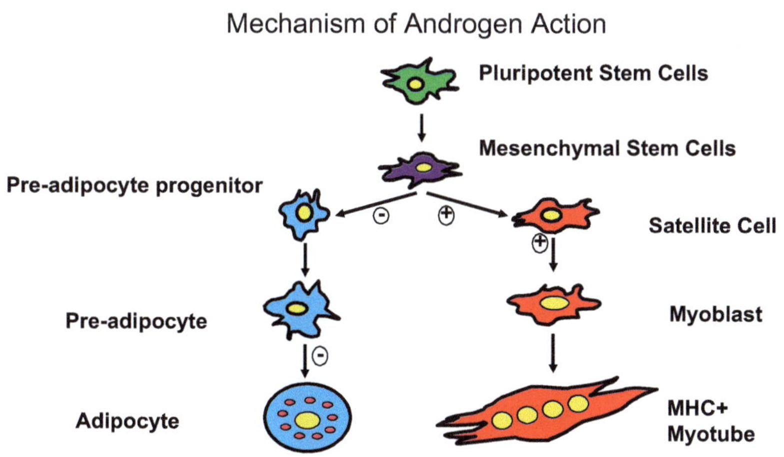

Fig. 7.2 Testosterone stimulates pluripotent cells to commit to a myogenic lineage and inhibits differentation to adiopogenic lineage (Adapted from [20])

Effects of ADT on Body Composition

Male hypogonadism results in declines in lean body mass and an increase in fat mass [12]. Changes in body composition are also well-recognized as adverse effects of ADT in men with PCa. Both cross-sectional and longitudinal studies have shown that ADT increases accumulation of fat mass while decreasing lean body mass, both worsening with duration of ADT exposure [10, 23, 24] (Fig. 7.3). One cross-sectional study evaluated body composition, bone mineral density and muscle strength in men with PCa undergoing long-term ADT (12–101 months) and compared it with men with PCa who had previously undergone only local therapy (i.e., surgery/radiation; non-ADT group) and with age-matched healthy men (controls). This study found that men undergoing ADT had higher fat mass, lower bone mineral density and reduced upper-and lower body muscle strength compared to the other groups [25]. Importantly, the subjects in the non-ADT group had greater muscle strength than controls, implying that hypogonadism was the likely etiology of this greater fat mass and lower muscle strength in the ADT group and not due to effects of the disease (PCa) itself.

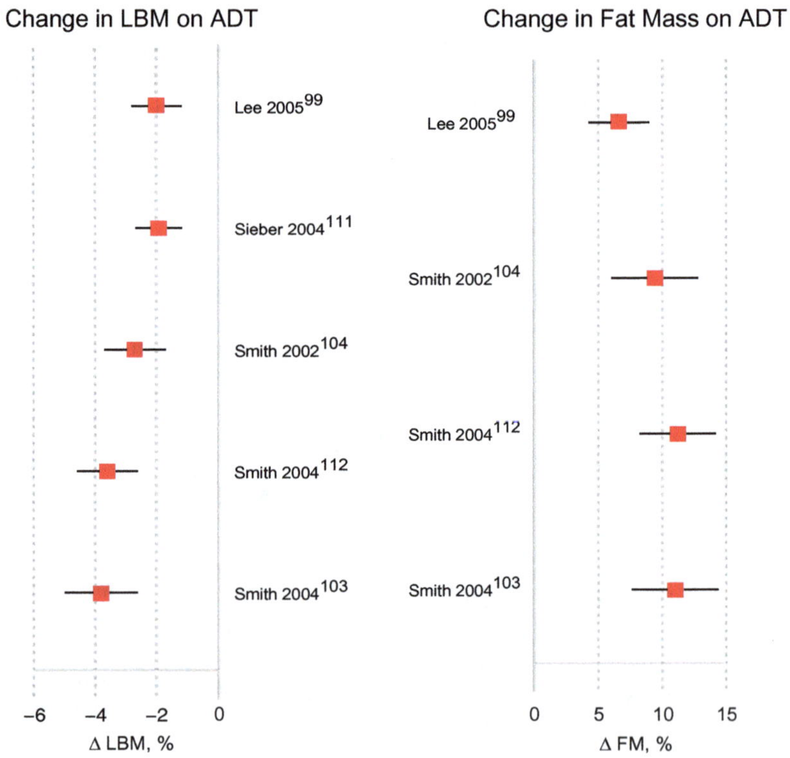

Fig. 7.3 (**a**) Change in LBM on ADT (**b**) Change in fat mass on ADT

One short term prospective study in 22 newly diagnosed men with PCa showed significant increases in fat mass (+1.7 kg) and decreases in lean body mass (−1.7 kg) after 3-months of ADT [26]. These findings have been confirmed in two long-term, prospective studies in men undergoing ADT for 48 weeks (+9.4% fat mass; −2.7% lean body mass) and 12-months (+6.6% fat mass; −2% lean mass) [23, 27]. Another 2-year prospective study compared body composition changes in 43 men on short-term ADT (less than 6 months), 67 men on chronic ADT (more than 6 months) and 53 age-matched healthy controls [28]. In this study, men undergoing short-term ADT had significant gains in body fat mass and loss in lean body mass that persisted at 12 (+1499.56 g fat mass; −929.74 g lean mass) and 24 months (+2167.15 g fat mass; −1785.81 g lean mass) after ADT completion compared to healthy controls. Similar to previously reported studies, these changes occurred early in the course of ADT and were most pronounced within the first year of initiation and continued to persist after the first year. Similarly, men on chronic ADT (mean duration 31 months) also experienced significant changes in body composition over 2 years of follow-up. Furthermore, there are some studies that suggest that hypogonadism related to ADT may also have differential effects on subcutaneous and visceral fat. One small study reported that ADT preferentially increased subcutaneous rather than visceral abdominal fat [23]. Larger prospective studies are required to confirm these findings.

A recent systematic review that investigated effects of ADT on lean mass from periods ranging from 3 to 24 months showed reductions in lean mass ranging between 1.4 and 3.86% with a mean annual reduction of −2.0% [29]. This 2.0% loss of lean mass per year in men undergoing ADT is substantial when compared to data in aging healthy older men who show a similar decrease in lean body mass but over a much longer period of time (1.9% decrease in lean body mass per decade) [30]. These changes in lean mass were not significantly related to changes in BMI.

In summary, ADT results in unfavorable changes in body composition. While the greatest changes in body composition occur during the first year in men on ADT, significant changes continue to occur even after 2 years [31]. The increase in fat mass from ADT correlates with higher insulin levels which in turn may lead to metabolic dysregulation, possibly via elaboration of adipokines and inflammatory cytokines [11, 26]. Furthermore, reduction in skeletal muscle mass from ADT may also result in decreased glucose uptake by muscle fibers, leading to insulin resistance, diabetes and increased risk for CVD in this population.

Metabolic Complications of ADT

It is well established that increased adiposity is a risk factor for insulin resistance, diabetes, dyslipidemia and metabolic syndrome [32]. Low serum testosterone levels in men are associated with obesity, insulin resistance, type 2 diabetes, dyslipidemia and metabolic syndrome [17, 33–35]. Similarly, men undergoing ADT have profound hypogonadism with testosterone levels in the castrate range potentially predisposing them to an even higher risk for developing these metabolic complications.

Insulin Resistance and Hyperglycemia After Short-Term (3–6 Months) ADT

Serum testosterone levels are positively associated with insulin sensitivity in men [36]; and testosterone replacement improves insulin sensitivity in hypogonadal men [37]. Acute withdrawal of testosterone in men with PCa who receive ADT is associated with the development of insulin resistance [38]; an early metabolic change that is correlated with increase in fat mass. In fact, several prospective studies have shown that men undergoing ADT develop insulin resistance within three months of initiation of ADT while no significant changes in insulin levels are seen in the non-ADT group [26, 39, 40]. In a 3-month prospective study of patients on ADT, Dockery and colleagues demonstrated a 63% increase in fasting insulin levels from baseline; however, there was no changes in fasting glucose [40]. Another 3-month intervention study using combined androgen blockade with leuprolide and bicalutamide reported a 26% increase in insulin levels that correlated with an increase in fat mass [39]; again, no change in fasting glucose was seen. Thus, the results of these short-term studies suggest that insulin resistance develops within a few months of starting ADT; however, the resulting hyperinsulinemia appears adequate to maintain normal serum glucose levels.

Insulin Resistance and Hyperglycemia After Long-Term (≥12 Months) ADT

Although euglycemia is maintained in the setting of insulin resistance with short-term ADT, longer duration of ADT can result in hyperglycemia and frank diabetes. In the last decade, some studies have evaluated long-term effects (≥12 months) of ADT on glucose metabolism. In a retrospective study of 44 patients with PCa undergoing ADT, fasting blood glucose levels initially remained unchanged at 6-months but then increased by 12-months after initiation of ADT [41]. In one cross-sectional study, 53 men with no history of diabetes were evaluated, including 18 men with PCa who received ADT for at least 12 months (ADT group), 17-age-matched men with nonmetastatic PCa who had undergone prostatectomy and/or radiotherapy and were not receiving ADT (non-ADT group) and 18 age-matched controls (control group) [38]. The mean duration of ADT was 45 months (range 12–101 months). In the ADT group, 15 men were being treated with GnRH analogs and 3 men had undergone orchiectomy. After adjustment for age and BMI, men in the ADT group had significantly higher fasting glucose, insulin and leptin levels compared to the both the non-ADT and control groups. Additionally, homeostatic model assessment for insulin resistance (HOMA-IR) was also significantly higher in the ADT group compared to non-ADT group and controls. Importantly, men in the ADT group had higher frequency (44%) of having fasting glucose levels meeting diagnostic criteria for diabetes mellitus (≥126 mg/dl) compared to men in the non-ADT (12%) and

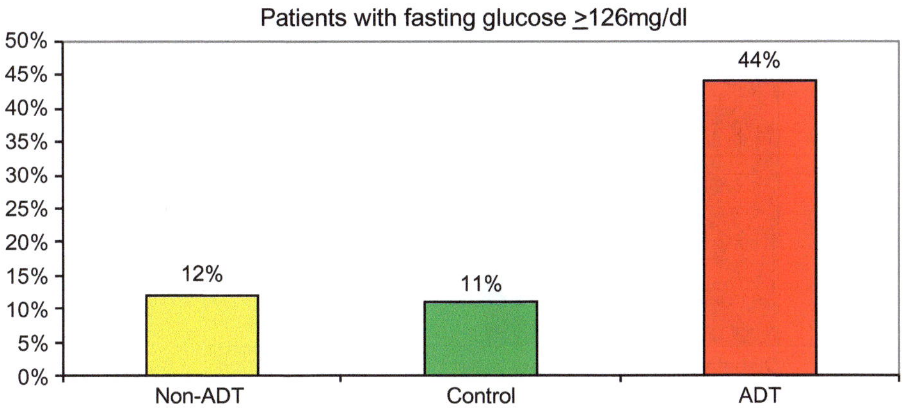

Fig. 7.4 ADT and DIABETES

control groups (11%) (Fig. 7.4). Furthermore, increases in fasting glucose, insulin, leptin and HOMA-IR negatively correlated with total and free testosterone levels. This study demonstrated that men with PCa receiving long-term ADT are at risk for development of insulin resistance and hyperglycemia independent of age and BMI and appears to be a direct result of androgen deprivation. However, it is important to appreciate that this study was cross-sectional in nature and that future prospective studies evaluating long-term effects of ADT on glucose metabolism are needed to establish causality. In a retrospective uncontrolled study in 396 patients receiving long-term ADT for PCa (median duration 60.1 months), of whom 319 did not have diabetes, 11.3% were diagnosed with new-onset diabetes [42]. This risk appeared to be stronger in patients with BMI $\geq$ 30 kg/m^2. Of the 77 patients with pre-existing diabetes mellitus in this study, 37 had worsening of their diabetes manifested by $\geq$10% increase in their serum HbA1c and/or fasting glucose levels. These results have been confirmed in a large prospective cohort study of 73,196 men with locoregional PCa undergoing ADT with GnRH agonists or orchiectomy [43]. In this study, men treated with ADT, regardless of modality, had significantly increased risk of incident diabetes (GnRH agonist: adjusted HR, 1.44; orchiectomy: adjusted HR 1.34) after median follow-up of 4.55 years (Fig. 7.5). These findings suggest that men with or without a history of diabetes already receiving or planning to start ADT may benefit from routine surveillance of glycemic control with appropriate screening, prevention and treatment measures.

Effect of ADT on Lipid Profile

Sex hormones are known to modulate serum lipoproteins. Epidemiologic studies have reported that testosterone levels are negatively related to total cholesterol, low-density lipoprotein (LDL) cholesterol and triglycerides in non-diabetic men

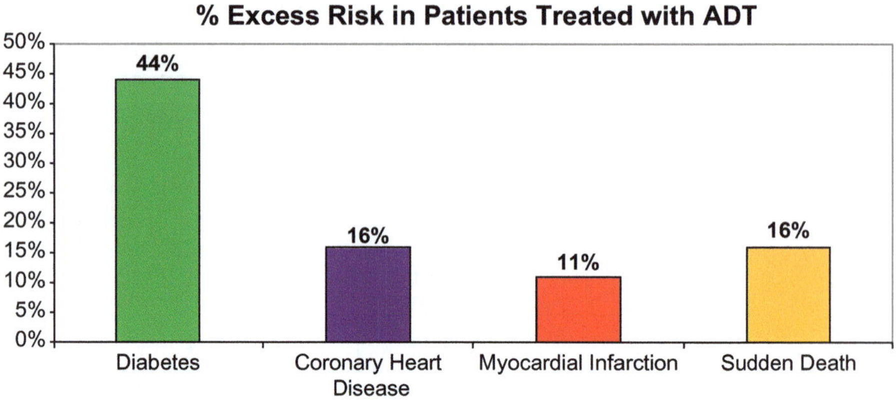

Fig. 7.5 ADT: Incident diabetes and CVD

[35]. This is further supported by the fact that low testosterone levels have been linked to altered lipoprotein lipase activity, leading to abnormal levels of LDL and triglycerides [40]. In longitudinal studies, the age-related decline in endogenous testosterone levels in men is associated with increase in serum triglycerides and decrease in serum HDL levels [44]. Furthermore, interventional studies have demonstrated that testosterone replacement in hypogonadal men results in improvements in lipid profile [45].

The effect of ADT on lipid profile has been evaluated in both cross-sectional and prospective studies. One short-term prospective study (3-months) of ADT showed significant increases in total and HDL cholesterol in the ADT group compared to non-ADT and non-cancer controls; while changes in LDL and triglycerides were non-significant [40]. Another study showed significant increases in serum triglycerides levels with ADT [39]. These findings are not universal as one prospective study did not demonstrate any significant changes in lipid profile after 3 months of ADT [26]; however, this study did not have a control group.

Long-term studies of ADT (≥12 months) have also reported similar changes in lipid profile. In one cross-sectional study of 44 men (16 undergoing ADT for at least 12-months, 14 age-matched eugonadal with non-metastatic PCa status post prostatectomy and/or radiotherapy and 14 age-matched eugonadal men not on ADT), men undergoing long-term ADT had higher total, LDL and non-HDL cholesterol compared to controls [46]. These findings are supported by a recent prospective study in 177 patients who demonstrated significant increases in total, LDL and HDL cholesterol after completing 1 year of ADT [47]. Another retrospective study in 44 men with PCa showed similar increases in total cholesterol, LDL cholesterol and triglycerides 12 months after initiation of ADT [41]. These changes in lipid metabolism were most prominent in the early ADT period consistent with the short-term studies described above. Interestingly, HDL cholesterol levels increased initially after the first 3-months of ADT in this study but then decreased after 12 months.

In summary, both short and long-term ADT in men with PCa leads to increases in total cholesterol, LDL-cholesterol and triglycerides; the specific lipoprotein changes are consistent in many but not all studies [48]. The HDL cholesterol also increased with ADT in some studies; however, the impact of these changes in various lipoproteins on CVD risk remains unclear. Long-term prospective studies are needed to determine whether alterations in lipoprotein levels resulting from ADT influences cardiovascular risk in men with PCa.

ADT and Metabolic Syndrome

Metabolic syndrome (MetS) is a risk factor for CVD, which confers a twofold increased risk for CVD [49]. MetS is an integrated measure of metabolic dysfunction comprised of central obesity, dyslipidemia, impaired glucose metabolism, and hypertension [50, 51]. Recent National Health and Nutrition Examination Survey (NHANES) data show that men have a higher prevalence of MetS than women, with higher proportions of men fulfilling criteria for the MetS components of hypertriglyceridemia, hypertension, low HDL and hyperglycemia [52]. Male hypogonadism has been shown to be an independent risk factor for the development of metabolic syndrome in population studies [53, 54]. This is significant given that the prevalence of MetS in patients with PCa is higher than the general population [55] and may be even higher after use of ADT.

The effect of ADT on development of the metabolic syndrome has been evaluated in both cross-sectional and prospective studies. A cross-sectional study evaluated the prevalence of metabolic syndrome in men with PCa undergoing long-term ADT with age and disease-matched controls [56]. In this study, more than half of men (55%) undergoing ADT had MetS compared with one fifth of men (22% and 20%) in the non-ADT and control groups, respectively; hyperglycemia and abdominal obesity appeared to be the major determinants of the higher prevalence of MetS in the ADT group (Fig. 7.6). In a case-control study, Valverde and colleagues reported that the prevalence of MetS in men was 21% after 6-months of ADT and increased to 36% after 12–18 months of treatment [57]. In a recent meta-analysis of nine studies published to date on risk of MetS following ADT for PCa, the investigators found a significant association between ADT and risk for MetS (RR 1.75) [58]. In this meta-analysis, diabetes was the most prevalent MetS component among ADT users (pooled relative risk 1.36). When examining specific components of the MetS, other studies have also suggested that the MetS phenotype associated with ADT is a pattern of metabolic alterations that is distinct from the classic MetS. In one open-label prospective study, 26 men with recurrent or locally advanced PCa were treated with leuprolide for 12-months [59]. In this study, leuprolide increased waist circumference and serum triglycerides (components of the MetS), but did not significantly alter blood pressure and paradoxically increased HDL cholesterol. In another prospective study, men with PCa undergoing ADT through surgical castration had significantly higher waist circumference,

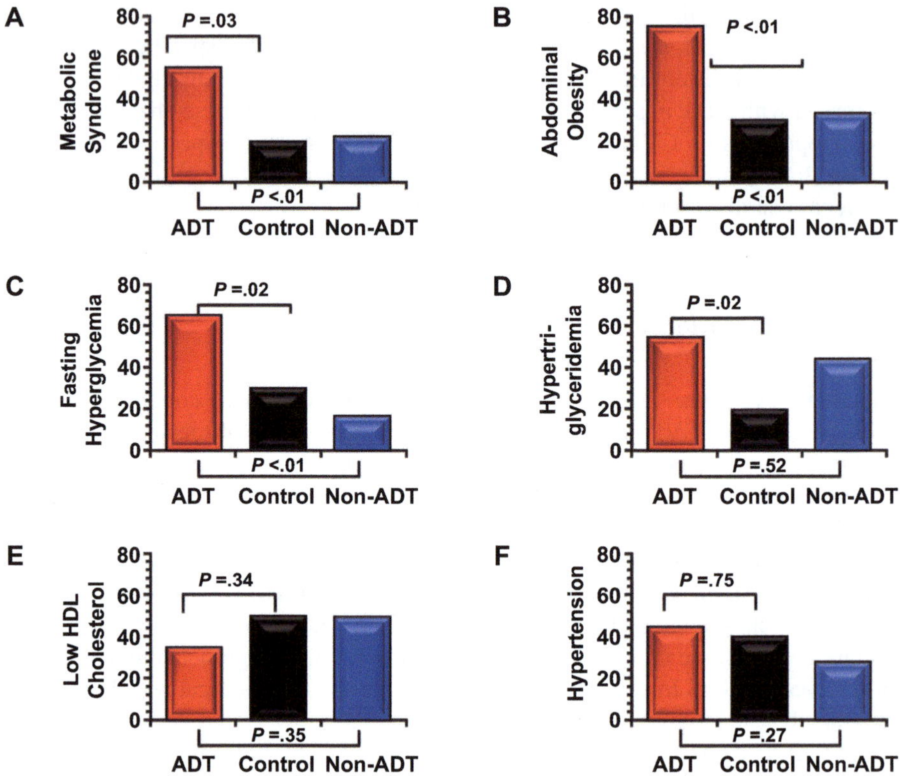

Fig. 7.6 Long-term ADT and metabolic syndrome

and levels of fasting glucose, fasting insulin, and HDL-cholesterol compared to both non-ADT and normal controls [60]. Classic MetS is typically characterized by central adiposity, insulin resistance, high triglycerides, low HDL cholesterol, hypertension, low adiponectin levels and elevated inflammatory markers [61, 62]. On the contrary, MetS in ADT is associated with increases in adiponectin and HDL cholesterol while not significantly changing C-reactive protein levels or blood pressure [62, 63].

In summary, several studies have shown that ADT for PCa increases risk for development of MetS. However, the metabolic phenotype in men undergoing ADT has some but not all the characteristics of the "classic" MetS. Furthermore, the severity of metabolic alterations of ADT may depend not only on the cumulative duration but also frequency of administration. A recent longitudinal study found that patients receiving intermittent ADT had lower rates of metabolic syndrome compared to those receiving continuous ADT over 12 months [64]. However, there is insufficient data to determine whether intermittent ADT administration has the potential to prevent or decrease these metabolic derangements. Larger long-term prospective studies are needed to better characterize the MetS phenotype in men undergoing different types of ADT for PCa as well as examining the implications of these metabolic effects on overall CVD risk.

Cardiovascular Disease

CVD is the most common cause of non-cancer death in patients with PCa [65]. Satariano and colleagues were the first to report that CVD was the second most common cause of death in men with PCa (after PCa-specific mortality) [66]. ADT is the standard treatment for patients with aggressive PCa and has resulted in decreased recurrence rates and improved survival [4]. However, despite its efficacy in the treatment of advanced and metastatic PCa, ADT, in some studies, has been associated with increased risk of coronary artery disease, myocardial infarction and sudden cardiac death [43].

Several studies have reported association of ADT use and increased risk of cardiovascular morbidity and mortality [67]. Saigal et al. reported that men undergoing ADT for at least 12 months had 20% higher risk of cardiovascular morbidity compared with men not receiving ADT [68]. Importantly, for many men, this risk occurred within the first year of treatment. Keating et al. showed that men undergoing ADT with GnRH agonist had higher risk of incident coronary heart disease, myocardial infarction and sudden cardiac death compared with non-ADT men over a median follow-up of 4.55 years (Fig. 7.5) [43]. Interestingly, men treated with ADT with orchiectomy did not demonstrate increased CVD risk in this study, likely attributable to the fact that few men (6.9%) underwent this treatment modality for their disease. A meta-analysis of randomized PCa trials showed that men aged 65 and older receiving ADT for as short as 6 months experienced shorter times to fatal myocardial infarction compared with age-matched men not receiving ADT and younger men [69]. Another study found that men undergoing ADT had 2.6 times the risk of cardiovascular mortality than non-ADT controls after adjusting for age and CVD risk factors [70]. In this study, the increased risk for CVD mortality was seen in both younger (<65 years) and older men (≥65 years).

Recent studies have suggested that the cardiovascular complications associated with ADT predominately occur in vulnerable subgroups of men with pre-existing CVD. Nanda and colleagues demonstrated that neoadjuvant hormone therapy use for localized or locally advanced PCa associated with increased risk of all-cause mortality among men with a history of coronary artery disease-induced congestive heart failure (CHF) or myocardial infarction (median follow-up 5.1 years); whereas, no significant risk was seen in men without comorbidity [71]. Another large prospective study of 5077 men with locally advanced PCa showed that use of ADT was associated with higher risk of cardiac-related mortality in those with CHF or prior MI [72].

In addition to CVD, ADT has also been associated in observational studies with thromboembolic events including deep vein thrombosis, pulmonary embolism, arterial thrombosis and stroke [73, 74]. Long-term randomized controlled studies are needed to determine potential effects of ADT on peripheral vascular disease.

Summary

ADT is associated with adverse changes in body composition and metabolic profile. Metabolic complications such as insulin resistance, diabetes, hyperlipidemia and MetS may be responsible for the increased cardiovascular morbidity and mortality seen in these men. The increased risk for these cardiometabolic complications becomes evident within months of beginning ADT. In 2010, the American Heart Association acknowledged the *potential* association between ADT and cardiovascular events [7]. In October 2010, the US Food and Drug Administration issued a safety warning requiring that the labeling of GnRH agonists include a statement disclosing "increased risk for diabetes and certain cardiovascular diseases (heart attack, sudden cardiac death and stroke) in men receiving these medications for treatment of prostate cancer" [67]. Thus, it is important for physicians to screen for various cardiovascular risk factors in men already receiving or planning to start ADT. Currently, there are no formal guidelines for the prevention and management of CVD in patients on ADT. However, findings from multiple studies suggest that these men may benefit from screening, treatment and prevention strategies for various cardiovascular risk factors. These men, especially those with preexisting CVD, should be counseled on lifestyle modification (diet, exercise, weight reduction, smoking cessation) and optimally treated for existing CVD risk factors such as diabetes, hyperlipidemia and hypertension [75]. In fact, a recent randomized controlled trial showed that a 12-week lifestyle intervention of supervised exercise training and dietary counseling led to improved endothelial function (measured by flow-mediated dilation) in men on long-term ADT for PCa [76]. The beneficial role of aspirin, statins and insulin sensitizers for the primary prevention of CVD in this population requires further study.

As androgen replacement is contraindicated in PCa, future prospective intervention trials assessing the role of novel anti-inflammatory agents, myostatin antagonists and anabolic agents such as SARMS (Selective Androgen Receptor Modulators—agents that act as agonists on muscle and metabolic tissues but spare the prostate) are needed to assess for potential targeted approaches in the prevention and treatment of cardiometabolic complications associated with ADT [77].

References

1. Siegel RL, Miller KD, Jemal A. Cancer statistics, 2017. CA Cancer J Clin. 2017;67(1):7–30.
2. Smith MR. Androgen deprivation therapy for prostate cancer: new concepts and concerns. Curr Opin Endocrinol Diabetes Obes. 2007;14(3):247–54.
3. Bubley GJ, et al. Eligibility and response guidelines for phase II clinical trials in androgen-independent prostate cancer: recommendations from the Prostate-Specific Antigen Working Group. J Clin Oncol. 1999;17(11):3461–7.
4. Messing EM, et al. Immediate hormonal therapy compared with observation after radical prostatectomy and pelvic lymphadenectomy in men with node-positive prostate cancer. N Engl J Med. 1999;341(24):1781–8.

5. Sharifi N, Gulley JL, Dahut WL. Androgen deprivation therapy for prostate cancer. JAMA. 2005;294(2):238–44.
6. Shahinian VB, et al. Increasing use of gonadotropin-releasing hormone agonists for the treatment of localized prostate carcinoma. Cancer. 2005;103(8):1615–24.
7. Levine GN, et al. Androgen-deprivation therapy in prostate cancer and cardiovascular risk: a science advisory from the American Heart Association, American Cancer Society, and American Urological Association: endorsed by the American Society for Radiation Oncology. CA Cancer J Clin. 2010;60(3):194–201.
8. Labrie F, et al. Gonadotropin-releasing hormone agonists in the treatment of prostate cancer. Endocr Rev. 2005;26(3):361–79.
9. Connolly RM, Carducci MA, Antonarakis ES. Use of androgen deprivation therapy in prostate cancer: indications and prevalence. Asian J Androl. 2012;14(2):177–86.
10. Storer TW, Miciek R, Travison TG. Muscle function, physical performance and body composition changes in men with prostate cancer undergoing androgen deprivation therapy. Asian J Androl. 2012;14(2):204–21.
11. Basaria S. Androgen deprivation therapy, insulin resistance, and cardiovascular mortality: an inconvenient truth. J Androl. 2008;29(5):534–9.
12. Spitzer M, et al. Risks and benefits of testosterone therapy in older men. Nat Rev Endocrinol. 2013;9(7):414–24.
13. Vermeulen A, Goemaere S, Kaufman JM. Testosterone, body composition and aging. J Endocrinol Invest. 1999;22(5 Suppl):110–6.
14. Basaria S, Dobs AS. Hypogonadism and androgen replacement therapy in elderly men. Am J Med. 2001;110(7):563–72.
15. Derby CA, et al. Body mass index, waist circumference and waist to hip ratio and change in sex steroid hormones: the Massachusetts Male Ageing Study. Clin Endocrinol (Oxf). 2006;65(1):125–31.
16. Ding EL, et al. Sex differences of endogenous sex hormones and risk of type 2 diabetes: a systematic review and meta-analysis. JAMA. 2006;295(11):1288–99.
17. Laaksonen DE, et al. Testosterone and sex hormone-binding globulin predict the metabolic syndrome and diabetes in middle-aged men. Diabetes Care. 2004;27(5):1036–41.
18. Wu FC, von Eckardstein A. Androgens and coronary artery disease. Endocr Rev. 2003;24(2):183–217.
19. Corona G, et al. Hypogonadism as a risk factor for cardiovascular mortality in men: a meta-analytic study. Eur J Endocrinol. 2011;165(5):687–701.
20. Bhasin S, et al. The mechanisms of androgen effects on body composition: mesenchymal pluripotent cell as the target of androgen action. J Gerontol A Biol Sci Med Sci. 2003;58(12):M1103–10.
21. Lin HY, et al. Increased hepatic steatosis and insulin resistance in mice lacking hepatic androgen receptor. Hepatology. 2008;47(6):1924–35.
22. Nathan L, et al. Testosterone inhibits early atherogenesis by conversion to estradiol: critical role of aromatase. Proc Natl Acad Sci USA. 2001;98(6):3589–93.
23. Smith MR, et al. Changes in body composition during androgen deprivation therapy for prostate cancer. J Clin Endocrinol Metab. 2002;87(2):599–603.
24. Smith MR. Changes in fat and lean body mass during androgen-deprivation therapy for prostate cancer. Urology. 2004;63(4):742–5.
25. Basaria S, et al. Long-term effects of androgen deprivation therapy in prostate cancer patients. Clin Endocrinol (Oxf). 2002;56(6):779–86.
26. Smith JC, et al. The effects of induced hypogonadism on arterial stiffness, body composition, and metabolic parameters in males with prostate cancer. J Clin Endocrinol. 2001;86(9):4261–7.
27. Lee H, et al. Changes in bone mineral density and body composition during initial and long-term gonadotropin-releasing hormone agonist treatment for prostate carcinoma. Cancer. 2005;104(8):1633–7.
28. van Londen GJ, et al. Body composition changes during androgen deprivation therapy for prostate cancer: a 2-year prospective study. Crit Rev Oncol Hematol. 2008;68(2):172–7.

29. Haseen F, et al. The effect of androgen deprivation therapy on body composition in men with prostate cancer: systematic review and meta-analysis. J Cancer Surviv. 2010;4(2):128–39.
30. Hughes VA, et al. Longitudinal changes in body composition in older men and women: role of body weight change and physical activity. Am J Clin Nutr. 2002;76(2):473–81.
31. Collins L, Basaria S. Adverse effects of androgen deprivation therapy in men with prostate cancer: a focus on metabolic and cardiovascular complications. Asian J Androl. 2012;14(2):222–5.
32. Grundy SM. Obesity, metabolic syndrome, and cardiovascular disease. J Clin Endocrinol Metabol. 2004;89(6):2595–600.
33. Muller M, et al. Endogenous sex hormones and metabolic syndrome in aging men. J Clin Endocrinol Metabol. 2005;90(5):2618–23.
34. Haffner SM, et al. Low levels of sex hormone-binding globulin and testosterone predict the development of non-insulin-dependent diabetes mellitus in men. MRFIT Research Group. Multiple Risk Factor Intervention Trial. Am J Epidemiol. 1996;143(9):889–97.
35. Haffner SM, et al. Relationship of sex hormones to lipids and lipoproteins in nondiabetic men. J Clin Endocrinol Metabol. 1993;77(6):1610–5.
36. Pitteloud N, et al. Increasing insulin resistance is associated with a decrease in Leydig cell testosterone secretion in men. J Clin Endocrinol Metabol. 2005;90(5):2636–41.
37. Marin P, et al. The effects of testosterone treatment on body composition and metabolism in middle-aged obese men. Int J Obes Relat Metab Disord. 1992;16(12):991–7.
38. Basaria S, et al. Hyperglycemia and insulin resistance in men with prostate carcinoma who receive androgen-deprivation therapy. Cancer. 2006;106(3):581–8.
39. Smith MR, Lee H, Nathan DM. Insulin sensitivity during combined androgen blockade for prostate cancer. J Clin Endocrinol Metabol. 2006;91(4):1305–8.
40. Dockery F, et al. Testosterone suppression in men with prostate cancer leads to an increase in arterial stiffness and hyperinsulinaemia. Clin Sci (Lond). 2003;104(2):195–201.
41. Saglam HS, et al. Fasting blood glucose and lipid profile alterations following twelve-month androgen deprivation therapy in men with prostate cancer. ScientificWorldJournal. 2012;2012:696329.
42. Derweesh IH, et al. Risk of new-onset diabetes mellitus and worsening glycaemic variables for established diabetes in men undergoing androgen-deprivation therapy for prostate cancer. BJU Int. 2007;100(5):1060–5.
43. Keating NL, O'Malley AJ, Smith MR. Diabetes and cardiovascular disease during androgen deprivation therapy for prostate cancer. J Clin Oncol. 2006;24(27):4448–56.
44. Zmuda JM, et al. Longitudinal relation between endogenous testosterone and cardiovascular disease risk factors in middle-aged men. A 13-year follow-up of former Multiple Risk Factor Intervention Trial participants. Am J Epidemiol. 1997;146(8):609–17.
45. Malkin CJ, et al. The effect of testosterone replacement on endogenous inflammatory cytokines and lipid profiles in hypogonadal men. J Clin Endocrinol Metab. 2004;89(7):3313–8.
46. Braga-Basaria M, et al. Lipoprotein profile in men with prostate cancer undergoing androgen deprivation therapy. Int J Impot Res. 2006;18(5):494–8.
47. Mitsuzuka K, et al. Influence of 1 year of androgen deprivation therapy on lipid and glucose metabolism and fat accumulation in Japanese patients with prostate cancer. Prostate Cancer Prostatic Dis. 2016;19(1):57–62.
48. Salvador C, et al. Analysis of the lipid profile and atherogenic risk during androgen deprivation therapy in prostate cancer patients. Urol Int. 2013;90(1):41–4.
49. Ford ES. Prevalence of the metabolic syndrome in US populations. Endocrinol Metab Clin North Am. 2004;33(2):333–50.
50. DeFronzo RA, Ferrannini E. Insulin resistance. A multifaceted syndrome responsible for NIDDM, obesity, hypertension, dyslipidemia, and atherosclerotic cardiovascular disease. Diabetes Care. 1991;14(3):173–94.
51. Reaven GM. Banting lecture 1988. Role of insulin resistance in human disease. Diabetes. 1998;37(12):1595–607.

52. Beltran-Sanchez H, et al. Prevalence and trends of metabolic syndrome in the adult U.S. population, 1999–2010. J Am Coll Cardiol. 2013;62(8):697–703.
53. Kupelian V, et al. Low sex hormone-binding globulin, total testosterone, and symptomatic androgen deficiency are associated with development of the metabolic syndrome in nonobese men. J Clin Endocrinol Metabol. 2006;91(3):843–50.
54. Laaksonen DE, et al. The metabolic syndrome and smoking in relation to hypogonadism in middle-aged men: a prospective cohort study. J Clin Endocrinol Metab. 2005;90(2):712–9.
55. Samper Ots PM, et al. SIMBOSPROST: Prevalence of metabolic syndrome and osteoporosis in prostate cancer patients treated with radiotherapy and androgen deprivation therapy: A multicentre, cross-sectional study. Rep Pract Oncol Radiother. 2015;20(5):370–6.
56. Braga-Basaria M, et al. Metabolic syndrome in men with prostate cancer undergoing long-term androgen-deprivation therapy. J Clin Oncol. 2006;24(24):3979–83.
57. Ropero Valverde J, Planas Morin J, Salvador Lacambra C, Trilla Herrera E, Placer Santos J, et al. Prevalence of metabolic syndrome in prostate cancer patients under androgen deprivation therapy: Interim results of a case-control study. Eur Urol Suppl. 2011;10:337.
58. Bosco C, et al. Quantifying the evidence for the risk of metabolic syndrome and its components following androgen deprivation therapy for prostate cancer: a meta-analysis. PLoS One. 2015;10(3):e0117344.
59. Smith MR, O'Malley AJ, Keating NL. Gonadotrophin-releasing hormone agonists, diabetes and cardiovascular disease in men with prostate cancer: which metabolic syndrome? BJU Int. 2008;101(11):1335–6.
60. Bo JJ, et al. Androgen deprivation therapy through bilateral orchiectomy: increased metabolic risks. Asian J Androl. 2011;13(6):833–7.
61. Smith MR, et al. Adipocytokines, obesity, and insulin resistance during combined androgen blockade for prostate cancer. Urology. 2008;71(2):318–22.
62. Smith MR, et al. Metabolic changes during gonadotropin-releasing hormone agonist therapy for prostate cancer: differences from the classic metabolic syndrome. Cancer. 2008;112(10):2188–94.
63. Morote J, et al. The metabolic syndrome and its components in patients with prostate cancer on androgen deprivation therapy. J Urol. 2015;193(6):1963–9.
64. Rezaei MM, et al. Metabolic syndrome in patients with prostate cancer undergoing intermittent androgen-deprivation therapy. Can Urol Assoc J. 2016;10(9-10):E300–5.
65. Epstein MM, et al. Temporal trends in cause of death among Swedish and US men with prostate cancer. J Natl Cancer Inst. 2012;104(17):1335–42.
66. Satariano WA, Ragland KE, Van Den Eeden SK. Cause of death in men diagnosed with prostate carcinoma. Cancer. 1998;83(6):1180–8.
67. Basaria S. Cardiovascular disease associated with androgen-deprivation therapy: time to give it due respect. J Clin Oncol. 2015;33(11):1232–4.
68. Saigal CS, et al. Androgen deprivation therapy increases cardiovascular morbidity in men with prostate cancer. Cancer. 2007;110(7):1493–500.
69. D'Amico AV, et al. Influence of androgen suppression therapy for prostate cancer on the frequency and timing of fatal myocardial infarctions. J Clin Oncol. 2007;25(17):2420–5.
70. Tsai HK, et al. Androgen deprivation therapy for localized prostate cancer and the risk of cardiovascular mortality. J Natl Cancer Inst. 2007;99(20):1516–24.
71. Nanda A, et al. Hormonal therapy use for prostate cancer and mortality in men with coronary artery disease-induced congestive heart failure or myocardial infarction. JAMA. 2009;302(8):866–73.
72. Ziehr DR, et al. Association of androgen-deprivation therapy with excess cardiac-specific mortality in men with prostate cancer. BJU Int. 2015;116(3):358–65.
73. Conteduca V, et al. The cardiovascular risk of gonadotropin releasing hormone agonists in men with prostate cancer: an unresolved controversy. Crit Rev Oncol Hematol. 2013;86(1):42–51.
74. Nguyen PL, et al. Adverse effects of androgen deprivation therapy and strategies to mitigate them. Eur Urol. 2015;67(5):825–36.

75. Bhatia N, et al. Cardiovascular Effects of Androgen Deprivation Therapy for the Treatment of Prostate Cancer: ABCDE Steps to Reduce Cardiovascular Disease in Patients With Prostate Cancer. Circulation. 2016;133(5):537–41.
76. Gilbert SE, et al. Effects of a lifestyle intervention on endothelial function in men on long-term androgen deprivation therapy for prostate cancer. Br J Cancer. 2016;114(4):401–8.
77. Basaria S, Bhasin S. Targeting the skeletal muscle-metabolism axis in prostate-cancer therapy. N Engl J Med. 2012;367(10):965–7.

Chapter 8
The Integration of Exercise and Dietary Lifestyle Interventions into Prostate Cancer Care

Ciaran M. Fairman, Alexander R. Lucas, Elizabeth Grainger, Steven K. Clinton, and Brian C. Focht

Abstract Prostate cancer (PCa) is among the most prevalent forms of cancer among American men. For many decades, androgen deprivation therapy and newer drugs inhibiting various aspects of aberrant androgen signaling, have been a mainstay of therapy and are increasingly incorporated into multimodality treatment plans for men with prostate cancer. Although improving rate of cure and promoting survival, the adverse effects of anti-androgen therapy place men at increased risk from loss of muscle mass, sarcopenic obesity, functional declines, and metabolic syndrome and its many sequela, such as cardiovascular disease. Consequently, there is growing interest in the feasibility and efficacy of implementing lifestyle interventions that have the potential to improve treatment outcomes and support quality of life and functional status men impacted by PCa patients. The purpose of the present chapter is to provide an overview of the current scientific evidence regarding the impact of dietary intervention and exercise, both separately and in combination, for men with PCa. Although the number of studies remains modest, current evidence demonstrates that exercise, diet, and combined exercise and dietary interventions

C.M. Fairman, M.S.
Kinesiology, Department of Human Sciences, The Ohio State University, 305 Annie and John Glenn Ave, Columbus, OH 43210, USA
e-mail: fairman.13@buckeyemail.osu.edu

A.R. Lucas, Ph.D.
Department of Social Sciences and Health Policy, Wake Forest School of Medicine, Medical Center Boulevard, Winston, Salem, NC 27157, USA
e-mail: arlucas@wakehealth.edu

E. Grainger, Ph.D., R.D • S.K. Clinton, M.D., Ph.D.
Division of Medical Oncology, College of Medicine, The Ohio State University, A 456 Starling-Loving Hall, 320 W 10th Ave, Columbus, OH 43210, USA
e-mail: Elizabeth.Grainger@osumc.edu; steven.clinton@osumc.edu

B.C. Focht, Ph.D., F.A.C.S.M., C.S.C.S. (✉)
Kinesiology, Department of Human Sciences, OSU Comprehensive Cancer Center, The Ohio State University, 305 Annie and John Glenn Ave, Columbus, OH 43210, USA
e-mail: focht.10@osu.edu

© Springer International Publishing AG 2018

E.A. Platz, N.A. Berger (eds.), *Energy Balance and Prostate Cancer*, Energy Balance and Cancer 14, DOI 10.1007/978-3-319-64940-5_8

can result in significant, clinically meaningful improvements in a variety of health, fitness, and quality of life outcomes among PCa patients. The emerging evidence supports the need for studies to optimize and personalize strategies integrating lifestyle exercise and dietary interventions into the multi-disciplinary treatment strategies that improve outcomes and quality of life for men with PCa.

Keywords Lifestyle Interventions • Dietary Interventions • Multidisciplinary Interventions • Behavioral Interventions • Individualized Diet and Exercise Adherence (IDEA-P) Trial

Prostate cancer (PCa) is the most common visceral malignancy in men in both Europe and North America [1]. The risk of PCa increases with advancing age, with over a 1000% increase from age 45 to 70, and the majority of men being diagnosed after 65 years of age [1]. Testosterone is a critical hormone regulating the normal development and function of the prostate, and this hormone plays a critical role in the carcinogenesis process. Thus, anti-androgen therapy has for decades played a key role in the treatment of advanced disease, and increasingly is utilized in multimodality therapy involving combination therapy with radiation, traditional chemotherapy, and novel biological treatments. Thus, the number of prostate cancer patients experiencing anti-androgen therapy to cure or prolong life continues to increase.

Regardless of the approach to reducing testosterone concentrations or antagonizing specific steps in androgen signaling, such as surgical castration or pharmacologic means, the impact is a complex syndrome that has many physiological and psychological effects on the patient. Of significant concern is the loss of lean muscle mass, increased fat mass, reduced muscle strength, and lower bone mineral density, that place men at greater risk for functional decline and frailty [2–9]. Emerging evidence also suggests that ADT increases risk for metabolic syndrome and its consequences, including cardiovascular disease (CVD) [9]. When we consider that many men in affluent nations have pre-existing obesity and cardiometabolic disorders prior to the diagnosis of prostate cancer, a cancer therapy that potentiates these conditions should be of major concern. As prolonged administration of ADT becomes increasingly common, particularly with the growing array of effective anti-androgens and multimodality treatment strategies in the adjuvant and neoadjuvant settings, many men will cope with lasting treatment-related physiological effects that meaningfully compromise their physical function and quality of life and heighten the risk of comorbid metabolic and cardiovascular events. In recent decades, we have increasingly appreciated the critical role of diet and exercise in maintaining health and preventing disease across the lifespan [10]. Furthermore, the utility of diet and exercise as part of a therapeutic plan for those with metabolic and cardiovascular disease is clear, yet poorly supported by our health care system.

Consequently, it is very clear that prostate cancer patients should be a critical target for defining the feasibility and efficacy of interventions that preserve or promote health and functional abilities through evidence based diet and exercise programs [2, 6, 11–18].

The objective of the present chapter is to provide a brief overview of the emerging studies that illustrate the effects of exercise and dietary interventions, both separately and in combination, among PCa patients/survivors. At the outset, we feel that the research in on this topic is in the very early phase of development, and that continued research to define effective interventions, to personalize strategies for diverse patient characteristics, and to insure durable efficacy are all critically needed. We also recognize that diet and fitness interventions must be individualized to manage energy balance and obesity issues relevant to each patient. Results from systematic reviews and findings of randomized controlled trials involving the use of energy balance interventions in PCa treatment are provided in this review. Implications of behavioral weight management approaches and how they can be implemented to guide the design and delivery of lifestyle interventions targeting men undergoing androgen deprivation therapy are also presented.

Exercise Interventions in the Treatment of PCa Patients and Survivors

In recent years, results from studies examining the effects of integrating exercise programs into the treatment and supportive care of PCa patients have emerged. Findings from multiple well-designed randomized controlled trials [19, 20] and systematic reviews [21, 22] demonstrate that exercise interventions consistently result in significant, clinically meaningful improvements in muscular strength, physical function, and quality of life in PCa patients. Thorsen et al. [22] conducted a systematic review of studies regarding physical activity in PCa patients focusing upon the outcomes, prevalence, and determinants of physical activity. Results of six intervention studies of modest size (404 men total) demonstrated that physical activity interventions yielded the most favorable improvements in muscular fitness, physical function, fatigue, and select quality of life outcomes. Findings from six cross-sectional studies (2121 men) evaluating physical activity participation revealed wide variability in prevalence of physical activity efforts, with 30–70% of PCa patients or survivors reporting engaging in regular physical activity programs.

Focht et al. [21] conducted a systematic review of nine studies (684 men) examining the effects of exercise on disablement process model outcomes among PCa patients undergoing ADT [21]. Consistent with the findings from intervention studies in the Thorsen et al. [22] review, exercise consistently yielded clinically meaningful improvements in an array of relevant physiologic, fitness, and patient-reported outcomes [22]. However, considerable heterogeneity in the magnitude of improvement in outcomes across the disablement process model domains was observed. For example, whereas the most pronounced improvements were observed for muscular strength (Cohen's *d* effect size = 0.74) and muscular endurance (*d* = 2.34), improvements in performance measures of physical function were accompanied by a moderate effect size (*d* = 0.46). It is particularly noteworthy that in contrast to change in muscular fitness and physical function, the exercise programs studied resulted in a small effect size improvement in body composition (*d* = 0.08), suggesting that ADT may make it more difficult to achieve this goal than in men with normal testosterone, a topic warranting additional research. Behavioral interventions that preserve or improve body composition are of particular value to PCa patients on ADT given the established adverse effects the treatment has on lean body mass, fat mass, and body composition. These early observations suggest that we must conduct studies of various exercise programs to better define optimal or desired outcomes regarding body composition in PCa patients. Nevertheless, we interpret the findings as underscoring the benefit of exercise interventions in preserving lean body mass and more favorable overall body composition in patients undergoing ADT. Notably, ADT has been associated with increases of approximately 8% body fat and 2% decrease in lean body mass across a year or more of treatment [23]. However, our systematic review demonstrated that PCa patients on ADT who received concomitant exercise therapy did not experience the deleterious effect upon body composition but rather exhibited small improvements in indices of body composition. Consequently, it was concluded that exercise interventions appear to have a protective effect by attenuating adverse changes in body composition that are consistently documented with administration of ADT [21]. It is important to acknowledge, the effect of exercise interventions upon body composition are influenced by the characteristics of the exercise training stimulus. Accordingly, it is possible that the intensity, volume, frequency, and length of the exercise interventions reviewed were inadequate to stimulate optimal improvement in body composition. Indeed, results from Galvão et al. [24] demonstrated that an intensive 12 week combined aerobic and strength training intervention resulted in an increase in nearly 2 kg of lean body mass in PCa patients undergoing prolonged ADT. Together, the findings demonstrate that exercise interventions resulted in meaningful improvements in muscular fitness and physical function outcomes. Such improvements in strength, endurance, and functional performance are of clinical relevance among aging men with PCa given their increased risk for loss of muscle mass, functional decline, and frailty.

Collectively, results from the exercise-PCa literature suggest that exercise interventions consistently yield significant, clinically meaningful improvements in a variety of relevant outcomes including muscular strength, muscular endurance, physical function, fatigue, and quality of life. However, while exercise alone did not consistently yield similar magnitude improvement in body composition, exercise interventions appear to attenuate adverse changes in body composition that are frequently observed in PCa patients on ADT. These findings are consistent with evidence from the behavioral weight management literature demonstrating that exercise alone does not result in the most favorable change in body weight and body composition outcomes [25]. Thus, from an energy balance perspective, while increased energy expenditure via exercise participation results in meaningful improvements in fitness, physical function, and patient reported outcomes, exercise alone may not produce optimal improvement in measures of obesity, body weight and/or body composition-related outcomes in PCa patients.

Dietary Interventions in the Treatment of PCa Patients and Survivors

Consistent with exercise-PCa research, there is growing interest in the role of dietary patterns and specific nutrients or foods in the prevention of PCa, as reviewed in the current Dietary Guidelines for America or the American Institute of Cancer Research recommendations [10, 26]. There is much less scientific literature regarding the optimal dietary patterns or the role of specific foods or nutrients relative to optimization of PCa treatment or in survivorship. It is reasonable to examine the literature on prostate prevention and propose hypotheses regarding how dietary patterns, foods, or nutrients impacting risk may also have potential benefits during therapy or for post therapy survivorship, but one should be cautious about making strong assumptions when study data is lacking. Much of the research in prevention has focused upon the association and/or effects of specific nutrients, vitamins and minerals, phytochemicals, and whole foods on PCa prevention and progression [10,26]. Currently, there is no convincing evidence for any one dietary component, food, or nutrient that can substantially impact prostate cancer risk [10, 26]. While are a number of variables under study associated with a lower risk, data is not substantial enough to support public health recommendations or interventions for higher risk individuals. Continued efforts examining diets rich in tomato products, soy, vitamin D, selenium, omega-3 fatty acids, energy balance, or dietary patterns such as a Mediterranean diet remain the focus of research in prostate cancer prevention. At the present time, advances in statistical analysis are providing epidemiologists with tools to examine more complex dietary patterns and their impact on risk and progression of PCa. Indeed, energy balance combined with other dietary variables may act in concert to impact health outcomes, such as prostate cancer risk. The complexity of PCa in humans, as reflected in its significant heterogeneity in response to therapy and duration of survivorship, may suggest a variety of disease subtypes, ranging from rather indolent to aggressive phenotypes. Continued efforts to subtype PCa by molecular tools and other biomarkers into unique subtypes will improve the precision of our nutritional research in the future.

Considerably less research has explored the effects of interventions designed to modify specific nutrients, foods, or overall dietary pattern/intake and energy balance on PCa outcomes [27]. A brief summary of limited evidence examining dietary interventions in PCa patients is provided in this section. Results from recent systematic reviews targeting body weight have yielded promising, yet inconsistent findings. Mohamad et al. [28] summarized the effects of six randomized trials investigating the effects of dietary interventions upon body weight and body composition among PCa patients. Results demonstrated that dietary interventions based upon a lower fat strategy or caloric restriction suggestetd superior improvements in body weight and body composition when compared to other dietary intervention approaches. Additionally, diet interventions alone produced more favorable weight loss relative to exercise interventions alone, a finding consistent with the majority of trials in behavioral weight management literature [25, 29, 30].

Similarly, in a systematic review of dietary interventions, Hackshaw-McGeagh et al. [31] indicated no convincing associations with prostate cancer outcome. While there is limited evidence that select nutrient and food intake is linked with more favorable PCa risk and progression, existing research on dietary interventions in PCa patients is characterized by heterogeneous methodology, outcome assessments, and often of limited statistical power [31]. Consequently, it was concluded the impact of dietary interventions cannot presently be reliably estimated and optimally powered, large scale randomized intervention trials are warranted to evaluate the extent to which various dietary interventions may yield preventative and therapeutic benefits.

It is critical to acknowledge that although associations between specific nutrients, foods or dietary patterns and PCa outcomes are inconsistent, there is accumulating evidence of the link between obesity and risk of advanced PCa [26], which is supported by many studies in experimental models [32, 33]. For example, adult weight gain was associated with significantly increased risk of fatal PCa in two large cohort studies [34, 35]. Additionally, a recent systematic literature review found that several different measures of obesity including body mass index, waist circumference and waist-hip ratio each demonstrated a dose-response relationship with risk of advanced prostate cancer [26]. Nonetheless, randomized controlled trials examining the extent to which dietary-induced modifications in energy balance and/or accompanying reduction in body weight results in favorable PCa outcomes remains limited. Presently, dietary recommendations for PCa patients and survivors emphasizes achieving/maintaining a healthy body weight through healthy dietary intake and regular physical activity participation, as would be appropriate for other patients at risk of metabolic syndrome and its complications. Thus, a dietary pattern advocated for prevention of prevalent chronic disease such as cardiovascular disease and diabetes including a nutrient dense diet that incorporates whole grains, fruit and vegetable intake, and lower levels of saturated fat consumption are currently recommended for PCa patients and survivors [26]. Consistent with this position, lifestyle recommendations from the expert panel of the World Cancer Research Fund/American Institute for Cancer Research (WCRF/AICR) encourages individuals to: (1) maintain a healthy body weight, (2) be as lean as possible without being underweight, (3) limit consumption of red meat, processed meat, sugary drinks, and energy dense foods, (4) promote increased intake of fruits, vegetables, whole grains, and legumes; and (5) participate in regular physical activity of at least 30 min/day [36].

In summary, there is mounting interest in the role of dietary interventions in the prevention of PCa, during therapy, and survivorship. A majority of the extant research in this line of inquiry has focused upon the role of specific nutrients, phytochemicals and individual foods in PCa prevention and progression [31, 37]. Although findings from this research are promising, they remain characterized by small sample sizes, heterogeneity in methods and outcome assessments, and select methodological limitations which detract from the ability to presently draw definitive conclusions regarding the therapeutic efficacy of diet and nutrition for PCa treatment. Finally, although epidemiological evidence demonstrates a link between obesity during specific stages of the life cycle and increased risk of aggressive PCa, the extent to which dietary-induced change in energy balance and body weight is effective for changing the course of disease has yet to be systematically investigated. Large-scale randomized controlled trials designed to delineate the effects of dietary-induced changes in energy balance and body weight are warranted to evaluate the efficacy of integrating dietary interventions in PCa treatment.

Combined Exercise and Dietary Interventions in the Treatment of PCa Patients and Survivors

Given the challenges faced by aging men in managing PCa symptoms and the adverse effects of traditional PCa treatments upon metabolic syndrome and other quality of life outcomes, it is appropriate to empower men and caregivers with knowledge regarding the benefits of regular exercise and healthy dietary habits [26, 38, 39]. The benefits of exercise for PCa patients and survivors on intermediate outcomes are clear [21, 22] and the evidence regarding the potential utility of dietary interventions on high-risk metabolic outcomes, is also promising. However, despite the potential utility of each of these approaches alone, *lifestyle interventions combining exercise and diet modification* likely represent the optimal approach for the management of PCa patients and survivors. As we noted previously, given the frequency of implementing ADT in PCa treatment, the adverse effects of this approach place patients at increased risk for weight gain, metabolic syndrome, sarcopenic obesity, cardiovascular disease, functional decline, and mobility disability.

It is well established within the behavioral weight management literature that modifying both energy expenditure through regular physical activity/exercise participation and energy intake via changes in dietary behavior are integral to successful behavioral weight management and more favorable change in body composition and various chronic disease risk factors [40–42]. Indeed, evidence from multiple large-scale lifestyle intervention trials demonstrate that combined exercise and dietary interventions result in superior improvements in weight management outcomes, mobility performance, and select cardiovascular and metabolic disease risk factors. Notably, findings from the ADAPT and IMPACT trials illustrated that a combined exercise and dietary weight loss intervention that elicited intentional weight loss resulted in superior improvements in weight loss, physical function, quality of life, and select inflammatory and biomarkers of chronic disease relative to exercise or diet alone among older overweight, obese knee osteoarthritis patients [29, 30, 43, 44]. Similarly, findings from the Cooperative Lifestyle Intervention Program (CLIP) trial also revealed that a community-based lifestyle exercise and dietary weight loss intervention yielded significantly greater improvement in weight loss, mobility performance, and quality of life relative to exercise alone or a successful aging control condition among obese older adults with cardiovascular disease and/or metabolic syndrome [45].

Collectively, these findings suggest lifestyle interventions designed to promote change in both exercise and dietary behavior yield superior changes for an array of outcomes that are of clinical relevance to PCa patients and survivors. Hence, the synergistic effects of combining exercise and diet could augment the beneficial impact of either approach alone for men with PCa. Research examining the impact of such combined lifestyle interventions in men with PCa remains relatively limited at the present time, thus care is required in presenting the state of science to patients. However, there is growing interest in the potential utility of implementing lifestyle, behavioral weight management intervention approaches with confidence that physical performance and function outcomes can be improved, and that biomarkers of metabolic syndrome including hemoglobin A1c, lipid profiles, and hypertension can be favorably impacted. In the following section of this chapter, we provide a summary of the extent studies investigating the effects of lifestyle interventions combining exercise and diet in the treatment of PCa patients.

Ornish et al. [46] conducted a valuable intervention study focusing upon a strict lifestyle program involving modifications in both exercise and dietary behavior among men with PCa. The objective of this two-arm randomized controlled trial was to compare the effects of an intensive lifestyle intervention with those of usual care among 93 early-stage PCa patients who had chosen active surveillance. The multi-component lifestyle intervention involved a shift to a vegan diet promoting consumption of fruit and vegetables, whole grains, legumes, and soy coupled with 6 days per week of 30 min of moderate intensity walking. In addition to the exercise and dietary components, men in the lifestyle intervention were encouraged to practice stress management techniques (i.e., gentle yoga, meditation, imagery, progressive muscle relaxation) daily, and adopt a supplement regimen of selenium, fish oil, and vitamins E and C. Prior to reviewing the results, it is important to place this study in context of current knowledge. Although supplement intake was promoted in the lifestyle intervention, the most recent WCRF/ AICR report recommends that individuals not rely on using supplements to prevent cancer or cancer progression [36]. Furthermore, a study of vitamin E and selenium for prostate cancer prevention, well known as the SELECT (selenium and alpha-tochopheral study) supported by the National Cancer Institute failed to detect any benefits for PCa prevention and highlighted several risks [47]. Assessments of serum PSA, serum stimulated LNCaP cell growth (a bioassay using an androgen-dependent cell line to evaluate changes in the growth promoting effects of human serum before and after an intervention), C-reactive protein (CRP), and testosterone were obtained at baseline and 12-month follow-up. No assessments of change in body weight, body composition, or physical function were reported. Six men assigned to usual care active surveillance withdrew and underwent standard of care PCa treatment. Conversely, no patients randomized to the lifestyle intervention began conventional treatment. This is not an unusual observation when men enroll in a randomized diet and exercise study and are then assigned to a control group that is perceived as less favorable. Men randomized to the intensive lifestyle intervention demonstrated successful adoption and adherence to changes in diet, exercise, and stress management strategies. Results revealed that lifestyle intervention patients demonstrated more favorable changes in PSA and that serum from participants promoted less LNCap cell growth *in vitro* relative to serum from men in the control arm after the completion of the 12 months of intervention than the usual care approach. Additionally, changes in diet and exercise behavior were significantly associated with change in PSA and LNCap cell growth at 12 month follow-up. At a 2 year follow-up assessment, 13 usual care patients (27%) and 2 lifestyle intervention (2%) patients had transitioned from active surveillance to conventional PCa treatment [48]. Results at the 2-year follow-up also revealed no difference in death, cardiac events, total PSA, or quality of life between the usual care and lifestyle intervention groups. However, ancillary analysis demonstrated that irrespective of treatment group assignment, patients that reported adopting and maintaining healthier lifestyle behaviors reported more favorable levels of quality of life, perceived stress, and sexual function [49]. While the intensive lifestyle intervention resulted in the significant benefits in biomarkers and a cell culture based bioassay relative to the usual care approach at 12 months, these improvements were not maintained at the subsequent 2 year follow-up assessment, when the intensity of intervention declines [48] What is the key "take-home" message from this study is that men with PCa, particularly that chose active surveillance for indolent cancer, are a logical target for large intervention studies focusing upon optimal dietary and physical activity interventions. It is also worthy of mention that the Ornish-type intervention in non-cancer patients has demonstrated impact on multiple cardiovascular outcomes [50]. Indeed, the significant competing mortality from cardiovascular and other chronic diseases in men with PCa, and potentially accentuated by hormone therapy, is a major concern.

The Reach Out to Enhance Wellness trial was a 2-arm randomized controlled trial comparing the effects of a home-based exercise and dietary weight loss intervention to those of a wait list control group in 641 overweight cancer survivors [51]. A total of 261 of the participants were PCa survivors. The home-based lifestyle intervention consisted of providing each participant with exercise and dietary instructional materials, self-monitoring logs, pedometers, resistance exercise bands, and telephone counseling sessions. Cancer survivors randomized into the lifestyle intervention were encouraged to accrue 30 min of daily aerobic exercise and 15 min of strength training using the resistance bands every other day. With regard to dietary recommendations, participants were encouraged to increase fruit and vegetable intake and decrease caloric and saturated fat intake with a long-term goal of producing loss of 10% of initial body weight. Results revealed that although the home-based weight loss intervention resulted in generally modest change in survivors' exercise and dietary behaviors, it did produce significantly greater weight loss relative to the control group. Additionally, the lifestyle intervention significantly attenuated the decline in physical functioning observed in the control group at 12 month follow-up [51]. Thus, the encouraging results suggest that strategies to provide a more intense intervention with greater compliance may improve on the benefits reported.

Analysis at 2 year follow-up, after the wait-list control group had also received the lifestyle intervention, demonstrated that both the lifestyle intervention and delayed treatment resulted in significant improvements in body mass index, self-reported diet quality and physical activity participation, and physical function when compared to baseline values. Collectively, these findings illustrate that a home-based exercise and diet intervention results in modest weight loss and significant benefits for select physical function and patient reported outcomes that are maintained for up to 2 years in a large sample of overweight cancer survivors [52].

Nobes et al. [53] compared the effects of a lifestyle exercise and dietary intervention combined with metformin with those receiving usual care in a sample of 40 PCa patients undergoing ADT. The lifestyle intervention involved providing patients with exercise and dietary advice designed to promote independent adoption of regular exercise and a low glycemic index diet. Additionally, patients in the lifestyle intervention received a daily 850 mg dose of metformin which was increased to twice daily doses after 2 weeks of the intervention. Assessments of various physiologic and biomarker outcomes were obtained at baseline and 3 and 6-month follow-up. Findings revealed the lifestyle intervention combined with metformin resulted in superior improvements in weight loss, abdominal circumference, and blood pressure relative to usual care at 3 months. This study suggests that novel combinations of pharmaceuticals with diet and exercise interventions should be considered for future large scale interventions.

Bourke et al. [54] compared the effects of a 12-week exercise and dietary intervention with those receiving standard-of-care treatment in 50 PCa patients undergoing ADT. The exercise component of the intervention involved two supervised exercise sessions per week comprised of 30 min of aerobic exercise at 55–85% of maximum heart rate and 2–4 sets of resistance exercises targeting the major muscle groups. In addition to supervised exercise, patients were encouraged to complete 1–2 independent exercise sessions per week. Men in the lifestyle intervention also received dietary advice via printed materials and bi-weekly healthy eating seminars. The dietary advice encouraged men to reduce their intake of saturated fat and refined carbohydrates and increase dietary fiber intake. Men in the usual care arm received normal contact and follow-up with their oncology nurse and urologist at their respective treatment clinic. Assessments of exercise and dietary behavior, fitness, anthropometrics, and patient reported outcomes were obtained at baseline, 12 weeks, and 6 months. The lifestyle intervention had acceptable recruitment (64%), adherence (95% to supervised sessions), and attrition (14% during the 12-week intervention) rates. Loss to follow-up at the 6-month assessment was considerably higher at 44% for the study. The lifestyle intervention yielded significant, meaningful improvements in adoption of exercise and dietary behavior, less fatigue, greater aerobic fitness, and improved muscular strength relative to usual care at 12 weeks.

Additionally, the improvements in these outcomes were maintained at 6-month follow-up. The findings from this randomized controlled pilot study indicated that a pragmatic lifestyle intervention resulted in significantly greater improvement in clinically relevant outcomes in PCa patients undergoing ADT.

In a larger scale follow-up trial, Bourke et al. [55] examined the effects of a 12 week lifestyle intervention they piloted in their prior investigation [54] in 100 men with locally advanced or metastatic PCa on long-term ADT. Assessments of exercise and dietary behavior, fitness, quality of life, and blood pressure were obtained at baseline and12 week and 6 month follow-ups. Results demonstrated that the lifestyle intervention yielded significant improvements in quality of life, fatigue, fitness, exercise participation, and favorable dietary outcomes. Furthermore, improvements in fatigue, exercise participation, and fitness observed at 12 weeks were found to persist to the 6-month follow-up. In addition to the primary trial outcomes, findings from an ancillary analysis of a subsample of 50 PCa patients revealed the lifestyle intervention produced significant improvements in vascular function (as assessed by flow-mediated dilation of the brachial artery), muscle mass, aerobic fitness, and exercise participation following the 12-week intervention. However, only the significant improvement in aerobic fitness was maintained at subsequent 6-months follow-up assessment. These findings replicate and extend previous work demonstrating the potential promise of a lifestyle intervention targeting change in both exercise participation and dietary intake in the supportive care of PCa patients on ADT [55].

O'Neill et al. [56] compared the effects of a 6 month home-based exercise and dietary intervention with those of a standard of care approach in 94 PCa patients undergoing ADT. Assessments of body composition (obtained via four site skinfold caliper measurement), functional performance (6 min walk time), fatigue, quality of life, and exercise and dietary behavior were obtained at baseline and 3-month and 6-month follow-up. The exercise component of the lifestyle intervention involved encouraging participants to engage in 30 min of home-based, self-directed moderate intensity walking 5 or more days per week. Patients were provided a pedometer and asked to record daily and weekly step counts. The dietary component of the lifestyle intervention individually tailored dietary recommendations emphasizing a shift toward intake recommended within the UK healthy eating guidelines. Specific aspects of the recommendations included increasing fruit and vegetable intake to ≥5 servings per day, decrease fat intake to ≤30% of total daily caloric intake with <10% from saturated fat, and limit consumption of processed meats, alcohol, and food high in salt and sugar. Overall, adherence to exercise (91%) and retention (96%) were excellent. Results revealed the lifestyle intervention resulted in superior weight loss and improvement in fat mass relative to standard of care. Additionally, the exercise and dietary intervention yielded significant increases in functional performance and successful adoption of change in exercise participation and dietary intake when compared to men receiving standard of care.

Collectively, the findings from the limited number of combined exercise and dietary interventions provide support for the utility of implementing this approach in the treatment of PCa patients and survivors. A lifestyle intervention approach may be particularly relevant for patients treated with ADT. A common adverse effect of ADT is an increase in weight and body fat in parallel with a decrease in muscle mass and strength, which in turn, place PCa patients at increased risk for functional decline, metabolic syndrome, and their respective complications. In addition to management of energy balance, diet composition is a critical risk factor for these pathologic processes and optimization of dietary patterns to those defined by Dietary Guidelines for Americans [10] and the WCRF/AICR [36] are desirable. Thus, the additive or synergistic benefits of concomitant change in both exercise and dietary behavior could represent an approach for offsetting the adverse effects experienced by PCa patients during ADT while also empowering patients to contribute to their health.

Although these findings underscore the potential value of implementing combined exercise and dietary interventions in the treatment of PCa patients, these studies also demonstrate the meaningful challenges associated with promoting adoption and adherence to exercise and dietary behavior change. Notably, select studies were characterized by very high attrition rates at post-treatment follow-up [54, 55]. Additionally, clinically meaningful improvements in various clinically-relevant outcomes accompanying the lifestyle intervention were not maintained at longer term follow-up in select studies [48, 55].

The deterioration of benefits following lifestyle interventions have been proposed to be directly related to poor post-treatment strategies, particularly reliance upon self-directed adherence to the defined exercise and dietary behavior change [57–59]. Thus, adherence to the desired behavior changes are essential determinants to achieve longer term efficacy regarding meaningful disease endpoints, and these findings underscore the pressing need to explore novel approaches to promoting successful adoption and maintenance of independent exercise and dietary behavior among PCa patients. One approach, a group-mediated cognitive behavioral (GMCB) lifestyle intervention based on social cognitive theory and the group dynamics literature [60], has recently produced superior adherence to exercise and dietary behavior change and also yielded significant improvements in a variety of clinically relevant outcomes for PCa patients in randomized trials targeting chronic disease patients [59, 61]. The GMCB intervention couples exercise and dietary behavior change with self-regulatory skills counseling in order to promote independent maintenance of lifestyle behavior change and to sustain intervention-induced improvements in relevant outcomes. Although these findings suggest an integrated lifestyle intervention holds promise for improving the utility of lifestyle exercise and dietary interventions targeting PCa patients, the feasibility and efficacy of implementing this approach in the treatment of PCa patients undergoing ADT has not been investigated.

Recognizing these challenges, we recently completed the Individualized Diet and Exercise Adherence (IDEA-P) trial [62, 63], a randomized controlled pilot trial designed to examine the feasibility and preliminary efficacy of a combined exercise and dietary intervention (EX+D), implementing a group-mediated cognitive behavioral (GMCB) lifestyle intervention approach, relative to standard-of-care control in the treatment of PCa patients undergoing ADT. A key component of our EX+D intervention is the use of the GMCB approach to promote the development and practice of the key behavioral self-regulatory skills, harness the social dynamics of small groups to support motivation for behavior change, and personalize the intervention to each PCa patient's needs to improve adoption, adherence, and intervention impact. We provide a detailed summary of the IDEA-P trial methodology and findings in the following section of the chapter.

The IDEA-P trial compared the effects of a 12 week lifestyle exercise and dietary intervention using the GMCB approach with those of standard of care treatment in 32 PCa patients undergoing ADT. The lifestyle intervention was specifically designed to facilitate exercise and dietary behavior change and promote adherence, independent of study staff, to these changes in lifestyle behavior. The exercise component of the EX+D intervention integrated a combination of resistance and aerobic exercise performed twice per week. All exercise sessions lasted 1 h in duration. The exercise prescription was tailored to each individual's baseline functional abilities and exercise tolerance/capacity. Consequently, resistance exercise load, volume, and volume-load and aerobic exercise duration and intensity was guided by each participant's exercise tolerance and gradually increased across the intervention to progress towards optimal, targeted prescription ranges.

Given that a primary goal of the intervention was to offset ADT-induced declines in muscle mass and strength, resistance exercise was the focal aspect of center-based training sessions. The resistance exercise stimulus involved performing 3 sets at each individual's 8 repetition maximum (RM; i.e., the most weight that an individual can lift for the specified number of repetitions) to 12RM at a rating of perceived exertion (1–10) ranging from 3 (Moderately Hard) to 6 (Hard) for 9 different exercises (leg extension, leg curl, chest press, lateral pull-down, overhead press, triceps extension, bicep curl, calf raises, and abdominal crunch). A 1–2 min rest interval was maintained between each set, and all sets were performed in a symptom-limited manner. The aerobic exercise stimulus consisted of 10–20 min of exercise performed at a rating of perceived exertion (1–10) ranging from 3 (Fairly Light) to 4 (Moderately Hard) on the participant's choice of a treadmill, stationary cycle, or elliptical trainer. Participants were also encouraged to gradually increase independent, home-based exercise participation and purposeful activity and decrease sedentary time in order to progress towards accruing a volume of physical activity consistent with national guidelines for health (i.e., 150 min of physical activity per week and 10,000 steps per day). The objective of the GMCB intervention was to integrate group-based cognitive behavioral counseling with exercise therapy to facilitate the development, practice, and mastery of key activity-related self-regulatory skills (i.e., self-monitoring, group and individual goal setting, barrier problem solving, action planning, relaxation/pain management strategies), while using group dynamics as an agent supporting behavior change, to promote exercise adherence, increased physical activity participation, modification in dietary intake, and reengagement in challenging ADLs. The GMCB approach concomitantly titrates away from supervised center-based exercise and dietary intervention emphasizing progressively more independent self-regulation of exercise and behavior and dietary intake [59, 64].

The fully integrated dietary component of the EX+D intervention included ten nutritional counseling sessions with a registered dietitian. The first eight counseling sessions were conducted in a group setting, once per immediately following a center-based exercise session during months 1–2. The two remaining sessions were conducted via biweekly phone calls during weeks 9–12. The dietary components of the intervention was modest in intensity, but certainly more than what is provided as standard of care in cancer clinics, and aimed to provide basic nutrition education to all participants, address contemporary topics in nutrition and cancer and provide individualized guidance toward adopting a healthy dietary pattern The nutrition intervention was designed consistent with the dietary objectives recommended by 2010–2015 Dietary Guidelines for Americans, the American Heart Association/American College of Cardiology [10, 65, 66], the WCRF/AICR [36] and the American Cancer Society [38, 67, 68]. The nutrition counseling also built upon many of the cognitive-behavioral self-management strategies utilized in the exercise intervention including self-monitoring, building self-efficacy, goal setting, and anticipating and overcoming barriers to dietary behavior change. Men randomized to the control arm received usual PCa treatment and standard disease management education, as well as additional educational literature describing the WCRF/AICR dietary and physical activity guidelines and education. Men receiving standard of care also received bi-weekly calls from clinic staff focusing upon routine aspects of PCa self-management.

Assessments of mobility performance (400 m walk and stair climb performance), muscular strength, body composition (body fat percentage, fat mass, and fat free mass), and exercise and dietary behavior were obtained at baseline, 2 months, and 3 months. The lifestyle intervention had acceptable recruitment (59%), adherence (88%), and retention (88%) rates. The lifestyle exercise and dietary intervention yielded significant, meaningful improvements in mobility performance, muscular strength, body weight, body composition, and exercise participation, and select aspects of dietary intake at 2 month follow-up. Additionally, men successfully sustained independent adherence to the exercise and dietary behavior change in Month 3 and the improvements in these outcomes were maintained at the 3 month follow-up assessment. Findings from the IDEA-P trial demonstrated that a personalized exercise and dietary intervention resulted in excellent retention and compliance and produced significant, clinically meaningful improvements in mobility performance, body composition, and muscular strength outcomes relative to standard of care in PCa patients undergoing ADT. In addition to the favorable outcomes observed in IDEA-P, the trial findings also suggest that the EX+D intervention was successful in promoting adoption and short-term maintenance of independent, self-regulated exercise and dietary behavior change. Therefore, the IDEA-P trial is one of the first studies demonstrating the feasibility and preliminary efficacy of a personalized GMCB-based lifestyle intervention in countering the well-established functional, musculoskeletal, and body composition changes associated with ADT. It is also particularly important to acknowledge that over 80% of men randomized to the lifestyle intervention in IDEA-P were classified as overweight or obese. Consequently, modest daily caloric restriction was a primary goal of the dietary portion of the intervention. It is notable that select patients in the intervention arm were not overweight and could be characterized as being more frail thus requiring dietary modification tailored to aid in efforts to maintain and/or increase lean body mass. This variation in weight status at baseline highlights the potential patient heterogeneity that can be evident when initiating lifestyle interventions and underscores the importance of personalizing the exercise and dietary intervention approaches to PCa patients' specific needs.

In summary, findings addressed in this section of the chapter provide accumulating and rather strong evidence supporting the benefits of lifestyle interventions designed to promote exercise and dietary-induced modifications in energy balance for PCa patients and survivors. Indeed, exercise and dietary interventions, both separately and in combination, result in consistent improvements in clinically-relevant outcomes and show promise for being integrated into the supportive care of PCa. Nonetheless, given the limited extant evidence, considerably more research is needed to define optimal, personalized lifestyle intervention approaches that promote sustained adherence and maximal lasting therapeutic benefits that, in turn, are balanced against cost to the health care system. Although we are biased in our belief that the time and effort of nutritionists and exercise/fitness professionals involved in lifestyle intervention delivery provides excellent cost/benefit value when measured against many of the expensive pharmaceutical interventions currently provide to PCa patients, this cost and value has yet to be clearly defined. Thus, it is critical that future inquiry addressing the efficacy of exercise and dietary interventions has focus upon delineating the cost effectiveness of integrating such lifestyle interventions in the treatment of PCa. In addition to combination diet and physical activity studies, we also feel that additional research documenting the independent effects of exercise and diet interventions are warranted to better delineate the potentially unique characteristics and benefits associated with each type of intervention, which in turn will assist in the design of future studies integrating strategies. For example, further inquiry designed to define the exercise stimulus characteristics (i.e., frequency, mode, intensity, duration, volume) that promote favorable change in body composition physiologic, fitness/function, and quality of life outcomes would be valuable. Advances in this area will inform best practices for the development and implementation of exercise prescription efforts for PCa patients. Similarly, additional research addressing the effects of dietary composition, dietary patterns, nutrient intake, and food factors will contribute to the enhanced knowledge and practice of promoting healthy dietary practices before, during, and following PCa treatment.

Provided the importance of promoting effective behavioral weight management among PCa patients, it is reasonable to suggest the synergistic benefits of lifestyle interventions targeting change in both exercise and dietary habits make this approach particularly promising as a supportive care intervention for PCa. Nonetheless, despite the promising findings, there are still few studies specifically examining combined exercise and dietary interventions in PCa patients and the limitations evident in the research must be acknowledged. Notably, many of the lifestyle intervention studies conducted to date in PCa patients have failed to employ blinded outcomes assessments or intention-to-treat analysis and are generally characterized by small sample sizes and relatively high rates of attrition and/or loss to follow-up [28, 62]. In light of the relatively limited extant research addressing the feasibility and efficacy of exercise and dietary interventions presently available, future well designed, optimally powered randomized controlled lifestyle intervention trials are necessary to elucidate the benefits of these approaches, define the optimal methods for designing and delivering such lifestyle interventions, and determine how to develop and extend the scalability and reach of these lifestyle interventions in order to successfully integrate exercise and diet more directly in the supportive care of PCa patients.

Considerations for Implementing Lifestyle Interventions in the Treatment of PCa: Lessons Learned from Behavioral Weight Management Research

Mounting evidence demonstrates the role of obesity in cancer recurrence and mortality [69, 70]. Additionally, the American Society of Clinical Oncology has suggested that obesity is poised to exceed tobacco use as the leading preventable cause of cancer in the U.S. [71]. Consistent with the emerging evidence supporting the myriad of benefits accompanying exercise and dietary interventions across the cancer control continuum, there is growing interest in the utility of implementing behavioral weight management approaches in the treatment of cancer patients and survivors. Indeed, it is now recommended that cancer survivors maintain as lean and healthy body weight as possible; strive to attain appropriate dietary portion control; increase intake of fruits, vegetables, and whole grains; limit consumption of alcohol, sugar, salt, and high caloric, low nutrient dense foods, and accrue 150 min of physical activity and 2 days of resistance and/or strength training per week [36, 38, 39, 72].

The efficacy of implementing lifestyle exercise and dietary weight loss interventions in the treatment of overweight or obese individuals as part of comprehensive behavioral disease prevention and health promotion efforts is well established in the behavioral weight management literature [42, 73–75]. As the study of the impact of lifestyle interventions combining exercise and dietary approaches in the treatment of PCa patients remains a relatively new area of inquiry, we contend there are important lessons from the behavioral weight management literature that can be applied to guide future lifestyle intervention research and practice targeting PCa patients and survivors.

In order to optimize the utility of lifestyle weight management approaches, it is critical to address the considerable behavioral challenges that overweight and obese individuals face when engaging in weight management efforts. From a conceptual position, Perri et al. [74] have proposed that successful behavioral weight management involves a continuous care approach. A central tenet of this approach is that obesity is viewed as a chronic condition that necessitates a flexible, behaviorally-based problem solving approach to treatment requiring patient vigilance, consistency and long-term, sustained health care provider support. Thus, flexible, collaborative approaches involving active engagement of the patient and extended support/contact with healthcare providers to facilitate maintenance of lifestyle behavior change are essential aspects of the continuous care model of behavioral weight management.

As it is the largest, long-term randomized controlled lifestyle weight management intervention conducted to date, findings from the Action for Health and Diabetes trial (Look AHEAD) can provide particularly relevant evidence to implement in guiding lifestyle interventions that may be relevant to our efforts targeting PCa patients and survivors [76]. Look AHEAD was a multi-center, 2-arm randomized controlled trial comparing the effects of an intensive lifestyle intervention with those of standard diabetes education/support in a sample of over 5000 obese adults with Type II diabetes. The lifestyle intervention was designed to produce a weight loss of 7% of initial body weight during the intensive phase of the intervention via modification of exercise/physical activity participation and dietary intake. The Look AHEAD findings demonstrated that weight loss and long-term weight loss maintenance can be successfully achieved through a lifestyle intervention focusing upon modification of physical activity and dietary behavior. Notably, patients randomized to the lifestyle intervention loss approximately 9% of initial body weight by 12 months. Across the extensive 8-year follow-up period, gradual weight regain was observed. However, patients largely maintained a 5% weight loss from years 4 to 8 of the trial. In fact, at 8-year follow-up, more than half the patients had sustained their year 1 weight loss and significantly greater proportions of the lifestyle intervention patients had maintained $\geq$5% total weight loss when compared to the standard diabetes support intervention.

In addition to weight loss, the lifestyle intervention resulted in superior improvements in fitness, glycemic control, and select cardiovascular disease risk factors [77]. Furthermore, the lifestyle intervention also elicited greater improvements in physical function [78], body composition [79], and quality of life [80]. Promoting adoption and adherence to exercise and dietary behavior change is integral to the success of lifestyle interventions [75, 81, 82]. The Look AHEAD lifestyle intervention's focus upon behavioral self-regulatory strategies appears to have been particularly critical in contributing to success in adhering to the lifestyle behavior changes required to successfully maintain weight loss. For example, patients in the lifestyle intervention reported greater use of weight control-related self-regulatory strategies such as increased frequency and volume of exercise, greater use of dietary restraint strategies, decreased caloric intake, regular self-weighing, and more frequent use of meal replacement shakes [76]. As many PCa patients are overweight or obese and have, or are at high risk for cardiovascular disease and metabolic syndrome, it should be recognized the weight loss, biomarkers of chronic disease, and patient-reported outcomes that were positively impacted by the lifestyle intervention in Look AHEAD are directly relevant for a considerable proportion of PCa patients and survivors.

Findings from the National Weight Control Registry (NWCR) also reinforce the importance of behavioral self-regulatory skills and weight control strategies in weight loss maintenance [83]. The NWCR is a 10-year prospective observational cohort study tracking over 10,000 adults who lost ≥30 lbs and maintained that weight loss for at least 1 year. Consistent with the results of the Look AHEAD trial, patients who were most successful in maintaining weight loss reported increased volume of exercise and physical activity participation, greater use of dietary restraint strategies, more frequent self-monitoring of exercise and dietary behaviors and body weight (self-weighing), and decreased caloric and dietary fat intake.

Collectively results from the Look AHEAD trial, NWCR, and evidence from the extant behavioral weight management literature demonstrate that lifestyle interventions promoting modification of exercise and dietary behaviors (i.e., increased exercise and physical activity participation and reduced caloric intake), the development, practice, and mastery of a toolbox of behavioral self-regulatory strategies, and the provision of ongoing, personalized support contribute to successful lifestyle-based weight management. These findings, together with the results of exercise and dietary interventions implemented, both separately and in combination, within PCa patients, underscore the potential utility of integrating behavioral lifestyle weight management intervention approaches in the treatment of PCa. Given both the relatively limited amount of lifestyle intervention research directly targeting men with PCa and that the majority of the behavioral weight management literature has been conducted in individuals who have not been diagnosed with cancer, the extent to which these approaches will be similarly beneficial for PCa patients has yet to be adequately delineated. Nonetheless, in light of the promising findings observed to date, the efficacy of implementing lifestyle interventions in the supportive care of PCa treatment warrants continued systematic inquiry. It is particularly relevant when we consider that many men live for years and/or decades following a diagnosis of PCa, and the value of instituting dietary and exercise programs that have lasting impact on survivorship, age associated disease morbidity, and competing mortality is likely substantial.

Summary and Future Directions

The findings addressed in this chapter demonstrate the benefits of exercise, diet, and combined exercise and dietary interventions for PCa patients and survivors and underscore the utility of integrating lifestyle interventions in the treatment of PCa. Despite these promising findings, the overall volume of research addressing lifestyle interventions in PCa patients remains relatively limited and further systematic inquiry is warranted to determine many key aspects regarding the therapeutic efficacy of lifestyle interventions for the treatment of men with or recovering from PCa.

As many of the trials conducted to date are characterized by relatively small sample sizes, and less than optimal intervention and follow-up durations, future optimally powered, large scale randomized lifestyle intervention trials incorporating longer duration interventions and follow-up periods are warranted. Research better delineating the independent and synergistic effects of exercise and dietary interventions is also important. A focal element of this inquiry should aim to explore the behavioral and physiological mechanisms through which lifestyle interventions contribute to improvements in clinically relevant outcomes and the extent to which the favorable changes in select fitness, anthropometric, functional, and quality of life outcomes are linked with improvement in salient indicators of PCa progression and other disease processes.

It is also necessary to determine the most effective methods for integrating lifestyle interventions directly into the care of PCa patients and survivors. Specifically, establishing the best practices to guide the design and delivery of lifestyle interventions, determine how, when, and in what settings to implement these approaches to optimize the reach, access, and therapeutic benefit of exercise and dietary approaches. In exploring the best practices for delivering lifestyle interventions it is critical to recognize any single prescription and/or approach is unlikely to be optimal for all patients or yield a uniform beneficial effect upon all relevant outcomes of interest. Therefore, while it is important to refine current understanding of the most effective ways to integrate lifestyle interventions into the treatment of PCa, flexible exercise and dietary prescription processes that personalize the content and characteristics of the intervention to one's individual needs, preferences, and tolerances should be viewed as an integral component of future inquiry determining the optimal lifestyle approaches.

Similarly, promoting successful adoption and long-term maintenance of the exercise and dietary behavior change are critical determinants of the efficacy of lifestyle interventions. The deterioration of benefits accompanying lifestyle interventions have been proposed to be directly related to poor post-treatment adherence to exercise and dietary behavior change [58, 59]. It has been proposed that high attrition and poor adherence observed in lifestyle interventions may be attributable to a failure to provide patients with the self-regulatory skills necessary to adopt and maintain independent lifestyle behavior change [58, 59]. Thus, given that adherence to the desired behavior changes is an essential determinant of the efficacy of lifestyle interventions, these findings underscore the pressing need to explore novel approaches to promoting successful adoption and maintenance of independent exercise and dietary behavior among patients with PCa. Therefore, a personalized lifestyle medicine and continuous care approach that assists patients in developing the behavioral skills necessary to maintain behavior adherence is essential.

In summary, the primary objective of this chapter was is to provide an overview of the extant research addressing the effects of interventions involving modification of energy balance interventions in PCa treatment. Results from studies examining exercise and dietary interventions, both separately and in combination among PCa patients and survivors revealed lifestyle interventions result in significant, clinically meaningful improvements in an array of outcomes. Taken collectively, this emerging evidence supports the utility of integrating lifestyle interventions as an adjuvant, supportive care intervention in the treatment of PCa patients and survivors.

References

1. Siegel RL, Miller KD, Jemal A. Cancer statistics, 2016. CA Cancer J Clin. 2016;66(1):7–30.
2. Basaria S, Lieb J, Tang AM, DeWeese T, Carducci M, Eisenberger M, Dobs AS. Long-term effects of androgen deprivation therapy in prostate cancer patients. Clin Endocrinol (Oxf). 2002;56(6):779–86.
3. Boxer RS, Kenny AM, Dowsett R, Taxel P. The effect of 6 months of androgen deprivation therapy on muscle and fat mass in older men with localized prostate cancer. Aging Male. 2005;8(3–4):207–12. doi:10.1080/13685530500361226.
4. Bylow K, Dale W, Mustian K, Stadler WM, Rodin M, Hall W, et al. Falls and physical performance deficits in older patients with prostate cancer undergoing androgen deprivation therapy. Urology. 2008;72(2):422–7. doi:10.1016/j.urology.2008.03.032.
5. Bylow K, Mohile SG, Stadler WM, Dale W. Does androgen-deprivation therapy accelerate the development of frailty in older men with prostate cancer?: a conceptual review. Cancer. 2007;110(12):2604–13. doi:10.1002/cncr.23084.
6. Chen Z, Maricic M, Nguyen P, Ahmann FR, Bruhn R, Dalkin BL. Low bone density and high percentage of body fat among men who were treated with androgen deprivation therapy for prostate carcinoma. Cancer. 2002;95(10):2136–44. doi:10.1002/cncr.10967.
7. Decal K, Sereika SM, Greenspan SL. Quality of life in prostate cancer patients taking androgen deprivation therapy. J Am Geriatr Soc. 2006;54(1):85–90. doi:10.1111/j.1532-5415.2005.00567.x.
8. Diamond TH, Higano CS, Smith MR, Guise TA, Singer FR. Osteoporosis in men with prostate carcinoma receiving androgen-deprivation therapy: recommendations for diagnosis and therapies. Cancer. 2004;100(5):892–9. doi:10.1002/cncr.20056.
9. Levine GN, D'Amico AV, Berger P, Clark PE, Eckel RH, Keating NL, et al. Androgen-deprivation therapy in prostate cancer and cardiovascular risk: a science advisory from the American Heart Association, American Cancer Society, and American Urological Association: endorsed by the American Society for Radiation Oncology. CA Cancer J Clin. 2010;60(3):194–201. doi:10.3322/caac.20061.
10. American College of Cardiology/American Heart Association Task Force on Practice Guidelines, Obesity Expert Panel, 2013. Executive summary: Guidelines (2013) for the management of overweight and obesity in adults: a report of the American College of Cardiology/American Heart Association Task Force on Practice Guidelines and the Obesity Society published by the Obesity Society and American College of Cardiology/American Heart Association Task Force on Practice Guidelines. Based on a systematic review from the The Obesity Expert Panel, 2013. Obesity (Silver Spring, Md.). 2014;22(Suppl 2):S5–39. doi:10.1002/oby.20821.
11. American Cancer Society. (2005). American Cancer Society. Atlanta.
12. American Cancer Society. (2006). American Cancer Society. Atlanta.
13. Courneya KS, Stevinson C, Vallance JKH. Exercise and psychosocial issues for cancer survivors. In: Handbook of sport psychology. Third ed. Hoboken, NJ: Wiley; 2007. p. 578–97. doi:10.1002/9781118270011.ch26.
14. Crawford ED. Epidemiology of prostate cancer. Urology. 2003;62(6 Suppl 1):3–12.
15. Holzbeierlein JM, McLaughlin MD, Thrasher JB. Complications of androgen deprivation therapy for prostate cancer. Curr Opin Urol. 2004;14(3):177–83.
16. Joly F, Alibhai SMH, Galica J, Park A, Yi Q-L, Wagner L, Tannock IF. Impact of androgen deprivation therapy on physical and cognitive function, as well as quality of life of patients with nonmetastatic prostate cancer. J Urol. 2006;176(6 Pt 1):2443–7. doi:10.1016/j.juro.2006.07.151.
17. Kornblith AB, Herr HW, Ofman US, Scher HI, Holland JC. Quality of life of patients with prostate cancer and their spouses. The value of a data base in clinical care. Cancer. 1994;73(11):2791–802.
18. Ruchlin HS, Pellissier JM. An economic overview of prostate carcinoma. Cancer. 2001;92(11):2796–810.

19. Galvão DA, Taaffe DR, Spry N, Joseph D, Turner D, Newton RU. Reduced muscle strength and functional performance in men with prostate cancer undergoing androgen suppression: a comprehensive cross-sectional investigation. Prostate Cancer Prostatic Dis. 2009;12(2): 198–203. doi:10.1038/pcan.2008.51.
20. Segal RJ, Reid RD, Courneya KS, Malone SC, Parliament MB, Scott CG, et al. Resistance exercise in men receiving androgen deprivation therapy for prostate cancer. J Clin Oncol. 2003;21(9):1653–9. doi:10.1200/JCO.2003.09.534.
21. Focht BC, Clinton SK, Devor ST, Garver MJ, Lucas AR, Thomas-Ahner JM, Grainger E. Resistance exercise interventions during and following cancer treatment: a systematic review. J Support Oncol. 2013;11(2):45–60.
22. Thorsen L, Courneya KS, Stevinson C, Fosså SD. A systematic review of physical activity in prostate cancer survivors: outcomes, prevalence, and determinants. Support Care Cancer. 2008;16(9):987–97. doi:10.1007/s00520-008-0411-7.
23. Haseen F, Murray LJ, Cardwell CR, O'Sullivan JM, Cantwell MM. The effect of androgen deprivation therapy on body composition in men with prostate cancer: systematic review and meta-analysis. J Cancer Surviv. 2010;4(2):128–39. doi:10.1007/s11764-009-0114-1.
24. Galvão DA, Taaffe DR, Spry N, Joseph D, Newton RU. Combined resistance and aerobic exercise program reverses muscle loss in men undergoing androgen suppression therapy for prostate cancer without bone metastases: a randomized controlled trial. J Clin Oncol. 2010;28(2):340–7. 10.1200/JCO.2009.23.2488
25. Wing RR. Physical activity in the treatment of the adulthood overweight and obesity: current evidence and research issues. Med Sci Sports Exerc. 1999;31(11 Suppl):S547–52.
26. World Cancer Research Fund International/American Institute for Cancer Research Continuous Update Project Report: Diet, Nutrition, Physical Activity, and Prostate Cancer. 2014. Available at: www.wcrf.org/sites/default/files/Prostate-Cancer-2014-Report.pdf
27. Demark-Wahnefried W, Rogers LQ, Alfano CM, Thomson CA, Courneya KS, Meyerhardt JA, et al. Practical clinical interventions for diet, physical activity, and weight control in cancer survivors. CA Cancer J Clin. 2015;65(3):167–89. doi:10.3322/caac.21265.
28. Mohamad H, McNeill G, Haseen F, N'Dow J, Craig LCA, Heys SD. The effect of dietary and exercise interventions on body weight in prostate cancer patients: a systematic review. Nutr Cancer. 2015;67(1):43–60. doi:10.1080/01635581.2015.976313.
29. Focht BC, Rejeski WJ, Ambrosius WT, Katula JA, Messier SP. Exercise, self-efficacy, and mobility performance in overweight and obese older adults with knee osteoarthritis. Arthritis Rheum. 2005;53(5):659–65. doi:10.1002/art.21466.
30. Messier SP, Loeser RF, Miller GD, Morgan TM, Rejeski WJ, Sevick MA, et al. Exercise and dietary weight loss in overweight and obese older adults with knee osteoarthritis: the Arthritis, Diet, and Activity Promotion Trial. Arthritis Rheum. 2004;50(5):1501–10. doi:10.1002/art.20256.
31. Hackshaw-McGeagh LE, Perry RE, Leach VA, Qandil S, Jeffreys M, Martin RM, Lane JA. A systematic review of dietary, nutritional, and physical activity interventions for the prevention of prostate cancer progression and mortality. Cancer Causes Control. 2015;26(11):1521–50. doi:10.1007/s10552-015-0659-4.
32. Boileau TW-M, et al. Prostate carcinogenesis in N-methyl-N-nitrosourea (NMU)-testosterone-treated rats fed tomato powder, lycopene, or energy-restricted diets. J Natl Cancer Inst. 2003;95(21):1578–86.
33. Mukherjee P, et al. Energy intake and prostate tumor growth, angiogenesis, and vascular endothelial growth factor expression. J Natl Cancer Inst. 1999;91(6):512–23.
34. Rodriguez C, Freedland SJ, Deka A, Jacobs EJ, McCullough ML, Patel AV, et al. Body mass index, weight change, and risk of prostate cancer in the Cancer Prevention Study II Nutrition Cohort. Cancer Epidemiol Biomarkers Prev. 2007;16(1):63–9. doi:10.1158/1055-9965.EPI-06-0754.
35. Wright ME, Chang S-C, Schatzkin A, Albanes D, Kipnis V, Mouw T, et al. Prospective study of adiposity and weight change in relation to prostate cancer incidence and mortality. Cancer. 2007;109(4):675–84. doi:10.1002/cncr.22443.

36. World Cancer Research Fund/American Institute for Cancer Research. Food, nutrition, physical activity, and the prevention of cancer: a global perspective. Washington DC: AICR; 2007.
37. Lin P-H, Aronson W, Freedland SJ. Nutrition, dietary interventions and prostate cancer: the latest evidence. BMC Med. 2015;13(1):3. doi:10.1186/s12916-014-0234-y.
38. Rock CL, Doyle C, Demark-Wahnefried W, Meyerhardt J, Courneya KS, Schwartz AL, et al. Nutrition and physical activity guidelines for cancer survivors. CA Cancer J Clin. 2012;62(4):243–74. doi:10.3322/caac.21142.
39. Rutledge L, Demark-Wahnefried W. Weight management and exercise for cancer survivors. Clin J Oncol Nurs. 2016;20(2):129–32. doi:10.1188/16.CJON.129-132.
40. Goldberg JH, King AC. Physical activity and weight management across the lifespan. Annu Rev Public Health. 2007;28(1):145–70. doi:10.1146/annurev.publhealth.28.021406.144105.
41. Jakicic JM, Otto AD. Treatment and prevention of obesity: what is the role of exercise? Nutr Rev. 2006;64(2 Pt 2):S57–61.
42. Wing RR. Cross-cutting themes in maintenance of behavior change. Health Psychol. 2000;19(1 Suppl):84–8.
43. Beavers KM, Beavers DP, Newman JJ, Anderson AM, Loeser RF, Nicklas BJ, et al. Effects of total and regional fat loss on plasma CRP and IL-6 in overweight and obese, older adults with knee osteoarthritis. Osteoarthritis Cartilage. 2015;23(2):249–56. doi:10.1016/j.joca.2014.11.005.
44. Messier SP, Mihalko SL, Legault C, Miller GD, Nicklas BJ, DeVita P, et al. Effects of intensive diet and exercise on knee joint loads, inflammation, and clinical outcomes among overweight and obese adults with knee osteoarthritis: the IDEA randomized clinical trial. JAMA. 2013;310(12):1263–73. doi:10.1001/jama.2013.277669.
45. Rejeski, W. J., Mihalko, S. L., Ambrosius, W. T., Bearon, L. B., & McClelland, J. W. (2011b). Weight loss and self-regulatory eating efficacy in older adults: the cooperative lifestyle intervention program. J Gerontol B Psychol Sci Soc Sci, 66(3), 279–286. 10.1093/geronb/gbq104
46. Ornish, D., Weidner, G., Fair, W. R., Marlin, R., Pettengill, E. B., Raisin, C. J., et al. (2005). Intensive lifestyle changes may affect the progression of prostate cancer. J Urol, 174(3), 1065–1069.– discussion 1069–70. 10.1097/01.ju.0000169487.49018.73
47. Dunn BK, et al. A nutrient approach to prostate cancer prevention: the Selenium and vitamin E Cancer Prevention Trial (SELECT). Nutr Cancer. 2010;62(7):896–918.
48. Frattaroli J, Weidner G, Dnistrian AM, Kemp C, Daubenmier JJ, Marlin RO, et al. Clinical events in prostate cancer lifestyle trial: results from two years of follow-up. Urology. 2008;72(6):1319–23. doi:10.1016/j.urology.2008.04.050.
49. Daubenmier JJ, Weidner G, Marlin R, Crutchfield L, Dunn-Emke S, Chi C, et al. Lifestyle and health-related quality of life of men with prostate cancer managed with active surveillance. Urology. 2006;67(1):125–30. doi:10.1016/j.urology.2005.07.056.
50. Ornish D, et al. Effects of stress management training and dietary changes in treating ischemic heart disease. JAMA. 1983;249(1):54–9.
51. Morey MC, Snyder DC, Sloane R, Cohen HJ, Peterson B, Hartman TJ, et al. Effects of home-based diet and exercise on functional outcomes among older, overweight long-term cancer survivors: RENEW: a randomized controlled trial. JAMA. 2009;301(18):1883–91. doi:10.1001/jama.2009.643.
52. Demark-Wahnefried W, et al. Reach out to enhance wellness home-based diet-exercise intervention promotes reproducible and sustainable long-term improvements in health behaviors, body weight, and physical functioning in older, overweight/obese cancer survivors. J Clin Oncol. 2012;30(19):2354–61.
53. Nobes JP, Langley SEM, Klopper T, Russell-Jones D, Laing RW. A prospective, randomized pilot study evaluating the effects of metformin and lifestyle intervention on patients with prostate cancer receiving androgen deprivation therapy. BJU Int. 2012;109(10):1495–502. doi:10.1111/j.1464-410X.2011.10555.x.
54. Bourke L, Doll H, Crank H, Daley A, Rosario D, Saxton JM. Lifestyle intervention in men with advanced prostate cancer receiving androgen suppression therapy: a feasibility study. Cancer Epidemiol Biomarkers Prev. 2011;20(4):647–57. doi:10.1158/1055-9965.EPI-10-1143.

55. Bourke L, Gilbert S, Hooper R, Steed LA, Joshi M, Catto JWF, et al. Lifestyle changes for improving disease-specific quality of life in sedentary men on long-term androgen-deprivation therapy for advanced prostate cancer: a randomised controlled trial. Eur Urol. 2014;65(5):865–72. doi:10.1016/j.eururo.2013.09.040.
56. O'Neill RF, Haseen F, Murray LJ, O'Sullivan JM, Cantwell MM. A randomised controlled trial to evaluate the efficacy of a 6-month dietary and physical activity intervention for patients receiving androgen deprivation therapy for prostate cancer. J Cancer Surviv. 2015;9(3):431–40. doi:10.1007/s11764-014-0417-8.
57. Ettinger WH, Burns R, Messier SP, Applegate W, Rejeski WJ, Morgan T, et al. A randomized trial comparing aerobic exercise and resistance exercise with a health education program in older adults with knee osteoarthritis. The Fitness Arthritis and Seniors Trial (FAST). JAMA. 1997;277(1):25–31.
58. Focht BC. Effectiveness of exercise interventions in reducing pain symptoms among older adults with knee osteoarthritis: a review. J Aging Phys Act. 2006;14(2):212–35.
59. Rejeski WJ, Brawley LR, Ambrosius WT, Brubaker PH, Focht BC, Foy CG, Fox LD. Older adults with chronic disease: benefits of group-mediated counseling in the promotion of physically active lifestyles. Health Psychol. 2003;22(4):414–23.
60. Bandura A. Self-efficacy: the exercise of control. 1st ed. New York: Worth; 1997.
61. Focht BC, Garver MJ, Devor ST, Dials J, Rose M, Lucas AR, et al. Improving maintenance of physical activity in older, knee osteoarthritis patients trial-pilot (IMPACT-P): design and methods. Contemp Clin Trials. 2012;33(5):976–82. doi:10.1016/j.cct.2012.04.012.
62. Focht BC, Lucas AR, Grainger E, Simpson C, Thomas-Ahner JM, Clinton SK. The Individualized Diet and Exercise Adherence Pilot Trial (IDEA-P) in prostate cancer patients undergoing androgen deprivation therapy: study protocol for a randomized controlled trial. Trials. 2014;15(1):354. doi:10.1186/1745-6215-15-354.
63. Focht BC, Lucas AR, Grainger E, Simpson C, Fairman CM, Thomas-Ahner JM, Monk JP, Mortazavi A, Clinton SK. Effects of a group-mediated exercise and dietary intervention in the treatment of prostate cancer patients undergoing androgen deprivation therapy: results from the IDEA-P trial. Ann Behav Med (In Press)
64. Rejeski WJ, Brubaker PH, Goff DC, Bearon LB, McClelland JW, Perri MG, Ambrosius WT. Translating weight loss and physical activity programs into the community to preserve mobility in older, obese adults in poor cardiovascular health. Arch Intern Med. 2011a;171(10):880–6. doi:10.1001/archinternmed.2010.522.
65. Eckel, R. H., Jakicic, J. M., Ard, J. D., de Jesus, J. M., Houston Miller, N., Hubbard, V. S., et al. (2014, July 1). 2013 AHA/ACC guideline on lifestyle management to reduce cardiovascular risk: a report of the American College of Cardiology/American Heart Association Task Force on Practice Guidelines. J Am Coll Cardiol. 63(25 Pt B):2960-2984 10.1016/j.jacc.2013.11.003
66. Jensen MD, Ryan DH, Apovian CM, Ard JD, Comuzzie AG, Donato KA, et al. 2013 AHA/ACC/TOS guideline for the management of overweight and obesity in adults: a report of the American College of Cardiology/American Heart Association Task Force on Practice Guidelines and The Obesity Society. J Am Coll Cardiol. 2014, July 1;63(25 Pt B):2985–3023. doi:10.1016/j.jacc.2013.11.004.
67. Melzack R. The short-form McGill Pain Questionnaire. Pain. 1987;30(2):191–7.
68. Mendoza TR, Wang XS, Cleeland CS, Morrissey M, Johnson BA, Wendt JK, Huber SL. The rapid assessment of fatigue severity in cancer patients: use of the Brief Fatigue Inventory. Cancer. 1999;85(5):1186–96.
69. De Pergola G, Silvestris F. Obesity as a major risk factor for cancer. J Obes. 2013;2013(8):291546–11. doi:10.1155/2013/291546.
70. Siegel RL, Miller KD, Jemal A. Cancer statistics, 2015. CA Cancer J Clin. 2015;65(1):5–29. doi:10.3322/caac.21254.
71. Ligibel JA, Alfano CM, Hershman D, Ballard RM, Bruinooge SS, Courneya KS, et al. Recommendations for obesity clinical trials in cancer survivors: American Society of Clinical Oncology Statement. J Clin Oncol. 2015;33(33):3961–7. doi:10.1200/JCO.2015.63.1440.

72. Demark-Wahnefried W, Case LD, Blackwell K, Marcom PK, Kraus W, Aziz N, et al. Results of a diet/exercise feasibility trial to prevent adverse body composition change in breast cancer patients on adjuvant chemotherapy. Clin Breast Cancer. 2008;8(1):70–9. doi:10.3816/CBC.2008.n.005.
73. Jakicic JM. The role of physical activity in prevention and treatment of body weight gain in adults. J Nutr. 2002;132:3826S–9S.
74. Perri MG, Nezu AM, Viegener BJ. Improving the long-term management of obesity. New Jersey: Wiley; 1992.
75. Perri MG, Sears SF, Clark JE. Strategies for improving maintenance of weight loss. Toward a continuous care model of obesity management. Diabetes Care. 1993;16(1):200–9.
76. Perri MG. Effects of behavioral treatment on long-term weight loss: lessons learned from the look AHEAD trial. Obesity (Silver Spring, Md). 2014;22(1):3–4. doi:10.1002/oby.20672.
77. Look AHEAD Research Group, Wing RR. Long-term effects of a lifestyle intervention on weight and cardiovascular risk factors in individuals with type 2 diabetes mellitus: four-year results of the Look AHEAD trial. Arch Intern Med. 2010;170(17):1566–75. doi:10.1001/archinternmed.2010.334.
78. Houston DK, Leng X, Bray GA, Hergenroeder AL, Hill JO, Jakicic JM, et al. A long-term intensive lifestyle intervention and physical function: the look AHEAD Movement and Memory Study. Obesity (Silver Spring, Md). 2015;23(1):77–84. doi:10.1002/oby.20944.
79. Pownall HJ, Bray GA, Wagenknecht LE, Walkup MP, Heshka S, Hubbard VS, et al. Changes in body composition over 8 years in a randomized trial of a lifestyle intervention: the look AHEAD study. Obesity (Silver Spring, Md). 2015;23(3):565–72. doi:10.1002/oby.21005.
80. Rubin RR, Wadden TA, Bahnson JL, Blackburn GL, Brancati FL, Bray GA, et al. Impact of intensive lifestyle intervention on depression and health-related quality of life in type 2 diabetes: the Look AHEAD Trial. Diabetes Care. 2014;37(6):1544–53. doi:10.2337/dc13-1928.
81. Focht BC, Brawley LR, Rejeski WJ, Ambrosius WT. Group-mediated activity counseling and traditional exercise therapy programs: effects on health-related quality of life among older adults in cardiac rehabilitation. Ann Behav Med. 2004;28(1):52–61. doi:10.1207/s15324796abm2801_7.
82. Focht BC, Knapp DJ, Gavin TP, Raedeke TD, Hickner RC. Affective and self-efficacy responses to acute aerobic exercise in sedentary older and younger adults. J Aging Phys Act. 2007;15(2):123–38.
83. Thomas JG, Bond DS, Phelan S, Hill JO, Wing RR. Weight-loss maintenance for 10 years in the National Weight Control Registry. Am J Prev Med. 2014;46(1):17–23. doi:10.1016/j.amepre.2013.08.019.

Chapter 9
Energy Balance-Based Strategies to Reduce Consequences of Prostate Cancer: How to Communicate with Men

Yonaira M. Rivera and Katherine Clegg Smith

Abstract As outlined in previous chapters, men with a history of prostate cancer face increased rates of morbidity associated with both their cancer and the side effects of its treatment. Prostate cancer and its treatment can result in altered body composition, increased fatigue, reduced physical activity, fitness and performance, which in turn create considerable and complex health risks. Moreover, obesity has been linked to cancer-related mortality and aggressive prostate cancer and poor prognosis, specifically. The benefits of energy balance among prostate cancer survivors include reduced fatigue, improved quality of life scores, and greater muscular strength.

Keywords Physical Activity • Weight Loss • Planned Behavior Therapy • Transtheoretical Model • Social Cognitive Theory • Energy Balance Messaging

Introduction

Prostate cancer and its treatment create health risks [1, 2], which are considerably exacerbated by obesity [3–5]. The proportion of men with a history of prostate cancer who are engaged in regular exercise points to a potential value in focusing on the promotion of effective behavior change among this population [1, 6, 7]. Some studies have indicated high interest in health promotion programs [6], suggesting that messages regarding the potential benefits of physical activity are being heard and acted upon at least by some men with a history of prostate cancer [8]. However, until now, most energy balance interventions in the U.S. have been designed for female breast cancer survivors or survivors in general, rather than specifically for

Y.M. Rivera, MPH • K.C. Smith, PhD (✉)
Department of Health, Behavior and Society, Johns Hopkins Bloomberg School of Public Health, 624 N Broadway, 7th Floor, Baltimore, MD 21205-1996, USA
e-mail: yrivera2@jhu.edu; katecsmith@jhu.edu

© Springer International Publishing AG 2018
E.A. Platz, N.A. Berger (eds.), *Energy Balance and Prostate Cancer*, Energy Balance and Cancer 14, DOI 10.1007/978-3-319-64940-5_9

prostate cancer survivors [9–11]. Interventions that are designed for women, or that do not specifically address the issues related to prostate cancer and the barriers that men often face in making changes in dietary and physical activity are unlikely to be optimally effective. Thus, it is important to identify appropriate strategies to communicate with prostate cancer survivors about ways to reduce their risk of cancer progression and improve outcomes. In this chapter, we outline many of the important factors to consider in planning for such an undertaking, and effective communication modalities to promote energy balance among men with a prostate cancer history.

Norms, attitudes and practices related to both diet and physical activity are not universal, and thus one might expect people's trajectory through behavior change to be shaped by factors such as social position, age and gender [12–14]. As such, it is important to consider the facilitators and barriers to any behavior change messaging for intervention implementation. Prior research has identified a range of potential barriers to achieving sustained and effective behavior change to achieve energy balance among prostate cancer survivors. For example:

- Older cancer survivors (age 65 and above) have been found to be less physically active than younger counterparts [15]; the average age at diagnosis for prostate cancer is approximately 66 years [16].
- Weight-based stigma, sedentary lifestyle and lack of work-life balance have been identified as barriers to weight-loss among men who are obese [17].
- Men have been found to be less motivated to partake in weight loss strategies focused on dietary modifications than physical activity [17, 18].
- Prostate cancer survivors' adherence to an exercise program was found to be lower for men with severe hormonal symptoms and low perceived ability to perform daily tasks and leisure activities [19].
- Among men with a history of prostate cancer, work demands and the cost of healthy food have been highlighted as barriers to dietary behavior changes [20].

Effective energy-balance messaging will require engagement with such factors to present meaningful objectives for change and address potential difficulties in attaining them.

Efficacy of Evidence-Based, Theory-Driven Energy Balance Interventions Among Prostate Cancer Survivors

Reviews of the energy balance intervention literature have indicated potential for improvements in an array of physical and mental health outcomes for cancer survivors [9]. Achieving these outcomes may be facilitated by the integration of behavioral theories in the development of interventions, allowing for a stronger assessment of factors influencing behavior change [21]. However, there is inconsistent evidence of the extent to which behavioral theories have informed and/or driven interventions to improve diet and exercise among cancer survivors [22]. This section explores the utilization of behavioral theories to develop and test energy balance interventions among cancer survivors.

Among the most popular theories in diet and physical activity interventions for cancer survivors are the Theory of Planned Behavior, Transtheoretical Model, and Social Cognitive Theory [22–25]. According to the Theory of Planned Behavior, behavioral intention is the most important direct influence on behavior change [26]; messages are therefore to be designed to create and maintain a positive intention towards the desired change. Intention to perform a behavior depends on several factors, including one's attitude toward changing a behavior, beliefs about others' perceived approval or disapproval of a behavior, and perceived control over the ability to enact behavior change. Somewhat in contrast, the Transtheoretical Model emphasizes the extent to which individuals balance the pros and cons of changing a behavior as they go through the six stages of change, spanning from precontemplation to termination of a behavior [27]. Lastly, Social Cognitive Theory posits that the interplay between individuals and their environments—known as reciprocal determinism—impacts personal and collective behaviors and emphasizes an individual's potential to facilitate changes in his or her environment [28]. While each theory conceptualizes behavior change in a somewhat different way, all three provide strong frameworks from which to design energy balance interventions that address barriers to physical activity and dietary change among prostate cancer survivors. Energy balance messaging for men with a history of prostate cancer should have at its foundation an understanding of men's attitudes towards any modifications of diet and/or physical activity being posed, as well as the extent to which success is seen as being within their control, the environment within which an individual change will occur, and the man's relationship to that environment. The benefits and potential negative implications of changes being promoted should be acknowledged and addressed, and considerations given not only to individual factors but also social context for making any changes.

Physical activity interventions that have at their foundation substantive behavior change theory have been shown to enhance effectiveness among breast cancer survivors [22]. Nevertheless, only a limited number of energy balance interventions targeting cancer survivors have explicitly integrated theoretical constructs; even fewer have measured these constructs to evaluate their effectiveness, and fewer still have been designed and implemented with prostate cancer survivors. Husebø and colleagues [25] conducted a systematic review and meta-analysis examining theoretical predictors of adherence to exercise programs targeting cancer survivors. Of the 12 studies reviewed, 9 utilized the Theory of Planned Behavior and 5 applied the Transtheoretical Model's stages of change for exercise (2 studies used both theories). Results from their meta-analysis indicated that exercise stage of change is a strong predictor of exercise adherence among cancer survivors, while perceived behavioral control and intention to engage in exercise were significantly correlated with exercise adherence. Interestingly, only one study focused exclusively on prostate cancer survivors; this study found intention and exercise stage of change to be statistically significant predictors of exercise adherence [29]. A more recent systematic review and meta-analysis assessing 12 diet and exercise interventions for cancer survivors utilizing Social Cognitive Theory as their theoretical framework established that, while findings support the theory's efficacy in changing behavior among cancer survivors, most trials failed to properly measure utilized constructs [23]. The review also identified self-efficacy—an individual's belief that he/she can achieve an outcome of interest [30]—as the only construct associated with positive behavior change in both diet and physical activity among reviewed studies that reported assessing the impact of theoretical constructs in their interventions. It is important to note that only 3 of the 12 randomized controlled trials in their analysis included prostate cancer survivors. Of these, only one diet-specific intervention was delivered exclusively to prostate cancer survivors [31].

As evidenced by the literature, there is a need for additional theoretically informed evidence as to how to promote energy balance among prostate cancer survivors. In light of this growing interest, a recent cluster randomized controlled trial conducted in Australia—known as the ENGAGE study—utilized Social Cognitive Theory to design a 12-week clinician referral-based exercise intervention targeting recently diagnosed prostate cancer survivors [32]. While primary and secondary outcomes focus on physical activity participation, physical functioning, quality of life, anxiety and depression, researchers are also interested in exploring the mediating effects of self-efficacy, outcome expectations, goals and socio-cultural factors on these outcomes. Results from the analysis of adherence predictors suggest the incorporation of behavioral change techniques informed by Social Cognitive Theory may explain high adherence levels (80.3%) among participants in the exercise training intervention arm of the study [19]. Designing intervention messaging around key aspects of the theory allows for a rigorous examination (and potential modification) of the effects of key components that is otherwise not possible.

Energy Balance Messaging for Prostate Cancer Survivors

Effectively communicating the importance of energy balance to prostate cancer survivors is an essential part of achieving positive outcomes and improved health. As such, messages should be tailored to meet men's interests and attitudes, and directed towards goals that are seen as most important and understood to be achievable. Although improved cancer prognosis as a result of weight loss may be critical to some prostate cancer survivors, discussing the benefits of energy balance from other vantage points may yield better outcomes among others. The following section discusses several messaging approaches.

A common theme in several studies focusing on dietary and exercise patterns among prostate cancer survivors is the importance of the concept of masculinity in understanding the behavioral patterns in question, as well as existing facilitators and barriers to change. Literature suggests dominant ideals of masculinity impact food choices and many times conflict with healthier eating habits, which in turn may contribute to poorer prostate cancer prognosis [33]. Among foods considered to be emblems of masculinity are red meat and dairy, both of which have been associated with an increased risk of prostate cancer [34]. Findings in a study exploring the influence of healthfulness on prostate cancer survivors' diets highlight the importance of understanding masculine dietary patterns, as these may impact receptiveness to dietary interventions [20]. Participants described a preference towards consuming red meat, and the idea of eating for pleasure rather than for health promotion, both of which may prove problematic for dietary interventions aimed at prostate cancer survivors. The relevance of certain food types to constructs of masculinity were echoed in a recent study assessing men's needs and interests, with 64% of men reporting daily dairy consumption and 26% reporting daily red meat consumption [35]. As such, messages should emphasize the importance of not only encouraging eating in moderation as a vehicle for weight loss, but also promoting healthy foods that taste good (identified as an important factor in men's dietary decisions) as alternatives to red meat and dairy [20].

Concepts of masculinity also impact how men view and engage in physical activity. Multiple studies suggest men view exercise as a more masculine approach to weight loss than dieting, as it allows for men to not only lose weight but also be more muscular, fitter and stronger [17, 18]. Lewis et al. [17] also note obese men's notion that weight loss is about "balancing energy in versus energy out," which should be achievable by increasing physical activity without necessarily changing one's diet. These qualitative findings were echoed in a recent study reporting that 64% of surveyed men have resorted to physical activity for weight loss [35], while only 21% of women in another study using a similar survey format reported using physical activity to lose weight [36]. Similar trends have been observed among prostate cancer survivors: when compared to female cancer survivors, male cancer survivors were 30% more likely to meet the American Cancer Society's weekly recommendations of moderate-to-vigorous physical activity (>150 min) [37]. Furthermore, when specifically looking at male cancer survivors, prostate cancer survivors were 35% more likely than colorectal cancer survivors to meet the same guidelines [37]; while this may partially be due to limitations in physical activity among colorectal cancer survivors [38, 39], it is also possible that prostate cancer survivors experiencing impotency or other treatment side-effects view physical activity as one way to maintain or enhance their masculinity. Interventions should therefore consider highlighting the masculine benefits of physical activity when developing energy balance messages for prostate cancer survivors.

Framing behavior change specifically in relation to one's cancer prognosis may not, however, always be the most impactful messaging strategy for men with a prostate cancer history. Age and life stage are also relevant considerations for messaging design. As people age, the meaning of a cancer diagnosis (and the associated impetus for behavior change to reduce likelihood of recurrence) is often different than it would have been earlier in life [40]. For some prostate cancer survivors, it may be more effective to promote the benefits of energy balance outside the purview of cancer, and instead focus on health in general or other chronic conditions. Co-morbidities are very prevalent among prostate cancer survivors in the U.S. [41]: data from the 2009 Behavioral Risk Factor Surveillance System survey indicate that 72% of men with a history of prostate cancer are overweight or obese, 20.1% had heart disease, 58.3% had hypertension, 53.9% had high cholesterol, and 23.7% had diabetes [37]. Studies have found that cancer often does not play a leading role in prostate cancer survivors' dietary habits; if there is a health consideration in how men eat, it is often related to another chronic condition such as heart disease [20, 42]. Research also notes that prostate cancer survivors are more likely to die of a co-morbid disease than of prostate cancer [41, 43, 44], which provides further support for the importance of a health promotional focus that does not consider prostate cancer in isolation, but rather gives explicit consideration to the entire health of the individual—and specifically to chronic co-morbidities.

As outlined, given the prevalence of co-morbidities, it may also be more effective for energy balance messages to focus on how diet and exercise can improve the life span of survivors in general, rather than specifically prioritizing implications for cancer. More diffuse "healthy lifestyle" messaging may also be particularly important for men with a prostate cancer history who do not identify with the term "cancer survivor," or those who have been cancer-free for a long time [45]. To these men, their experience with prostate cancer may no longer be salient; hence, energy balance messages that are focused on other benefits to diet and exercise may be more likely to be impactful.

Sexual function is also an important issue to prostate cancer survivors, with short and long-term effects of treatment including erectile dysfunction, testicular atrophy, loss of libido, penile shortening and an altered orgasm experience [46–48]. These effects have been noted to impact notions of masculinity, further impacting distress caused by sexual dysfunction [49]. While sexual dysfunction has been acknowledged as important to prostate cancer survivors in general [48], younger prostate cancer survivors have been reported to be more concerned about treatment impact on their sexuality [50]. Although interventions exploring the benefits of exercise on sexual function among prostate cancer survivors are scarce, a recent randomized controlled trial among prostate cancer patients undergoing androgen deprivation therapy reported men participating in 12 weeks of bi-weekly sessions of moderate to high intensity resistance and aerobic exercise maintained their sexual activity levels, while those in the control group experienced decreased libido [51]. Researchers suggested the effect of exercise on sexual activity was mediated by improved quality of life. As such, highlighting emerging findings of the benefits exercise may have on sexual function may be another way to deliver energy balance messages to prostate cancer survivors (particularly younger ones) that motivates them to increase physical activity levels [48].

The benefits of physical activity may also appeal to prostate cancer survivors who are more concerned about their current quality of life, rather than balancing energy intake as a distal goal. Studies report that cancer survivors engaging in physical activity have higher quality of life than those not meeting recommended levels [7, 52]. Quality of life was also statistically significantly higher among prostate cancer survivors receiving androgen deprivation therapy who were randomized to a 12-week resistance exercise training intervention compared to controls [5]. Meanwhile, findings from the ENGAGE study suggest that cancer-specific quality of life factors (such as role functioning, sexual activity, hormonal symptoms and education level) may predict adherence to physical activity programs for prostate cancer survivors [19]. Messages emphasizing the benefits of exercise on quality of life outcomes may thus posit themselves as more salient for a broad range of survivors desiring to improve their quality of life post treatment.

Effective Communication Modalities

In addition to identifying how to best tailor messages that promote energy balance among prostate cancer survivors, it is crucial to select appropriate modalities to communicate these messages. The communication modality will shape how information is received: When is a message conveyed? Where? And, in what form? The conveyance modality will also shape the potential influence of any delivered message, as engagement with messages is influenced by both message source and substance [53, 54].

In-person communication via healthcare providers continues to be a useful modality to reach and influence cancer survivors, particularly as not all populations have equal access to or engagement with messages conveyed via mass media [55]. Literature supporting the role of healthcare provider communication in behavior change among cancer survivors highlights providers' abilities to influence changes in physical activity levels and dietary behaviors, given their direct contact with prostate cancer survivors throughout treatment and the care continuum [56]. Especially important is the immediate post-diagnostic period, often referenced as the "teachable moment", when cancer survivors may be more motivated to change health behaviors due to the salience of their diagnosis [6, 42]. Healthcare providers and other practitioners may thus capitalize on this short timeframe to intervene with tailored energy balance messages.

It is important to note that as yet, energy balance interventions are not a routine part of survivorship care (in general, not just for prostate cancer survivors); the literature indicates that the doctor-patient interaction is often a missed interventional opportunity regarding physical activity as a part of healthy survivorship [1, 2, 57, 58]. A survey conducted at a Canadian cancer center highlights that 70% of cancer survivors reported not receiving exercise counseling throughout their cancer care continuum—although 90% stated a desire to participate in an exercise program post-diagnosis [58]. These findings may be indicative of the time constraints providers face during patient encounters. The 2007 Institute of Medicine (IOM) report on implementing survivorship care planning called for the inclusion of lifestyle recommendations within documentation that is intended to create the foundation for healthy survivorship beyond acute treatment [59]. To the extent that survivorship care plans become a routine part of care coordination for all cancer patients, so this may be an important mechanism by which to provide both information regarding the reasons why energy balance is key to healthy survivorship, as well as demonstrated effective mechanisms to achieve meaningful change.

Recent literature has suggested a central role for healthcare professionals beyond just physicians in communication about energy balance [60, 61]. For example, researchers in the Australian ENGAGE study assessed the efficacy of clinician referrals to a supervised exercise program for prostate cancer survivors [60]. The program used postgraduate clinical exercise physiology students (supervised by accredited exercise physiologists) to delivery two supervised, 50-min sessions per week at local gym and advised participants on a weekly home-based session. Among participants enrolled in the experimental arm of the study, 80% indicated the clinician's referral to the exercise program influenced their decision to participate. Another way to assist patient-provider communication regarding energy balance is by leveraging the efforts of nurses and other care team members. Webb, Foster and Poulter [61] describe the development of a training intervention designed to improve nurses' capability, opportunity and motivation in delivering very brief advice on physical activity to cancer survivors. This program is based on the Behaviour Change Wheel, a theoretical model describing eight steps to designing behavior change interventions [62]. The program teaches nurses to 'Ask, Advise and Act': *ask* patients about physical activity levels and whether they are aware of the health benefits; *advise* on the benefits of physical activity, based on the patient's needs; and *act* by providing support and referring to local services or other resources. Although this study is still ongoing, nurses' promotion of physical activity through brief advice may successfully influence cancer survivors, given their regular interaction through treatment and follow-up visits [63].

When we consider behavioral modifications for men as a path to achieving energy balance, it is also important to adopt a socio-ecological approach and consider the individual within a familial, cultural and structural context. Partners have been reported to be very influential in decision making that affects patient care [20, 50, 64]. Davison and colleagues [50] discussed decision-making among prostate cancer survivors and partners at the time of diagnosis, reporting that the majority of both groups preferred collaborative roles in making medical decisions. Communication strategies may thus be more successful if tailored to the dyad or the broader familial context, rather than men alone. There is also strong reason to focus on female spouses beyond medical decision-making in order to understand and impact men's dietary behaviors. While familial norms have changed significantly over the past 30 years, women still tend to take primary responsibility for daily food preparation [65]. Prior research has found that wives of men with a prostate cancer history play a key role in shaping the diets of their husbands [20], with the majority of men relying on their spouses to prepare their meals [35]. It may sometimes be most efficacious to direct dietary messaging for prostate cancer survivorship towards both spouses and the men themselves, given histories and structures for food preparation within households.

Targeting partners as part of an energy balance communication modality may also be effective, particularly when combined with strategies targeting quality of life issues. For example, Song and colleagues [66] developed a web-based educational intervention targeting quality of life among prostate cancer survivors and their partner. The interactive website included seven modules for couples to review, among which was a mandatory module focusing on working as a team. In addition to reporting that the website was informative and easy to use, participants also stated that the program provided couples with new ways to work together and strengthen their relationship during a time of hardship. While this intervention was developed to assist with quality of life issues, these communication skills can be transferred to messages educating couples about the benefits of exercise in improving both quality of life and disease prognosis.

Another communication modality that may assist in delivering energy balance messages is the utilization of peer groups. Peer support groups have been used for some time as a way to improve depression and self-efficacy, including among prostate cancer survivors who had recently undergone a radical prostatectomy [67]. Weber et al.'s study [67] demonstrated that men who participated in an eight-week peer support intervention had higher self-efficacy and lower depression over time than those not partnered with a peer mentor. This provides some support for the idea that utilizing peer support groups may be a beneficial mechanism for promoting energy balance activities among prostate cancer survivors, especially given findings that suggest group-based exercise is better at improving prostate cancer survivors' physical fitness and quality of life than home-based exercise programs [2].

It may not always be feasible to communicate with prostate cancer survivors about energy balance strategies in person. In such scenarios, telephone and/or mail may be a useful strategy to communicate with men to maintain healthy physical activity levels and dietary behaviors. Parsons and colleagues [31] used the Social Cognitive Theory and motivational interviewing techniques to develop a 6-month telephone-based dietary counseling program tailored to prostate cancer survivors aged 50 to 80. At the end of the intervention, vegetable consumption and carotenoid concentrations had increased in the intervention arm [31]. Another telephone-based intervention designed using the Social Cognitive Theory was the Reach out to Enhance Wellness (RENEW) trial, a 12-month home-based telephone counseling program with mailed materials developed to promote physical activity and diet quality among long-term breast, prostate and colorectal cancer survivors aged 65 years or older [68]. Results indicate statistically significant changes in physical activity levels and dietary behaviors between intervention and control groups, with intervention participants reporting a mean weight loss more than double that reported by controls. It is important to note that, compared to individuals not recruited for this study, participants were younger, female (breast cancer survivors), and had a more proximal cancer diagnosis [68]. Given in-person dialogue has been reported to be preferred among older audiences [69, 70], the RENEW trial's findings may suggest that in-person communication modalities may be more effective than telephone and/or mail communication among some older men. Nonetheless, these communication modalities have the capacity of reaching a large number of prostate cancer survivors in cost-effective ways, as do newer technologies (such as social media and texting), which are further discussed below.

Moving Forward

As outlined in other chapters in this volume, the evidence base regarding energy balance and prostate cancer survivorship is complex, yet clearly pertinent for effective health promotion in this population. The following section provides recommendations for future energy balance interventions for men with a history of prostate cancer. One of the challenges regarding messaging for such interventions is that much of the evidence of the impact of weight loss on cancer survival is focused on women with breast cancer [9]. There is a need for greater specificity of efficacy of interventions (weight loss as well as physical activity) for specific survivor subgroups [9]. There is also a need for a more robust evidence base on the benefits of physical activity for prostate cancer survivors by intensity, duration and frequency, as well as studies that consider the nature of treatment undergone [2].

Our review of the literature did not reveal much in the way of cultural tailoring of energy balance messaging for subpopulations of men with a history of prostate cancer. There is also a gap in the evidence base regarding the extent to which behavior change messaging is more efficacious if it is targeted by gender and cultural factors. Cultural awareness has been shown to be key to developing and implementing impactful screening programs for underserved populations [71] and it might be assumed that such tailoring would also be beneficial for sustainable and impactful energy balance interventions during survivorship. This is particularly important among minority groups with a higher burden of obesity and other co-morbid conditions that may result from poor energy balance. For example, a recent study assessing racial and ethnic differences in health behaviors among prostate cancer survivors highlights that African American men had higher prevalence of obesity and diabetes than White and Hispanic survivors [72]. However, the study did not have sufficient power to detect differences between groups other than African Americans and Whites, further highlighting the importance of exploring factors impacting energy balance among other prostate cancer survivor subpopulations.

Understanding the cultural and historical context of care provision is also key to designing efficacious messaging and interventions. Prior research with African American men with a history of prostate cancer illustrated an initial level of mistrust with the healthcare system and a desire for providers to address them with respect and as knowledgeable participants in their care [73]. Meanwhile, a study of coping strategies of low-income, immigrant Mexican men with a prostate cancer diagnosis highlighted the importance of relying on God and doctors as sources of support for many men with this shared cultural heritage [74]. Studies such as these are illustrative of the importance of seeking to understand the specific facets that may be important for underserved groups in making meaningful behavior change. Cultural understanding can form the foundation for appropriate program design and message tailoring that will assist not only in recruiting participants in energy balance clinical trials, but also in creating and sustaining interventions that embed energy balance messaging into issues important to these communities.

Interventions focusing on the effects of exercise on masculinity and sexual functioning are also needed. As highlighted by Cormie and colleagues [48], exercise as a way to lessen the effects of prostate cancer treatment on sexual dysfunction has both strong theoretical rationale and budding empirical support [51]. This is an issue of importance to not only prostate cancer survivors, but also their partners. A recent study by Wootten et al. [64] focusing on prostate cancer highlighted the role that partners have in helping with influencing how the survivor adapts to and copes with a prostate cancer diagnosis. Partners stated the importance of supporting men who feel a loss in masculinity, particularly as they face challenges with communication constrains. Researchers suggest psychosocial interventions could focus on dyadic communication, sexuality and intimacy issues, support and communication pertaining loss of masculinity, social support and coping strategies (including discussions about thoughts and emotions). As such, future research should consider developing exercise interventions both assessing the impact of exercise on improving sexual function and notions of masculinity, while also integrating partners as a means of support.

The utilization of technology to promote energy balance is another important area for further research [9, 75]. As technology continues to advance and the digital divide shrinks, mobile apps, text messaging, social media and other mHealth platforms may help facilitate behavioral change interventions that reach multiple audiences that are difficult to access. Such interventions have already been used to promote weight loss among overweight and obese men [76], improve quality of life among couples with a prostate cancer survivor [66], and, more recently, assess the feasibility of text messaging to increase prostate cancer screening awareness among African American men [77]. These technologies present as areas of opportunity to engage hard-to-reach prostate cancer survivors, such as those living in rural areas with limited transportation, as well as men from racial/ethnic minorities or other underserved groups. However, technology-driven interventions may not be appropriate for all: results from a recent survey assessing men's needs and interests for a technology-driven weight loss intervention reported that while the Internet (88%) and email (91%) were commonly used among men over the age of 60, text messaging (49%) and smartphone app utilization (22%) was substantially lower [35]. Future research exploring mHealth avenues must therefore assess the readiness of its intended audiences in adopting new technologies prior to delivery of energy balance messages.

References

1. Bellizzi KM, Rowland JH, Jeffery DD, McNeel T. Health behaviors of cancer survivors: examining opportunities for cancer control intervention. J Clin Oncol. 2005;23(34):8884–93.
2. Keogh JW, MacLeod RD. Body composition, physical fitness, functional performance, quality of life and fatigue benefits of exercise for prostate cancer patients: a systematic review. J Pain Symptom Manage. 2012;43(1):96–110.

3. Ligibel JA, Alfano CM, Courneya KS, Demark-Wahnefried W, Burger RA, Chlebowski RT, et al. American Society of Clinical Oncology position statement on obesity and cancer. J Clin Oncol. 2014;32(31):3568–74.
4. Cao Y, Ma J. Body mass index, prostate cancer–specific mortality, and biochemical recurrence: a systematic review and meta-analysis. Cancer Prev Res. 2011;4(4):486–501.
5. Segal RJ, Reid RD, Courneya KS, Malone SC, Parliament MB, Scott CG, et al. Resistance exercise in men receiving androgen deprivation therapy for prostate cancer. J Clin Oncol. 2003;21(9):1653–9.
6. Demark-Wahnefried W, Peterson B, McBride C, Lipkus I, Clipp E. Current health behaviors and readiness to pursue life-style changes among men and women diagnosed with early stage prostate and breast carcinomas. Cancer. 2000;88(3):674–84.
7. Blanchard CM, Courneya KS, Stein K. Cancer survivors' adherence to lifestyle behavior recommendations and associations with health-related quality of life: results from the American Cancer Society's SCS-II. J Clin Oncol. 2008;26(13):2198–204.
8. Kwon S, Hou N, Wang M. Comparison of physical activity levels between cancer survivors and non-cancer participants in the 2009 BRFSS. J Cancer Surviv. 2012;6(1):54–62.
9. Alfano CM, Molfino A, Muscaritoli M. Interventions to promote energy balance and cancer survivorship. Cancer. 2013;119(S11):2143–50.
10. Ballard-Barbash R, Siddiqi SM, Berrigan DA, Ross SA, Nebeling LC, Dowling EC. Trends in research on energy balance supported by the National Cancer Institute. Am J Prev Med. 2013;44(4):416–23.
11. Demark-Wahnefried W, Rogers LQ, Alfano CM, Thomson CA, Courneya KS, Meyerhardt JA, et al. Practical clinical interventions for diet, physical activity, and weight control in cancer survivors. CA Cancer J Clin. 2015;65(3):167–89.
12. Segar M, Jayaratne T, Hanlon J, Richardson CR. Fitting fitness into women's lives: effects of a gender-tailored physical activity intervention. Womens Health Issues. 2002;12(6):338–47.
13. Albarracín D, Gillette JC, Earl AN, Glasman LR, Durantini MR, Ho MH. A test of major assumptions about behavior change: a comprehensive look at the effects of passive and active HIV-prevention interventions since the beginning of the epidemic. Psychol Bull. 2005;131(6):856.
14. Noar SM, Benac CN, Harris MS. Does tailoring matter? Meta-analytic review of tailored print health behavior change interventions. Psychol Bull. 2007;133(4):673.
15. Gjerset GM, Fosså SD, Courneya KS, Skovlund E, Thorsen L. Exercise behavior in cancer survivors and associated factors. J Cancer Surviv. 2011;5(1):35–43.
16. American Cancer Society. Key statistics for prostate cancer. 2016. Retrieved from http://www.cancer.org/cancer/prostatecancer/detailedguide/prostate-cancer-key-statistics.
17. Lewis S, Thomas SL, Hyde J, Castle DJ, Komesaroff PA. A qualitative investigation of obese men's experiences with their weight. Am J Health Behav. 2011;35(4):458–69.
18. Barker R, Cooke B. Diet, obesity and being overweight: a qualitative research study. Health Educ J. 1992;51(3):117–21.
19. Craike M, Gaskin CJ, Courneya KS, Fraser SF, Salmon J, Owen PJ, et al. Predictors of adherence to a 12-week exercise program among men treated for prostate cancer: ENGAGE study. Cancer Med. 2016;5(5):787–94.
20. Coa KI, Smith KC, Klassen AC, Thorpe RJ, Caulfield LE. Exploring important influences on the healthfulness of prostate cancer survivors' diets. Qual Health Res. 2015;25(6):857–70.
21. Glanz K, Rimer BK, Viswanath K, editors. Health behavior and health education: theory, research, and practice. 4th ed. San Francisco, CA: Jossey-Bass; 2008.
22. Bluethmann SM, Bartholomew LK, Murphy CC, Vernon SW. Use of theory in behavior change interventions: an analysis of programs to increase physical activity in posttreatment breast cancer survivors. Health Educ Behav. 2016;44(2):245–53. doi:10.1177/1090198116647712.
23. Stacey FG, James EL, Chapman K, Courneya KS, Lubans DR. A systematic review and meta-analysis of social cognitive theory-based physical activity and/or nutrition behavior change interventions for cancer survivors. J Cancer Surviv. 2015;9(2):305–38.

24. Green HJ, Steinnagel G, Morris C, Laakso EL. Health behaviour models and patient preferences regarding nutrition and physical activity after breast or prostate cancer diagnosis. Eur J Cancer Care. 2014;23(5):640–52.
25. Husebø AML, Dyrstad SM, Søreide JA, Bru E. Predicting exercise adherence in cancer patients and survivors: a systematic review and meta-analysis of motivational and behavioural factors. J Clin Nurs. 2013;22(1-2):4–21.
26. Ajzen I. The theory of planned behavior. Organ Behav Hum Decis Process. 1991;50(2):179–211.
27. Prochaska JO, Velicer WF. The transtheoretical model of health behavior change. Am J Health Promot. 1997;12(1):38–48.
28. Bandura A. Social foundations of thought and action: a social cognitive theory. Englewood Cliffs, NJ: Prentice-Hall, Inc; 1986.
29. Courneya KS, Segal RJ, Reid RD, Jones LW, Malone SC, Venner PM, et al. Three independent factors predicted adherence in a randomized controlled trial of resistance exercise training among prostate cancer survivors. J Clin Epidemiol. 2004;57(6):571–9.
30. Bandura A. Self-efficacy mechanism in human agency. Am Psychol. 1982;37(2):122–47.
31. Parsons JK, Newman VA, Mohler JL, Pierce JP, Flatt S, Marshall J. Dietary modification in patients with prostate cancer on active surveillance: a randomized, multicentre feasibility study. BJU Int. 2008;101(10):1227–31.
32. Livingston PM, Salmon J, Courneya KS, Gaskin CJ, Craike M, Botti M, et al. Efficacy of a referral and physical activity program for survivors of prostate cancer [ENGAGE]: rationale and design for a cluster randomised controlled trial. BMC Cancer. 2011;11(1):1.
33. Mróz LW, Chapman GE, Oliffe JL, Bottorff JL. Men, food, and prostate cancer: gender influences on men's diets. Am J Mens Health. 2011;5(2):177–87.
34. Mandair D, Rossi RE, Pericleous M, Whyand T, Caplin ME. Prostate cancer and the influence of dietary factors and supplements: a systematic review. Nutr Metab. 2014;11(1):1.
35. Schleper A, Sullivan DK, Thrasher JB, Holzbeierlein JM, Klemp J, Befort C, Hamilton-Reeves JM. Weight management to reduce prostate cancer risk: a survey of men's needs and interests. Cancer Clin Oncol. 2016;5(1):43.
36. Befort CA, Austin H, Klemp JR. Weight control needs and experiences among rural breast cancer survivors. Psychooncology. 2011;20(10):1069–75.
37. LeMasters TJ, Madhavan SS, Sambamoorthi U, Kurian S. Health behaviors among breast, prostate, and colorectal cancer survivors: a US population-based case-control study, with comparisons by cancer type and gender. J Cancer Surviv. 2014;8(3):336–48.
38. Jansen L, Herrmann A, Stegmaier C, Singer S, Brenner H, Arndt V. Health-related quality of life during the 10 years after diagnosis of colorectal cancer: a population-based study. J Clin Oncol. 2011;29(24):3263–9.
39. Krouse RS, Herrinton LJ, Grant M, Wendel CS, Green SB, Mohler MJ, et al. Health-related quality of life among long-term rectal cancer survivors with an ostomy: manifestations by sex. J Clin Oncol. 2009;27(28):4664–70.
40. Hannum SM, Clegg Smith K, Coa K, Klassen AC. Identity reconstruction among older cancer survivors: age and meaning in the context of a life-altering illness. J Psychosoc Oncol. 2016:1–16.
41. Bradley CJ, Dahman B, Anscher M. Prostate cancer treatment and survival: evidence for men with prevalent comorbid conditions. Med Care. 2014;52(6):482.
42. Demark-Wahnefried W, Aziz NM, Rowland JH, Pinto BM. Riding the crest of the teachable moment: promoting long-term health after the diagnosis of cancer. J Clin Oncol. 2005;23(24):5814–30.
43. Chamie K, Daskivich TJ, Kwan L, Labo J, Dash A, Greenfield S, Litwin MS. Comorbidities, treatment and ensuing survival in men with prostate cancer. J Gen Intern Med. 2012;27(5):492–9.
44. Lund L, Borre M, Jacobsen J, Sørensen HT, Nørgaard M. Impact of comorbidity on survival of Danish prostate cancer patients, 1995–2006: a population-based cohort study. Urology. 2008;72(6):1258–62.

45. Smith KC, Klassen AC, Coa KI, Hannum SM. The salience of cancer and the "survivor" identity for people who have completed acute cancer treatment: a qualitative study. J Cancer Surviv. 2016;10(3):457–66.
46. Sadovsky R, Basson R, Krychman M, Morales AM, Schover L, Wang R, Incrocci L. Cancer and sexual problems. J Sex Med. 2010;7(1pt2):349–73.
47. Bober SL, Varela VS. Sexuality in adult cancer survivors: challenges and intervention. J Clin Oncol. 2012;30(30):3712–9.
48. Cormie P, Newton RU, Taaffe DR, Spry N, Galvão DA. Exercise therapy for sexual dysfunction after prostate cancer. Nat Rev Urol. 2013;10(12):731–6.
49. Zaider T, Manne S, Nelson C, Mulhall J, Kissane D. Loss of masculine identity, marital affection, and sexual bother in men with localized prostate cancer. J Sex Med. 2012;9(10):2724–32.
50. Davison BJ, Gleave ME, Goldenberg SL, Degner LF, Hoffart D, Berkowitz J. Assessing information and decision preferences of men with prostate cancer and their partners. Cancer Nurs. 2002;25(1):42–9.
51. Cormie P, Newton RU, Taaffe DR, Spry N, Joseph D, Hamid MA, Galvao DA. Exercise maintains sexual activity in men undergoing androgen suppression for prostate cancer: a randomized controlled trial. Prostate Cancer Prostatic Dis. 2013;16(2):170–5.
52. Courneya KS. Exercise in cancer survivors: an overview of research. Med Sci Sports Exerc. 2003;35(11):1846–52.
53. Silk KJ, Atkin CK, Salmon CT. Developing effective media campaigns for health promotion. In: Thompson TL, Parrott R, Nussbaum JF, editors. The Routledge handbook of health communication. New York: Routledge; 2011. p. 203–20.
54. Atkin CK, Rice RE. Theory and principles of public communication campaigns. In: Rice RE, Atkin CK, editors. Public communication campaigns. London: Sage; 2013. p. 3–19.
55. Clayman ML, Manganello JA, Viswanath K, Hesse BW, Arora NK. Providing health messages to Hispanics/Latinos: understanding the importance of language, trust in health information sources, and media use. J Health Commun. 2010;15(suppl 3):252–63.
56. Jones LW, Courneya KS, Fairey AS, Mackey JR. Effects of an oncologist's recommendation to exercise on self-reported exercise behavior in newly diagnosed breast cancer survivors: a single-blind, randomized controlled trial. Ann Behav Med. 2004;28(2):105–13.
57. Roberts CS, Baker F, Hann D, Runfola J, Witt C, McDonald J, et al. Patient-physician communication regarding use of complementary therapies during cancer treatment. J Psychosoc Oncol. 2006;23(4):35–60.
58. Dorsay JP, Cheifetz O. Cancer and exercise: a survey of patients' knowledge and preferences. Arch Phys Med Rehabil. 2008;89:e27.
59. Institute of Medicine. Implementing survivorship care planning. Washington, DC. 2007.
60. Livingston PM, Craike MJ, Salmon J, Courneya KS, Gaskin CJ, Fraser SF, et al. Effects of a clinician referral and exercise program for men who have completed active treatment for prostate cancer: a multicenter cluster randomized controlled trial (ENGAGE). Cancer. 2015;121(15):2646–54.
61. Webb J, Foster J, Poulter E. Increasing the frequency of physical activity very brief advice for cancer patients. Development of an intervention using the behaviour change wheel. Public Health. 2016;133:45–56.
62. Michie S, van Stralen MM, West R. The behaviour change wheel: a new method for characterising and designing behaviour change interventions. Implement Sci. 2011;6(1):1.
63. Murphy JL, Girot EA. The importance of nutrition, diet and lifestyle advice for cancer survivors–the role of nursing staff and interprofessional workers. J Clin Nurs. 2013;22(11–12):1539–49.
64. Wootten AC, Abbott JM, Osborne D, Austin DW, Klein B, Costello AJ, Murphy DG. The impact of prostate cancer on partners: a qualitative exploration. Psychooncology. 2014;23(11):1252–8.
65. Allen P, Sachs C. Women and food chains: The gendered politics of food. Int J Sociol Food Agric. 2012;15(1):1–23.
66. Song L, Rini C, Deal AM, Nielsen ME, Chang H, Kinneer P, Palmer MH. Improving couples' quality of life through a web-based prostate cancer education intervention. Oncol Nurs Forum. 2015, March;42(2):183–92.

67. Weber BA, Roberts BL, Resnick M, Deimling G, Zauszniewski JA, Musil C, Yarandi HN. The effect of dyadic intervention on self-efficacy, social support, and depression for men with prostate cancer. Psychooncology. 2004;13(1):47–60.
68. Morey MC, Snyder DC, Sloane R, Cohen HJ, Peterson B, Hartman TJ, et al. Effects of home-based diet and exercise on functional outcomes among older, overweight long-term cancer survivors: RENEW: a randomized controlled trial. JAMA. 2009;301(18):1883–91.
69. Witham MD, McMurdo ME. How to get older people included in clinical studies. Drugs Aging. 2007;24(3):187–96.
70. Norton MC, Breitner J, Welsh KA, Wyse BW. Characteristics of nonresponders in a community survey of the elderly. J Am Geriatr Soc. 1994;42(12):1252–6.
71. Ashing-Giwa K. The recruitment of breast cancer survivors into cancer control studies: a focus on African-American women. J Natl Med Assoc. 1999;91(5):255.
72. Li J, Thompson TD, Richards TB, Steele CB. Peer reviewed: racial and ethnic differences in health behaviors and preventive health services among prostate cancer survivors in the United States. Prev Chronic Dis. 2016;13:E95.
73. Allen JD, Kennedy M, Wilson-Glover A, Gilligan TD. African-American men's perceptions about prostate cancer: implications for designing educational interventions. Soc Sci Med. 2007;64(11):2189–200.
74. Maliski SL, Husain M, Connor SE, Litwin MS. Alliance of support for low-income Latino men with prostate cancer: god, doctor, and self. J Relig Health. 2012;51(3):752–62.
75. Alfano CM, Bluethmann SM, Tesauro G, Perna F, Agurs-Collins T, Elena JW, et al. NCI funding trends and priorities in physical activity and energy balance research among cancer survivors. J Natl Cancer Inst. 2016;108(1):djv285.
76. Patrick K, Calfas KJ, Norman GJ, Rosenberg D, Zabinski MF, Sallis JF, et al. Outcomes of a 12-month web-based intervention for overweight and obese men. Ann Behav Med. 2011;42(3):391–401.
77. Le D, Holt CL, Saunders DR, Wang MQ, Coriolan A, Savoy AD, et al. Feasibility and acceptability of SMS text messaging in a prostate cancer educational intervention for African American men. Health Informatics J. 2015;22(4):932–47.

Index

© Springer International Publishing AG 2018

E.A. Platz, N.A. Berger (eds.), *Energy Balance and Prostate Cancer*, Energy Balance and Cancer 14, DOI 10.1007/978-3-319-64940-5

MIX
Papier aus verantwortungsvollen Quellen
Paper from responsible sources
FSC® C105338
www.fsc.org

If you have any concerns about our products,
you can contact us on
ProductSafety@springernature.com

In case Publisher is established outside the EU,
the EU authorized representative is:
Springer Nature Customer Service Center GmbH
Europaplatz 3, 69115 Heidelberg, Germany

Printed by Libri Plureos GmbH
in Hamburg, Germany